Progress in Advanced Structural and Functional Materials Design

Tomoyuki Kakeshita
Editor

Progress in Advanced Structural and Functional Materials Design

Springer

Editor
Tomoyuki Kakeshita
Division of Materials and Manufacturing Science
Graduate School of Engineering
Osaka University
Osaka, Japan

ISBN 978-4-431-54063-2 ISBN 978-4-431-54064-9 (eBook)
DOI 10.1007/978-4-431-54064-9
Springer Tokyo Heidelberg New York Dordrecht London

Library of Congress Control Number: 2012954004

Printed on acid-free paper

Springer is part of Springer Science+Business Media (www.springer.com)

Preface

This book is based on educational and research achievements under the Global COE Program "Center of Excellence for Advanced Structural and Functional Materials Design," which was conducted between FY 2007 and 2011 at Osaka University, Japan. The Global COE Program was initiated to contribute to both fundamental and applied research in various fields of materials science and engineering. Under this program, we targeted a wide range of hard condensed materials (e.g., crystalline materials such as metals, ceramics, and semiconductor materials) and studied aspects such as physical properties, functional mechanisms, manufacturing processes, material structure, characterization of both bulk and nanostructures, evaluation of functionality, welding processes, and material recycling flow.

To accomplish the aim of the program, researchers from the following divisions, institutes, and centers at Osaka University collaborated: the Division of Materials and Manufacturing Science, the Department of Adaptive Machine System, the Center for Atomic and Molecular Technologies, the Joining and Welding Research Institute, the Institute of Scientific and Industrial Research, and the Research Center for Ultra-High Voltage Electron Microscopy. Through enhanced collaboration among researchers from the above-mentioned departments, we designed and developed advanced materials with a strong emphasis on their production and application.

Advanced materials studied under the Global COE Program included structural materials used in buildings and transportation, functional and intelligent materials essential for micromachines, semiconductor optoelectronics, and spintronics devices (e.g., ultra-high-density data-storage media and lasers for advanced information technologies), as well as biomaterials used in the medical and social welfare fields. We classified research on these advanced materials into the following three projects: (a) Advanced Materials Research Project for Structural Applications; (b) Advanced Materials Research Project for Combined Structural and Functional Applications; and (c) Advanced Materials Research Project for Functional Applications.

This book describes selected topics investigated under the Global COE Program. Every chapter is aimed at an understanding of the most advanced research in materials science by describing its fundamentals and details. Because both general explanations and cutting-edge commentaries on each topic are given in this book, it provides a large amount of useful information to interested readers as well as to materials scientists and engineers who wish to understand the direction of future development in the materials science fields of metals, alloys, ceramics, and semiconductors, among others. In particular, this book deals with the special fusion area of structural and functional materials such as medical bone materials. These contents are unique features for a materials science textbook. Each chapter is a complete unit in itself; thus, readers can peruse any chapter they choose without having to refer to other chapters.

We are grateful for the financial support for the Global COE Program from the Ministry of Education, Culture, Sports, Science and Technology, Japan. This book is dedicated to students who harbor ambitions of designing new materials by themselves.

Tomoyuki Kakeshita
Leader, "Center of Excellence for
Advanced Structural and Functional
Materials Design," Global COE Program

Contents

Part I Advanced Materials Research Project for Structural Applications

1 **Advanced Materials Design with Forming** 3
Hiroshi Utsunomiya and Ryo Matsumoto

2 **Fabrication of Porous Metals with Slender Directional Pores** 15
Hideo Nakajima

3 **Modeling of Arc Welding Process** 27
Yoshinori Hirata

4 **Advanced Materials Design Using Lasers** 43
Tomokazu Sano and Akio Hirose

5 **Advanced Material Designs Using Friction Stir Welding Technique** 59
Hidetoshi Fujii

6 **Advanced Analysis of Surface Films Formed on Passive Metals and Alloys Using X-ray Photoelectron Spectroscopy** 69
Shinji Fujimoto

7 **Advanced Numerical Simulations of Micro-, Macro-, and Mega-Scale Structurization** 83
Masahito Mochizuki

8 **Advanced Analysis of Solidification by X-ray Imaging** 93
Hideyuki Yasuda and Tomoya Nagira

Part II Advanced Materials Research Project for Combined Structural and Functional Applications

9 **Advanced Materials Design by Microstructure Control Under Magnetic Field** 107
Tomoyuki Kakeshita and Takashi Fukuda

10 **Eco-Friendly Materials Recycling Processing** 119
Toshihiro Tanaka and Masanori Suzuki

11 **Advanced Materials Design by Electrochemical Approach: Self-Organizing Anodization** 127
Hiroaki Tsuchiya

12 **Advanced Materials Design by Irradiation of High Energy Particles** 137
Takeshi Nagase

13 **Advanced Analysis and Control of Bone Microstructure Based on a Materials Scientific Study Including Microbeam X-ray Diffraction** 155
Takayoshi Nakano, Takuya Ishimoto, Naoko Ikeo, and Aira Matsugaki

14 **Advanced Materials Design by Controlling Transformation Temperature Using Magnetic Field** 169
Takashi Fukuda and Tomoyuki Kakeshita

15 **Advanced Materials Design for Fe-Based Shape Memory Alloys Through Structural Control** 181
Hiroyuki Y. Yasuda

Part III Advanced Materials Research Project for Functional Applications

16 **Fabrication of Photonic Crystals by Stereolithography Technique** 195
Soshu Kirihara

17 **Design, Fabrication, and Properties of Nanomaterials Using Ultrathin Film Techniques** 213
Yu Shiratsuchi

18 **Advanced Materials Design via Low-Damage Plasma Processes** 225
Yuichi Setsuhara

19 **Advanced Analysis of Magnetic Structure in Materials** 237
Tomoyuki Terai and Tomoyuki Kakeshita

20 Advanced Materials Design by Lithography Technique 249
Ryoichi Nakatani

21 Advanced Materials Design of Rare-Earth-Doped Semiconductors by Organometallic Vapor Phase Epitaxy 261
Yasufumi Fujiwara, Yoshikazu Terai, and Atsushi Nishikawa

22 Advanced Analysis of Defect Formations and Phase Transformations in Nanoparticles by In Situ Transmission Electron Microscopy 273
Hidehiro Yasuda

Index 283

Part I
Advanced Materials Research Project for Structural Applications

Chapter 1
Advanced Materials Design with Forming

Hiroshi Utsunomiya and Ryo Matsumoto

Abstract The microstructures and properties of industrial metals can be controlled by bulk deformation processes. First, the fundamentals of rolling and forging for microstructure control are explained. Current efforts to reduce the fuel consumption of transportation systems focus on weight reduction. This can be achieved through the use of lighter parts. The replacement parts may be made of (a) low-density materials, (b) porous materials, or (c) hollow structured materials. They should be stronger and stiffer than the original parts. The new parts require higher specific strengths (strength/density). Therefore, weight reduction and strengthening are important. In this chapter, three approaches are investigated by the authors: (1) the forming of magnesium alloys, (2) the forming of porous metals, (3) a new forming method using the servo press.

Keywords Forging • Forming • Magnesium alloy • Microstructure • Porous metals • Rolling • Servo press

1.1 Introduction

Energy saving, CO_2 emissions and sustainability are current major concerns in global engineering and industrial manufacturing. A reduction in weight is necessary for a reduction in the fuel consumption of transportation systems (e.g., automotives and aircrafts). This can be achieved by the use of lighter structures or parts made of the following:

1. Lightweight materials (low-density materials)
2. Porous materials
3. Hollow structured materials

H. Utsunomiya (✉) • R. Matsumoto
Division of Materials and Manufacturing Science, Graduate School of Engineering, Osaka University, 2-1 Yamadaoka, Suita, Osaka 565-0871, Japan
e-mail: uts@mat.eng.osaka-u.ac.jp

T. Kakeshita (ed.), *Progress in Advanced Structural and Functional Materials Design*, DOI 10.1007/978-4-431-54064-9_1, © Springer Japan 2013

However the solution is not simple. Applications of the above materials decrease weight, but they also decrease mechanical strength or stiffness. Therefore, materials of higher specific strength (strength/density) are needed. For example, if the density of the replacement is half that of the original and the strength is also half (the specific strength is the same), a material of double thickness is needed to support the same axial load. No reduction in weight is realized by the use of the low-density material. A weight reduction itself is not particularly beneficial, but an increase in specific strength is very important. In that sense, metal forming is a useful process because it creates a product shape and improves the microstructure and mechanical properties. In this chapter, a few approaches that have been investigated by the authors are presented.

1.2 Controlling the Microstructures of Materials by Forming

There are many kinds of bulk forming processes, as illustrated in Fig. 1.1. The aims of forming processes are to form materials with the designed shape and to control the microstructures and properties of materials.

1.2.1 Rolling

Rolling is the most important production process for metals because of its high productivity. Roughly 90% of commercial metals are processed by rolling. The dimensions, microstructures, properties, and surfaces of metals are controlled.

In flat rolling, the width change (lateral spreading) is negligible, and hence, the deformation is close to the plane-strain condition. The reduction in thickness, r, is normally used to describe the degree of deformation.

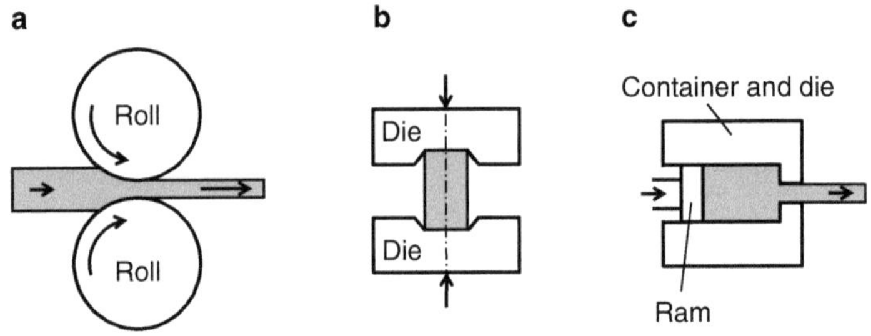

Fig. 1.1 Typical forming processes. (**a**) rolling, (**b**) forging, (**c**) extrusion

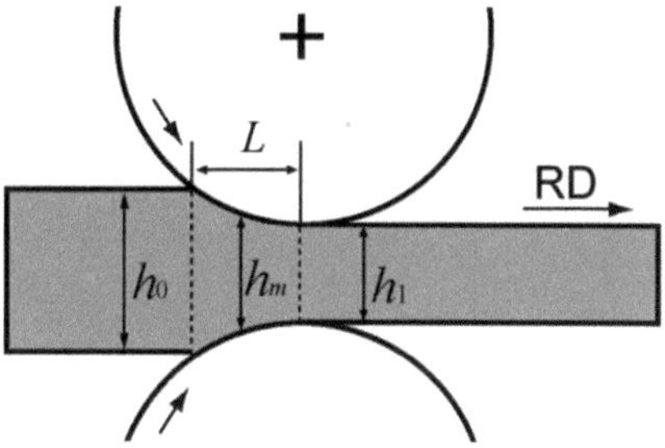

Fig. 1.2 Geometry of roll bite

$$r = \frac{h_0 - h_1}{h_0} = 1 - \frac{h_1}{h_0}$$

where h_0 is the initial thickness and h_1 is the thicknesses after rolling (Fig. 1.2).

If uniform deformation without shear is assumed, the equivalent plastic strain of plane-strain rolling is

$$\bar{\varepsilon} = -\frac{2}{\sqrt{3}} \ln\left(\frac{h_1}{h_0}\right) = -\frac{2}{\sqrt{3}} \ln(1 - r)$$

$2/\sqrt{3}$ is a multiplier to the strain in uni-axial deformation. For example, if sheet thickness is halved ($r = 50\%$) by rolling, the equivalent plastic strain is 0.80.

The contact length between the sheet and the rolls is an important geometric parameter, as shown in Fig. 1.2. The projected contact length, L, is given by

$$L = \sqrt{R(h_0 - h_1)}$$

where R is the radius of rolls.

The aspect ratio of the roll bite, L/h_m, is a key geometrical parameter in rolling. The mean thickness, h_m, can be calculated as

$$h_m = \frac{(h_0 + 2h_1)}{3}$$

Hydrostatic pressure is high and friction has stronger effects on deformation when L/h_m is substantially greater than unity (this is normally the case in sheet rolling). On the other hand, if L/h_m is less than unity (as in the case of brake-down rolling), the elastic constraint is significant, and hence, tensile stress may be generated on the mid plane.

The strain rate and sheet temperature are the most important factors in controlling microstructure and properties during hot rolling. The mean strain rate can be estimated from the equivalent plastic strain and rolling duration t.

$$\dot{\varepsilon} = \frac{\bar{\varepsilon}}{t} \cong \frac{\bar{\varepsilon}}{(L/v)}$$

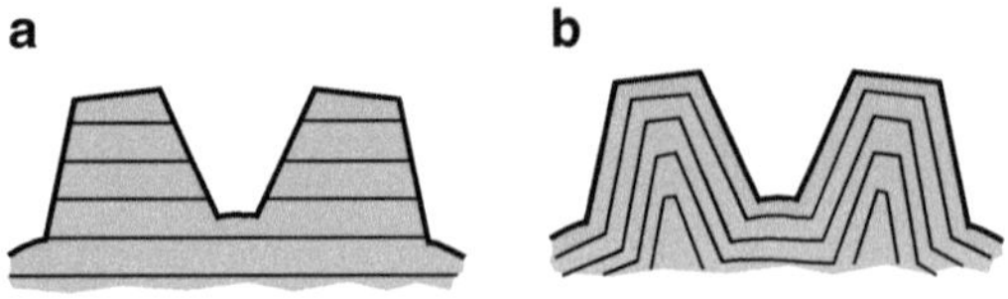

Fig. 1.3 Schematic illustrations of metal flows in (**a**) machining and (**b**) forging

where t is approximated as a passing time of the contact length L at roll speed v. In high-speed rolling, the roll speed, v, is around 1,000 m/min, and the typical strain rate is $10^3\ s^{-1}$. The deformation is that fast in impact tests.

Sheet temperature may change significantly during rolling. Heat generated by plastic deformation and frictional work on the interface raises the sheet temperature. On the other hand, heat transfers to cold rolls decrease the temperature. If the rolling speed increases, both plastic work and frictional work increase due to the positive strain-rate-sensitivity of flow stress. Nonetheless, the heat transfer to rolls apparently decreases because of the shorter contact time, t. Therefore, the sheet temperature is normally higher in high-speed rolling.

1.2.2 Forging

Forging is a process which a billet is formed by a set of dies on a press or a hammer. Unlike the rolling process, the forging process produces discrete parts. Typical forged products are connecting rods, crankshafts, bolts, and many other automotive parts. In the forging process, the billet is dominantly deformed by compressive force. Since the metal flow (see Fig. 1.3) and microstructure can be controlled by forging conditions such as the die shape, forging temperature, and forging speed, the forged parts show good mechanical properties.

In hot forging (forging above the recrystallization temperature), large deformation can be achieved by a small force; however, disadvantages include oxidation of the billet surface due to the heating process or poor dimensional accuracy of surface finishing. On the other hand, in cold forging (forged at room temperature), large force and good ductility of the billet are required; however, the forged parts have good dimensional accuracy and better mechanical properties. Precision forging, including net-shape or near-net-shape forging, is one of most important technical targets in forging industries.

1.3 Forming of Magnesium Alloys

1.3.1 Magnesium Alloy

Magnesium alloys are lightweight and relatively strong materials, as indicated by the data in Table 1.1. However, they are not widely used because of low deformability at low temperatures (<500 K) due to the *hcp* structure and inactiveness of

Table 1.1 Comparison of specific strength in industrial materials

Material	Density (g/cm^3)	Tensile strenth (MPa)	Specific strength (kN m/kg)
Mid steel (JIS: SPCC)	7.8	330	42
High tensile strength steel	7.8	980	126
Aluminium alloy (AA6061-T6)	2.7	310	115
Magnesium alloy (AZ31B-O)	1.78	255	143
Titanium alloy (Ti–6A1–4V)	4.43	980	221
Nickel super alloy (INCONEL 718)	8.3	1,270	153

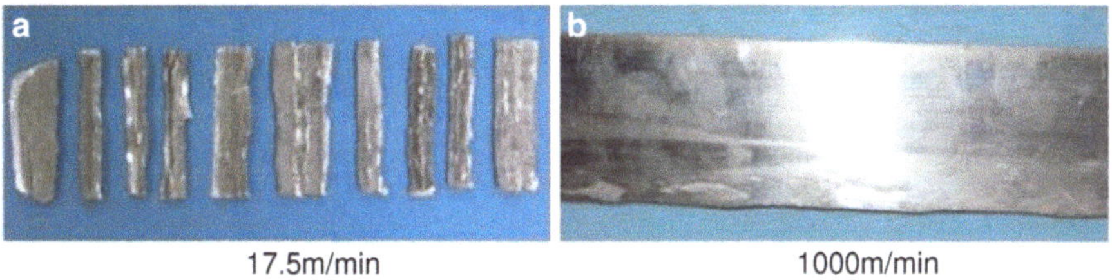

Fig. 1.4 Appearance of AZ31 rolled 50% at 473 K

non-basal slip systems. They are mostly shaped by gravity-casting, die-casting or Thixomolding®. Wrought magnesium products are currently limited; however, they are expected to be used in quantity for automotive parts in the near future.

1.3.2 High-Speed Rolling of Magnesium Alloys

Magnesium sheets are usually produced from cast slabs by rolling. In cold rolling, the applicable reduction in thickness is less than 10%. A multi-pass operation with small reduction accompanied by intermediate annealing is employed to suppress edge cracks or fractures of the material and to maintain workability in this process. Rolls are often heated to minimize the temperature drop. Because of all these procedures, the fabrication of magnesium alloy sheets is less productive and magnesium alloy sheets are more expensive than other metal sheets.

The authors proposed high-speed rolling for production of magnesium alloy sheets [1, 2]. The appearances of the AZ31B (Mg–3% Al–1% Zn) sheets rolled to 50% at 473 K are compared in Fig. 1.4. The magnesium alloy is fragmented into small pieces at low speeds. On the other hand, at 1,000 m/s, an unfractured sheet is obtained at high speed. It is even possible to reduce the thickness by up to 60% at 473 K. It is also possible to reduce it to 60% at room temperature without fracturing, although the rolled sheet shows many regular cracks running

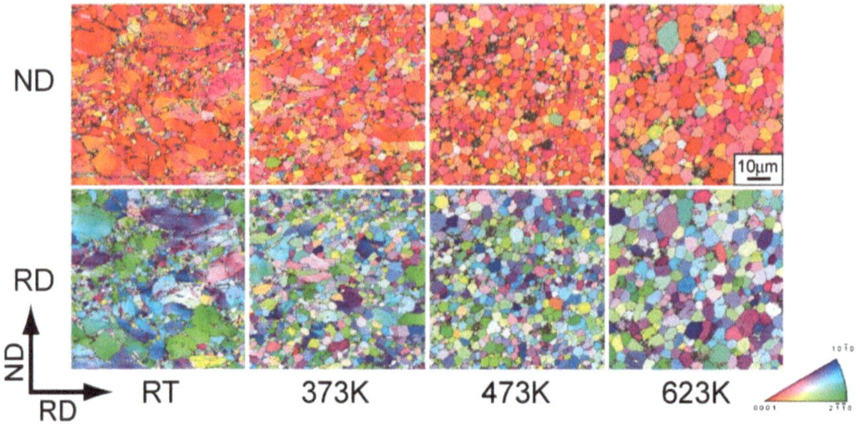

Fig. 1.5 IPF map on longitudinal section of AZ31 rolled at 2,000 m/min as a function of rolling temperature

in a transverse direction. It is notable that high-speed rolling significantly improves deformability and that a heavy reduction (>50%) is obtainable using a single-pass operation, even at the low temperature of 473 K.

The warm high-speed rolled sheet shows a fine-grained microstructure. The finest equiaxed structure is observed with a 50% reduction at 473 K. The mean grain size (the mean intercept length) is 2.2 μm. The size of the dynamically recrystallized grains increases with an increase in rolling temperature, as shown in Fig. 1.5. On the other hand, many deformation twins are found in the cold rolled sheet. A basal texture develops in all the high-speed rolled sheets [3, 4]. Grain refinement is effective for the improvement of the mechanical properties of the magnesium alloys. Sheets rolled at 473 K generally show a good balance of strength and elongation. For instance, the rolled sheets with 44% reduction show a tensile strength of 293 MPa and an elongation of 25%.

The higher material temperature during rolling is thought to be a major reason for the excellent workability in high-speed rolling [1, 5]. Plastic work and frictional work on the interface cause a temperature rise, while the heat transfer to cold rolls causes a temperature drop. It is predicted that when the roll speed is 200 m/min, the temperature change is negligible, and hence, isothermal rolling is virtually achieved. If the roll speed is above 200 m/min, the temperature increases in the roll bite to prevent deterioration of rollability. The microstructure change during the reheating process before rolling may be an additional reason, as an increase in rollability lowers the heating temperature and makes the microstructure finer.

It is concluded that high-speed rolling is a promising process for producing fine-grained magnesium alloy sheets with well-balanced mechanical properties. The adiabatic nature of high-speed rolling is the primary reason for the improvement in rollability of magnesium alloys.

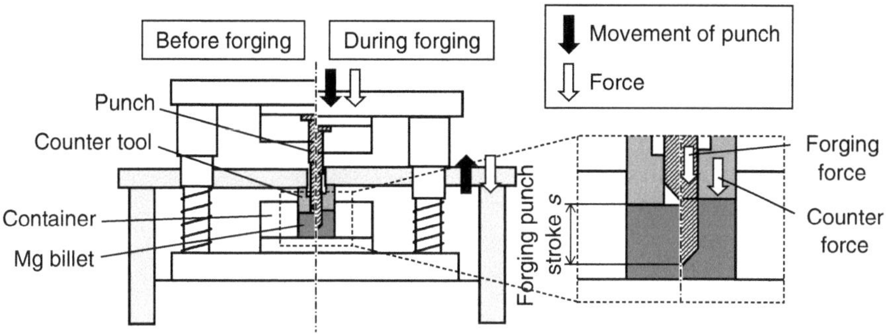

Fig. 1.6 Cold die forging of magnesium billet against counter punch pressure [6]

1.3.3 Cold Forging of Magnesium Alloy

Deformation under high pressure is thought to improve the formability of the magnesium alloy at room temperature, because the application of hydrostatic pressure is known to improve the ductility of metal. The authors proposed a die forging method against counter punch pressure, as shown in Fig. 1.6 [6]. Counter pressure is applied to the billet in a downward direction from the exit surface of the billet during forging by a counter tool located outside of the punch. Applying counter pressures of 100–200 MPa improves the critical punch stroke for cracking by about 20% compared with that of forging without counter pressure. Furthermore, the grain of the forged billet with counter pressure is finer than that without counter pressure. This method can be applied to the cold piercing of magnesium alloys [7]. Thus cold forming against counter punch pressure is one of effective methods of improving the formability of magnesium alloys at room temperature.

1.4 Forming of Porous Metals

Porous metal and metallic foams are emerging lightweight materials. Unidirectional casting of molten metal, heat treatment with a bubbling agent, and sintering of powder containing space holders are the major fabrication processes used [8]. Forming technology is important for using porous metals in industries because cutting and joining porous metals are difficult processes. Gasar and the lotus-type porous metal have one-dimensional elongated pores. The porous metal is promising because of its lightness and anisotropic mechanical properties [9]. The cold-working process may improve the strength of porous metals by strain hardening. However, the deformation behaviors of porous metals may not be similar to those of conventional nonporous metals, because their volumes do not remain constant.

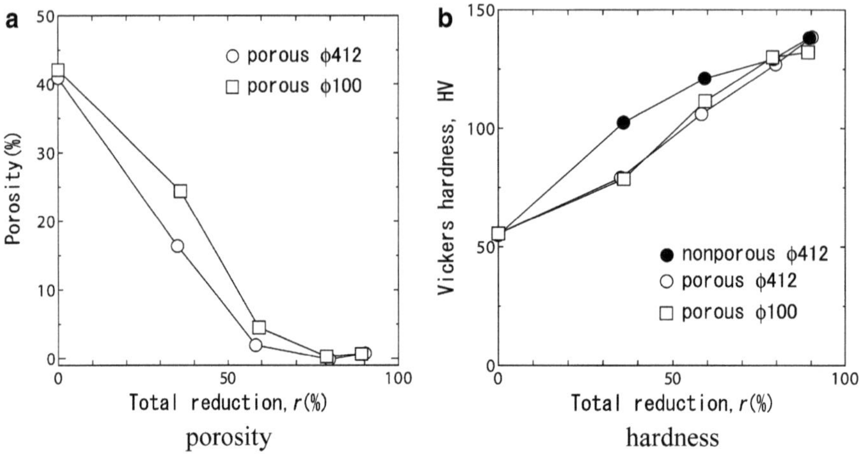

Fig. 1.7 Porosity and hardness as a function of total reduction in thickness [10]

In the experiment [10], cast porous copper with a porosity of 40.9%, was sectioned in length to produce plates that were 10 mm thick, 30 mm wide, and 150 mm long. The plates were cold-rolled by multi-pass operations under well-lubricated conditions such that the elongating direction of the pores was parallel to the rolling direction. The thickness was reduced to 1 mm by two pass schedules: (A) 20% per pass with rolls 412 mm in diameter, and (B) 10.6% per pass with rolls 100 mm in diameter. Mean stress is a key parameter that affects pore closure.

Changes in the (a) porosity and (b) hardness of the solid parts are shown in Fig. 1.7. The porosity decreases almost linearly with increasing total reduction up to 60%. The densification is retarded in pass schedule (B), with smaller rolls and draughts per pass. Pores are mostly closed when the total reduction reaches 80%. In Fig. 1.7b, strain hardening of the porous metal is apparent for all cases. Although nonporous copper shows a reduced slope of the curve, i.e., a lower hardening rate, porous copper shows an almost linear increase in hardness. Porous copper shows an increase in hardness from HV55 to HV140.

The change in the cross section (on the plane perpendicular to the rolling direction) is shown in Fig. 1.8 [10]. In the as-cast slab, the pores were generally circular and the area fraction by image processing was 44.1%. Rolling causes the pores to deform from circles into ovals, in general. However, the deformation is neither proportional nor uniform. Some pores are apparently closed, whereas others change very slightly. At a reduction of 36%, the area fraction of pores in schedule (A) is 25.0%, while that in schedule (B) is 32.6%. When the total reduction is 60%, most pores are closed. The retardation of densification in schedule (B) is confirmed.

It is clear that the pore deformation is much greater than that of the copper. However the deformation of copper is not negligible, even at the small total reduction of 36%, and it is sensitive to the pass schedule. The copper matrix can be significantly strengthened by cold rolling, which can improve the specific strength of the porous metal with decreasing porosity.

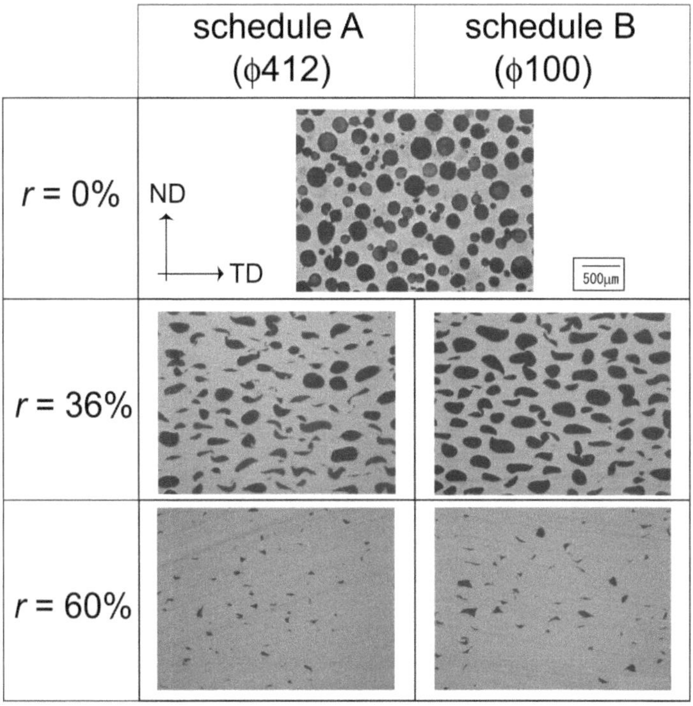

Fig. 1.8 Change in pore morphology on cross section [10]

1.5 New Forming Methods Using Servo Press

1.5.1 Servo Press

Many types of servo presses have recently been developed by several press builders, mainly in Japan and Germany [11]. The mechanical servo press provides the flexibility of the press ram, i.e., the speed and position of the ram can be controlled with high accuracy. The servo press is attracting attention in metal forming industries as a result. New forming processes using servo presses have been developed to form products with complicated shapes and/or high dimensional accuracy in both academic and industrial fields.

1.5.2 Warm Forging of Magnesium Alloys

Magnesium alloys are used for lightweight structural and functional parts, and therefore, the billet is usually thin, and the temperature of the billet is easily cooled down during the transfer process from the furnace to the press. Furthermore,

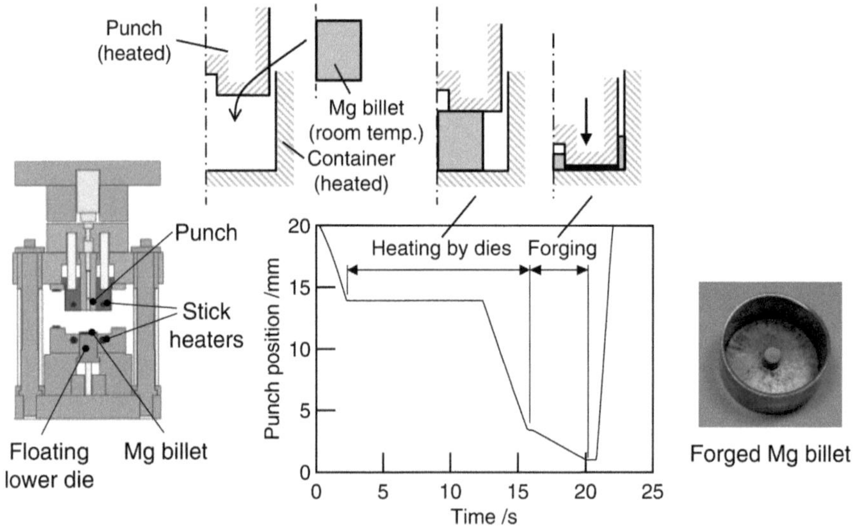

Fig. 1.9 Die forging method of magnesium alloy using servo press [12]

the flow stress of the magnesium alloy changes greatly with forming temperature. For these reasons, controlling the temperatures of the billet and the tool is critically important. A forging method for magnesium alloys using the servo press [12] is shown in Fig. 1.9. The Mg billet is sandwiched between high-temperature dies (473–673 K) at room temperature for several seconds, and then, it is directly heated by the dies to almost the same temperature as them. This method also has the advantage of preventing billet oxidation.

1.5.3 Forming of Deep Hole with Retreat and Advance Pulse Ram Motion

One of the major solutions for reducing the weight of a component is to employ lightweight structures such as hollow components. Since long and/or complex shaped hollow components are not easily produced by metal forming, the establishment of forming methods for components with hollow shapes is a crucial technical target. An extrusion method with retreat and advance pulse ram motion is proposed for the backward extrusion of deep holes, as shown in Fig. 1.10 [13]. In this method, a punch having an internal channel for lubricant flow is pushed into the billet in a manner combining pulsed and stepwise modes for supplying liquid lubricant to the punch nose. The internal pressure in the cavity formed in the previous forming steps is depressurized by the retreat action of the punch, and the lubricant is sucked into the cavity through the internal channel. When a sufficient

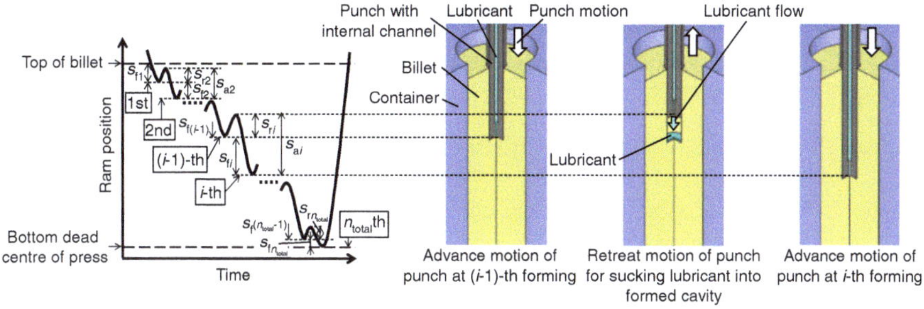

Fig. 1.10 Retreat and advance pulse ram motion of punch with internal channel for lubricant in forming for a high aspect ratio hole [13]

amount of the lubricant has been supplied to the cavity during the retreat motion of the punch, the formation of a hole can be carried out by maintaining good lubrication, thus forming a deep hole with good surface quality.

1.6 Summary

The dimensions and microstructures of materials can be controlled by bulk deformation processes. The fundamentals of rolling and forging are explained as tools for designing materials performance. Currently, a reduction in the weight of parts is required to reduce the fuel consumption of transportation systems. This can be achieved by the use of lighter structures or parts, such as (1) lightweight (low density) materials, (2) porous materials, or (3) hollow structured materials. Several bulk deformation processes of lightweight materials are presented in this chapter. It is demonstrated that metal forming is a powerful and useful tool for advanced materials design because it can control the shape, microstructure (including pore morphology), mechanical properties, and surface finish of materials with high productivity and flexibility.

Acknowledgments The authors are grateful to Prof. Testuo Sakai and Prof. Jerzy Szpunar for their kind and useful advice and to Mr. Jyoji Miyamoto for specimen preparation and experimental assistance. This work was supported by the Global COE program (Project: Centre of Excellence for Advanced Structural and Functional Materials Design) from MEXT, Japan.

References

1. Utsunomiya H, Sakai T, Minamiguchi S, Koh H (2006) High-speed heavy rolling of magnesium alloy sheets. In: Luo AA et al (eds) Magnesium technology. TMS, San Antonio, pp 201–204
2. Sakai T, Utsunomiya H, Minamiguchi S, Koh H (2006) Single-pass large draught rolling of magnesium alloy sheets by high-speed rolling. In: Pekguleryuz MO et al (eds) Magnesium technology in the global age. CIM, Montreal, pp 205–215

3. Koh H, Sakai T, Utsunomiya H, Minamiguchi S (2007) Deformation and texture evolution during high-speed rolling of AZ31 magnesium sheets. Mater Trans 48:2023–2027
4. Li H, Hsu E, Szpunar J, Utsunomiya H, Sakai T (2008) Deformation mechanism and texture and microstructure evolution during high-speed rolling of AZ31B Mg sheets. J Mater Sci 43:7148–7156
5. Sakai T, Hashimoto A, Hamada G, Utsunomiya H (2011) Deformation and evolution of microstructure and texture during high speed heavy rolling of AZ31 magnesium alloy sheet. In: Sillekens WH et al (eds) Magnesium technology. TMS, San Antonio, Warrendale, PA, USA, pp 369–372
6. Matsumoto R, Kubo T, Osakada K (2008) Improvement of forgeability of a commercial AZ31B magnesium alloy in cold backward extrusion with counter pressure. Mater Trans 49:1000–1005
7. Matsumoto R, Kubo T, Osakada K (2006) Cold piercing of magnesium alloy billet with high aspect ratio. Int J Mach Tools Manuf 46:459–466
8. Ashby MF, Evans A, Fleck NA, Gibson LJ, Hutchinson JW, Wadley HNG (2000) Metal foams – a design guide. Butterworth-Heinemann, Oxford, UK, pp 6–23
9. Nakajima H (2007) Fabrication, properties and application of porous metals with directional pores. Prog Mater Sci 52:1091–1173
10. Utsunomiya H, Yukimoto T, Sakai T, Suzuki S, Nakajima H (2010) Pore closure in multi-pass cold rolling of lotus-type porous copper. Steel Res Int 81:158–161
11. Osakada K, Mori K, Altan T, Groche P (2011) Mechanical servo press technology for metal forming. CIRP Ann Manuf Technol 60:651–672
12. Matsumoto R, Osakada K (2004) Development of warm forging method for magnesium alloy. Mater Trans 45:2838–2844
13. Matsumoto R, Sawa S, Utsunomiya H, Osakada K (2011) Prevention of galling in forming of deep hole with retreat and advance pulse Ram motion on servo press. CIRP Ann Manuf Technol 60:315–318

Chapter 2
Fabrication of Porous Metals with Slender Directional Pores

Hideo Nakajima

Abstract Lotus-type porous metals with aligned slender cylindrical pores are fabricated by unidirectional solidification from the melt with a dissolved gas such as hydrogen, nitrogen or oxygen. The gas atoms can be dissolved into the melt via a pressurized gas atmosphere or thermal decomposition of gaseous compounds. Three types of solidification techniques have been developed: mold casting, continuous zone melting and continuous casting techniques. The last technique is superior from the viewpoint of mass production of lotus metals.

Keywords Hydrogen • Nitrogen • Porosity • Porous metals • Solidification

2.1 Principle of Fabrication of Lotus-Type Porous Metals

Porous and foamed metals exhibit various characteristics that differ from bulk metals, including possessing a low density and large surface area. These metals are expected to be used as lightweight materials, catalyst carriers, electrodes, vibration and acoustic energy damping materials, impact energy absorption materials, etc. [1]. However, porous and foamed metals all suffer from deteriorating mechanical properties such as strength, stiffness, and fatigue due to the inhomogeneous pore number density distribution and pore size. Many methods, including powder metallurgy and the melt route, have been used to develop porous materials. Among these materials, lotus-type porous metals have attracted much attention because their slender cylindrical pores aligned in one direction [2, 3]. These metals are fabricated by a unidirectional solidification process using gas from a pressurized

H. Nakajima (✉)
The Institute of Scientific and Industrial Research, Osaka University, Ibaraki, Osaka 567-0047, Japan

The Wakasa Wan Energy Research Center, 64-52-1 Nagatani, Tsuruga, Fukui 914-0192, Japan
e-mail: nakajima@sanken.osaka-u.ac.jp; hnakajima@werc.or.jp

T. Kakeshita (ed.), *Progress in Advanced Structural and Functional Materials Design*,
DOI 10.1007/978-4-431-54064-9_2,

gas atmosphere such as hydrogen (gasar method) [3] or thermal decomposition of gas compounds such as hydrides [4]. The pores evolved from the insoluble gas when the molten metal dissolving the gas is solidified. Compared to conventional porous metals, which have nearly spherical and isotropic pores, these metals exhibit superior mechanical properties [5].

This article reviews recent developments in the fabrication techniques of lotus metals. Our group also investigated various properties and applications of lotus metals, whose details are described in elsewhere [2, 5].

2.2 Mold Casting Technique

Figure 2.1 shows schematic drawings of the mold casting technique; a metal inside a crucible is melted by an induction heating in a high-pressure gas atmosphere [2, 3]. The gas is dissolved up to the equilibrium gas concentration into the molten metal under a given gas pressure according to the Sieverts' law. The melt saturated with gas is poured into the mold. When some part of the mold is cooled down by a chiller or circulated water, the melt can be solidified unidirectionally from the vicinity of the cooling part. The elongated pores can evolve and grow by the influence of the unidirectional solidification. The pore growth direction can be controlled by changing the location of the cooling part. When the bottom of the mold is water-cooled, the molten metal is unidirectionally solidified upwards from the bottom part so that the directional pores grow in the upward direction. When the lateral side of the mold is cooled down, the solidification takes place inwardly from the surrounding and thus, the pore distribution becomes radial.

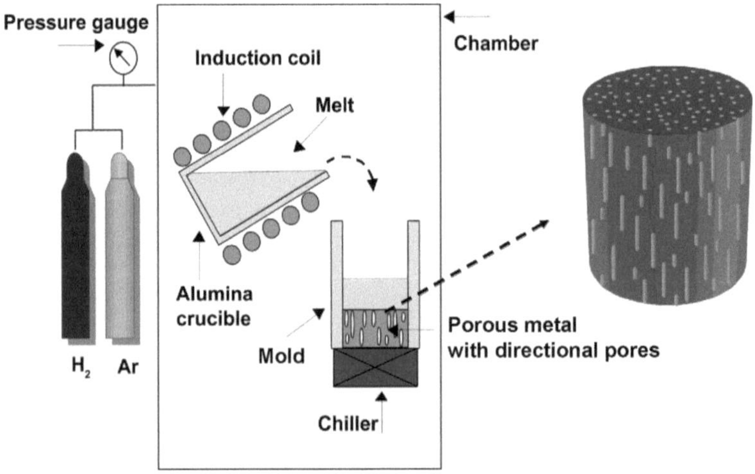

Fig. 2.1 Mold casting technique for fabrication of lotus and gasar-type porous metals. Reproduced from Nakajima H 2007 Fabrication, properties and application of porous metals with directional pores. Prog. Mater. Sci. **52**, 1091–1173, with permission from Elsevier

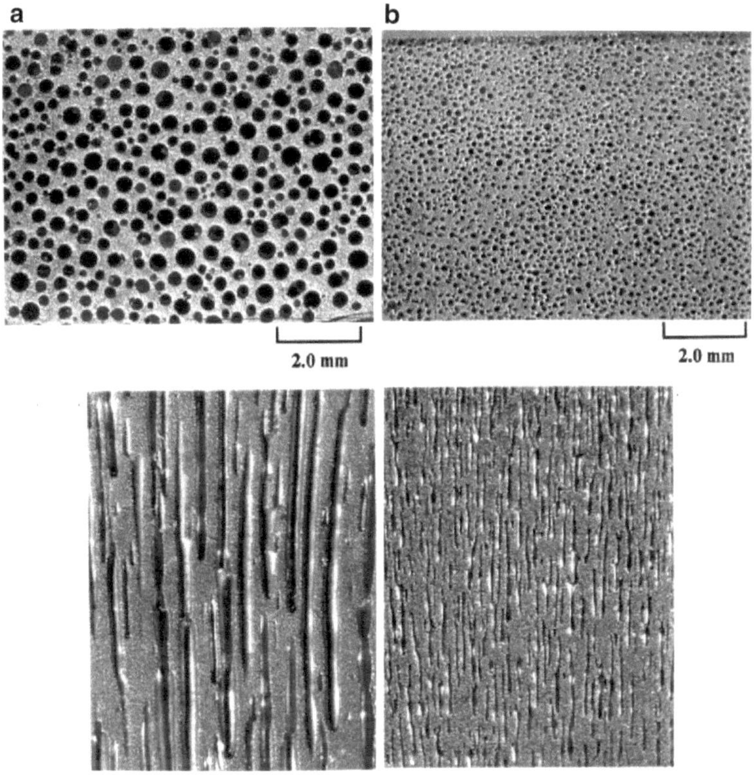

Fig. 2.2 Typical examples of optical micrographs on the cross-sections of lotus copper fabricated at different hydrogen pressure. The above is the cross-sections perpendicular to the solidification and the below is the cross-sections parallel to the solidification. (**a**) 0.4 MPa hydrogen, porosity 44.9%, and (**b**) 0.8MPa hydrogen, porosity 36.6%. Reproduced from Nakajima H 2007 Fabrication, properties and application of porous metals with directional pores. Prog. Mater. Sci. **52**, 1091–1173, with permission from Elsevier

The lotus metals are characterized by pore growth direction, pore size and porosity. The parameters to control the pore morphology can be listed up as

- The melt temperature
- The solidification rate
- The dissolving gas pressure during melting and solidification
- The inert gas pressure during melting and solidification.

Figure 2.2 shows typical examples of optical micrographs on the cross-sections (above) and the longitudinal sections (below) of lotus copper. The mold casting technique is usually used to produce copper and magnesium. Since these metals exhibit high thermal conductivity, the solidification proceeds with almost constant rate through the whole of ingot. Thus, lotus metals with uniform pore size and porosity can be produced by this technique.

2.3 Continuous Zone Melting Technique

The mold casting technique cannot be applied to fabricate lotus metals and alloys with low thermal conductivity such as stainless steel. For the metals and alloys with low thermal conductivity, although the heat from the melt is easily dissipated to the water-cooled plate during the solidification process the cooling becomes slower at the upper part of the solidified ingot where is far from the cooling part and thus the pores become coarse. As a result only lotus metals with non-uniform pore size and porosity can be produced as illustrated in Fig. 2.3. In order to overcome the shortcoming, a novel technique was invented by the present author to fabricate pore-elongated lotus metals even with low thermal conductivity [6]. Figure 2.4a

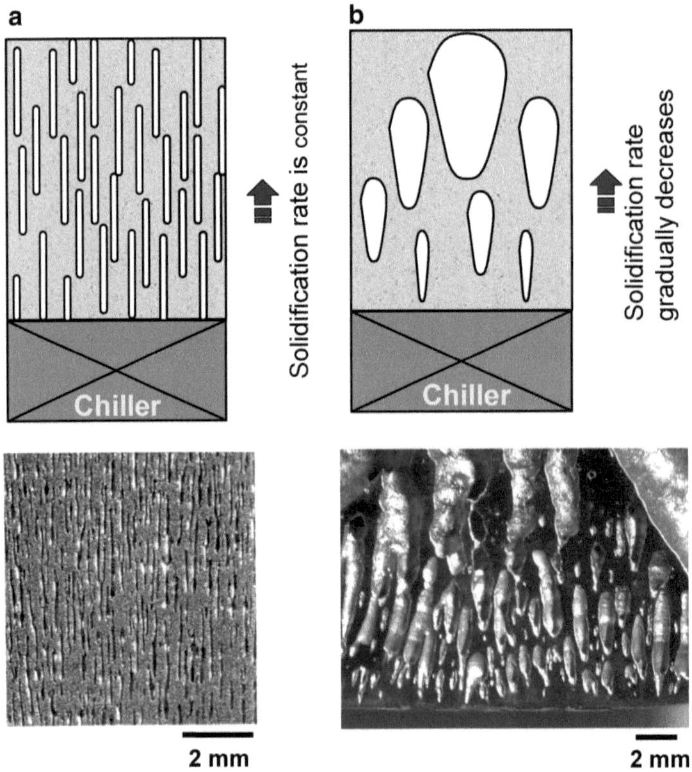

Fig. 2.3 Comparison of the evolution of pores in lotus metals fabricated by mold casting technique in gas atmosphere. The above is schematic drawings of pore evolution during the unidirectional solidification. The below is optical micrographs of the sectional views parallel to the solidification direction. The *left* is lotus copper and the *right* is stainless steel. (**a**) The uniform pore size and porosity are observed in copper and magnesium with high thermal conductivity, and (**b**) various pore size and porosity are found in stainless steel with low thermal conductivity. The magnitude of the thermal conductivity affects the solidification velocity of the melt. Reproduced from Nakajima H 2007 Fabrication, properties and application of porous metals with directional pores. Prog. Mater. Sci. **52**, 1091–1173, with permission from Elsevier

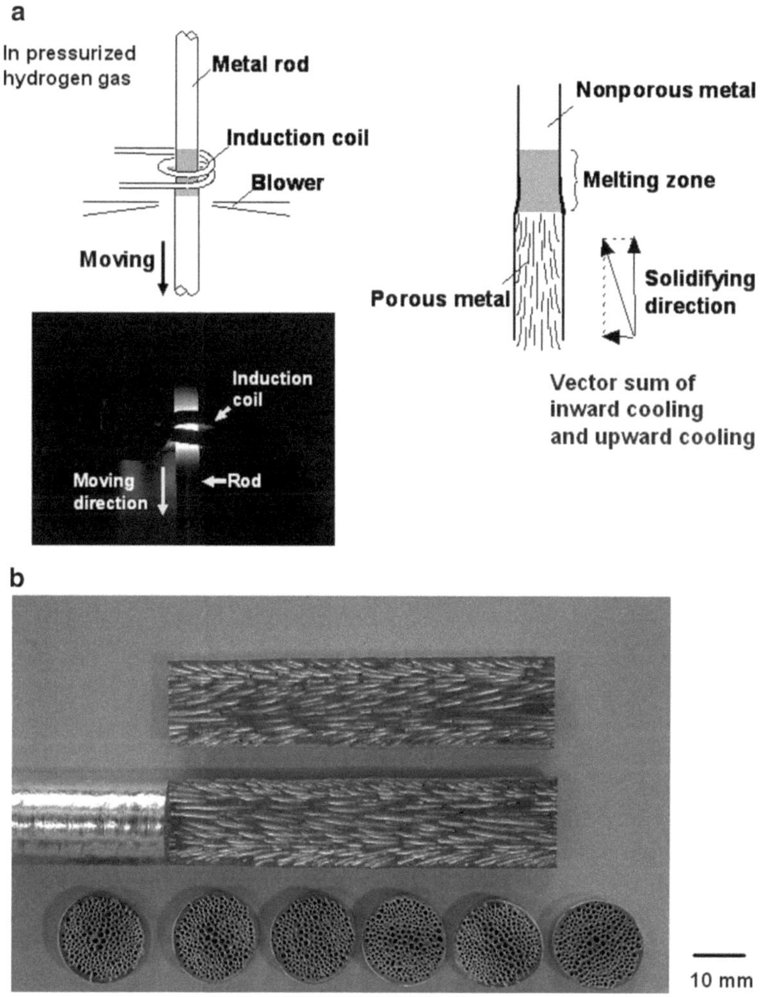

Fig. 2.4 (**a**) Schematic drawings and a photograph of the overview for the melting part of continuous zone melting technique. (**b**) Rod and sections of lotus stainless steel fabricated by the continuous zone melting technique in 2.0 MPa hydrogen atmosphere. The transference velocity of the rod is 330 μm^{-1}. Resulting porosity and average pore size are 40% and 320 μm, respectively, both of which are almost uniform in the whole part of the ingot. Reproduced from Nakajima H 2007 Fabrication, properties and application of porous metals with directional pores. Prog. Mater. Sci. **52**, 1091–1173, with permission from Elsevier

illustrates the schematic setup of the continuous zone melting technique, which consists of radio-frequency induction coil, blowers, specimen rod and movable specimen holders; the induction coil is used for zone (restricted) area melting of the rod specimen, while the blower is effective for further cooling of the melt metal. These components are placed into a high-pressure chamber filled with gases such as hydrogen (or nitrogen) and argon. While a part of the specimen rod is melted by induction heating, the hydrogen (or nitrogen) gas is absorbed into the melt up to the gas equilibrium solubility in the pressurized gas atmosphere according to Sieverts' law. Concurrently the specimen rod is moved downward at a given velocity. In the lower part of the melt zone, solidification takes place simultaneously. Then, directional elongated pores are evolved by precipitation of insoluble gas of hydrogen (or nitrogen) in the solidified specimen. If the transference velocity is kept constant, the solidification velocity becomes constant so that the pore size can be constant. Although the stainless steel exhibits a low thermal conductivity so that lotus stainless steel with homogeneous pore size and porosity is impossible by the mold casting technique as shown in Fig. 2.3, lotus stainless steel with homogeneous pore size and porosity is successfully fabricated by continuous zone melting technique. This technique has an advantage that the solidification velocity is controllable by changing the lowering speed of the specimen rod. Figure 2.4b shows a sectional view of lotus stainless steel fabricated by this technique.

2.4 Continuous Casting Technique

When lotus metals are put to practical use, mass production is indispensable. Since previous methods like mold casting and continuous zone melting techniques are not suitable, the present author et al. developed a new continuous casting technique, by which long plate or rod can be fabricated as shown in Fig. 2.5 [7]. This fabrication apparatus consists of a crucible with a rectangular hole on the crucible bottom, a dummy bar for preventing the melt flow through the hole, and induction heating coil and a mold with water-cooled plate. These are installed in a high-pressure chamber. The metal is melted in the crucible by radio-frequency heating in high-pressure mixture gas. After enough time to make hydrogen dissolve into the molten metal, the molten metal is pulled down through the cooled mold at a given velocity. In the mold, the molten metal is solidified simultaneously. Then, directional elongated pores are evolved by precipitation of insoluble gas of hydrogen (or nitrogen) in the solidified specimen.

The average pore diameter and the porosity are plotted against the transference velocity as shown in Fig. 2.6. The average pore diameter decreases with increasing transference velocity, while the porosity is not much different. The pores which are considered to nucleate heterogeneously grow by the hydrogen rejected in the solid–liquid interface and hydrogen diffusion from the solid copper to the pores. It can be understood that the amount of hydrogen diffusing from liquid to the pores increases with decreasing transference velocity. For this reason, the formed pores at lower velocity become larger than those at higher velocity. As the transference velocity increases, the pore size decreases but the number density of pores increases.

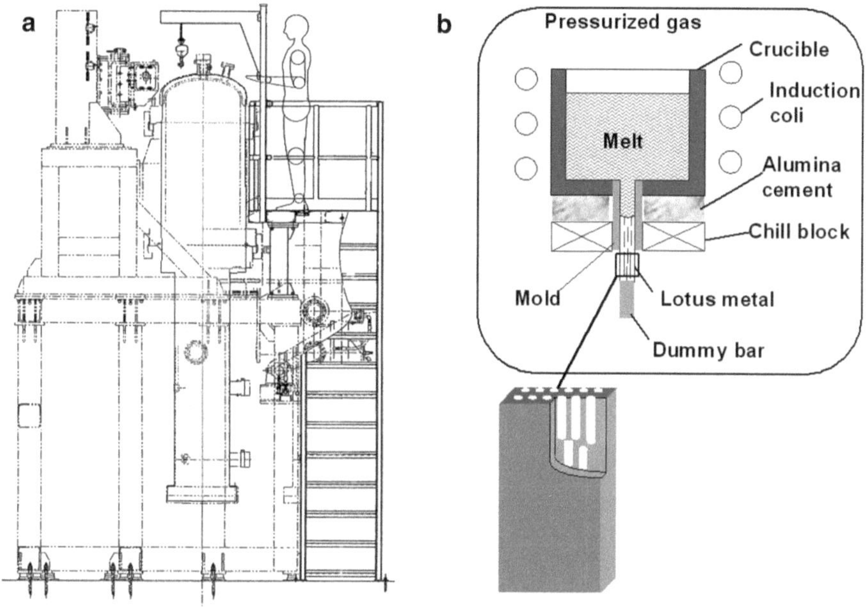

Fig. 2.5 Schematic drawings of fabrication apparatus of lotus metals by the continuous casting technique. (**a**) Large crucible and induction heating coil are located in the *upper part* of the chamber, while the mold with cooling part and movable mechanism of the solidified metal rod with pinch roll are installed in the *bottom part* of the chamber. (**b**) Schematic drawing of the details inside the chamber. The dummy bar is connected together with the melt at the mold. Reproduced from Nakajima H 2007 Fabrication, properties and application of porous metals with directional pores. Prog. Mater. Sci. **52**, 1091–1173, with permission from Elsevier

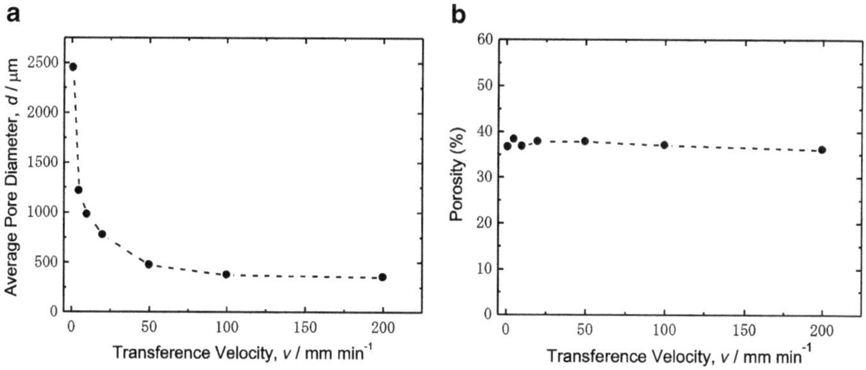

Fig. 2.6 (**a**) Average pore diameter and (**b**) porosity versus transference velocity of lotus copper fabricated in mixture gas of hydrogen 0.25 MPa and argon 0.15 MPa by continuous casting technique. Reproduced from Park JS, Hyun SK, Suzuki S, Nakajima H 2007 Effect of transference velocity and hydrogen pressure on porosity and pore morphology of lotus-type porous copper fabricated by a continuous casting technique. Acta Mater. **55**, 5646–5654, with permission from Elsevier

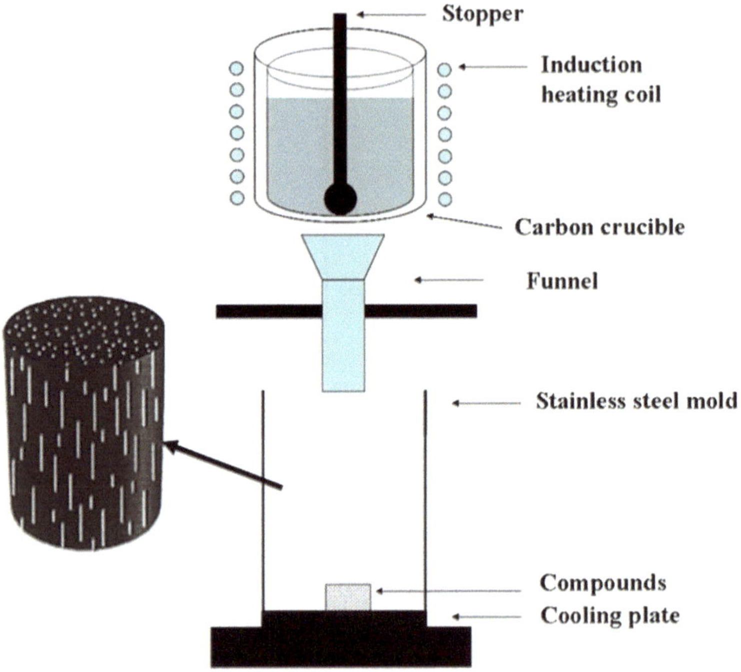

Fig. 2.7 Mold casting technique for fabrication of lotus aluminum by thermal decomposition technique

2.5 Thermal Decomposition Method

Although the fabrication techniques mentioned above are quite advanced, one large technical barrier remains; high pressure hydrogen gas must be used. Employing high pressure hydrogen gas has inherent risks because it may lead to inflammable and explosive accidents if oxygen is mixed. Therefore, a technique that does not require high pressure hydrogen to fabricate lotus metals is highly desirable. In order to overcome this difficulty, the present author et al. proposed an alternative, but simple method to fabricate lotus metals by a thermal decomposition method (TDM) of compounds containing gas elements in a non-hydrogen atmosphere under nearly atmospheric pressure or vacuum [4].

First a metal copper 200 g is melted by radio-frequency induction heating in a crucible under an argon atmosphere. Then the melt is poured into the mold, which has a copper bottom plate cooled by water. A few pellets of titanium hydride, which ranges from 0.075 and 0.25 g in mass, are set on the bottom plate of the mold. Unidirectional solidification occurs in the mold so that lotus copper is obtained, as illustrated in Fig. 2.7. Figure 2.8 shows the optical micrographs of the cross-sectional views of lotus copper parallel and perpendicular to the solidification direction. The pore growth direction is coincident to the direction of the

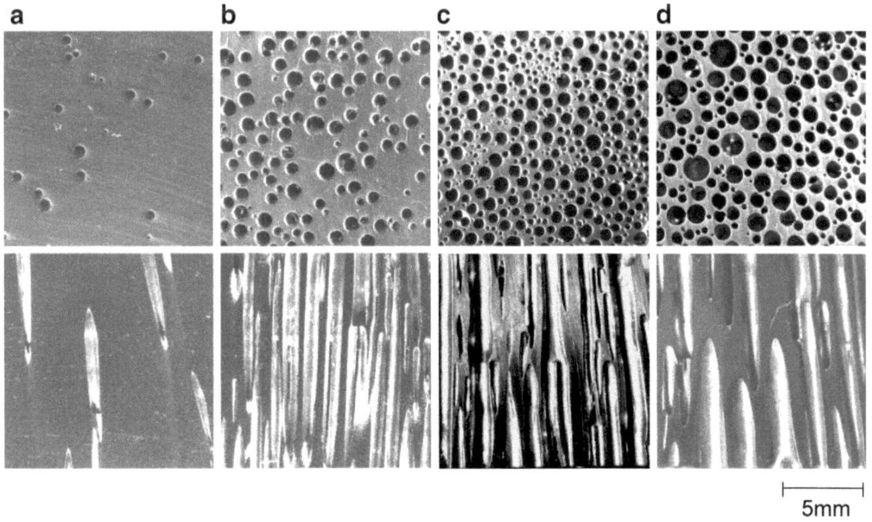

Fig. 2.8 Optical micrographs pf cross-sectional views of lotus copper (*upper views*) perpendicular and (*lower*) parallel to the solidification direction. Mass of titanium hydride added to the mold is (**a**) 0.075 g, (**b**) 0.10 g, (**c**) 0.125 g, and (**d**) 0.25 g. Melting and subsequent solidification were carried out in 0.1 MPa argon atmosphere. Reproduced from Nakajima H, Ide T 2008 Fabrication of porous copper with directional pores through thermal decomposition of compounds. Metall. Mater. Trans. **39A**, 390–394, with permission from Springer

unidirectional solidification, which is consistent with that of the conventional high pressure gas methods (PGM). This result suggests that the principle mechanism of this pore evolution is similar to that of PGM; when a molten metal dissolving a gas is solidified, the insoluble gas leaves the solid and evolves into gas pores in the solid metals. When titanium hydride is decomposed into hydrogen and titanium, the latter is very reactive element, which easily reacts with residual oxygen in the molten copper. Consequently, titanium oxide particles are formed and dispersed, which may serve as the nucleation sites for the hydrogen pores in the solid–liquid interface during unidirectional solidification. It is well known that the pores evolve by heterogeneous nucleation in metal melts in the presence of small amounts of foreign particles. Thus, it is expected that the pore size and porosity become homogeneous by uniformly distributed nucleation sites. Therefore, TDM exhibits another advantage to produce lotus metals with more homogeneous pore size and porosity than those by PGM, which does not provide intentional nucleation sites.

2.6 Fabrication of Lotus Aluminum Through Thermal Decomposition Method

Lotus metals are fabricated by using the gas solubility gap between liquid and solid. Although hydrogen in aluminum has a solubility gap at the melting point, the hydrogen concentration is low so that high porosity of lotus aluminum cannot be

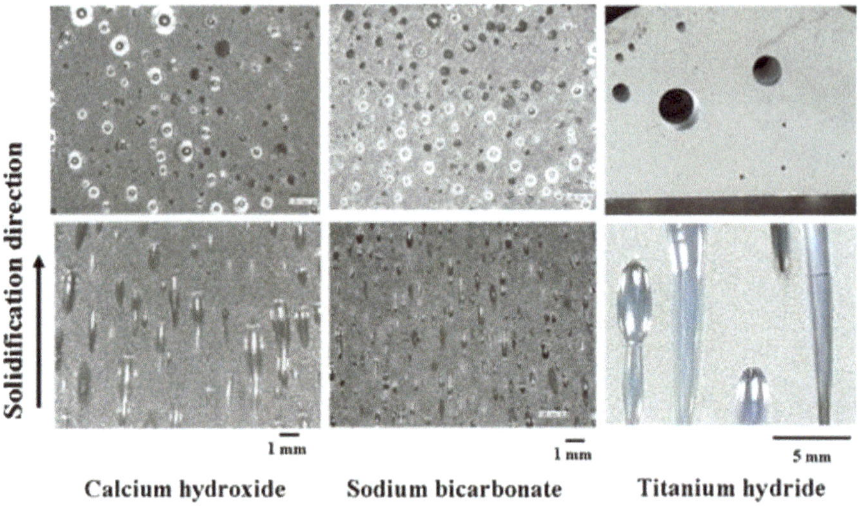

Fig. 2.9 Optical micrographs of lotus aluminum fabricated by mold casting technique with different compounds in vacuum at 1,023 K. The *upper* and *lower* micrographs are the cross sections perpendicular and parallel to the solidification direction, respectively. Reproduced from Kim SY, Park JS, Nakajima H 2009 Fabrication of lotus-type porous aluminum through thermal decomposition method. Metall. Mater. Trans. **40A**, 937–942, with permission from Springer

obtained by the conventional PGM of hydrogen. According to our recent investigation, lotus aluminum with a porosity as high as 10 pct can be fabricated by unidirectional solidification in hydrogen pressure less than atmospheric pressure [8]. The lower the hydrogen pressure is, the higher the porosity is. Kim et al. [8] was undertaken fabrication of lotus aluminum in vacuum using the thermal decomposition of gas-forming compounds.

Figure 2.9 shows the cross sectionals views of microstructure of lotus aluminum parallel and perpendicular to the solidification direction. The pore morphologies perpendicular to the solidification direction are shown in the upper photos, while those parallel to the solidification direction are shown in the lower photos. In all specimens, the aligned pores parallel to the solidification direction were observed. It is considered that the cylindrical gas pores are evolved by TDM from the compounds during solidification of aluminum containing hydrogen gas.

Table 2.1 compiles the decomposition reactions of three compounds in the aluminum melt. Calcium hydroxide and sodium bicarbonate decompose into vapor and compounds and then, the vapor decomposes to hydrogen and metallic oxide. On the other hand, titanium hydride decomposes into hydrogen and titanium. These decomposed gas elements can dissolve in aluminum melt. When the melt is solidified, lotus aluminum can be produced.

Figure 2.10a shows the pore structure on cross sections of lotus aluminum perpendicular (upper) and parallel (lower) to the solidification direction. The lotus aluminum was fabricated using calcium hydroxide in vacuum or under argon

Table 2.1 Decomposition reaction and temperature of gaseous compounds. Reproduced from Kim SY, Park JS, Nakajima H 2009 Fabrication of lotus-type porous aluminum through thermal decomposition method. Metall. Mater. Trans. **40A**, 937–942, with permission from Springer

Reactions	Decomposition temperature [K]	Gas atoms or molecules to be dissolved and bubbled
$Ca(OH)_2 \rightarrow CaO + H_2O$	853	H
$H_2O \rightarrow$ metallic oxide + 2H		
$2NaHCO_3 \rightarrow Na_2CO_3 + H_2O + CO_2$	473	H, CO, O
$H_2O \rightarrow$ metallic oxide + 2H		
$TiH_2 \rightarrow Ti + 2H$	723	H

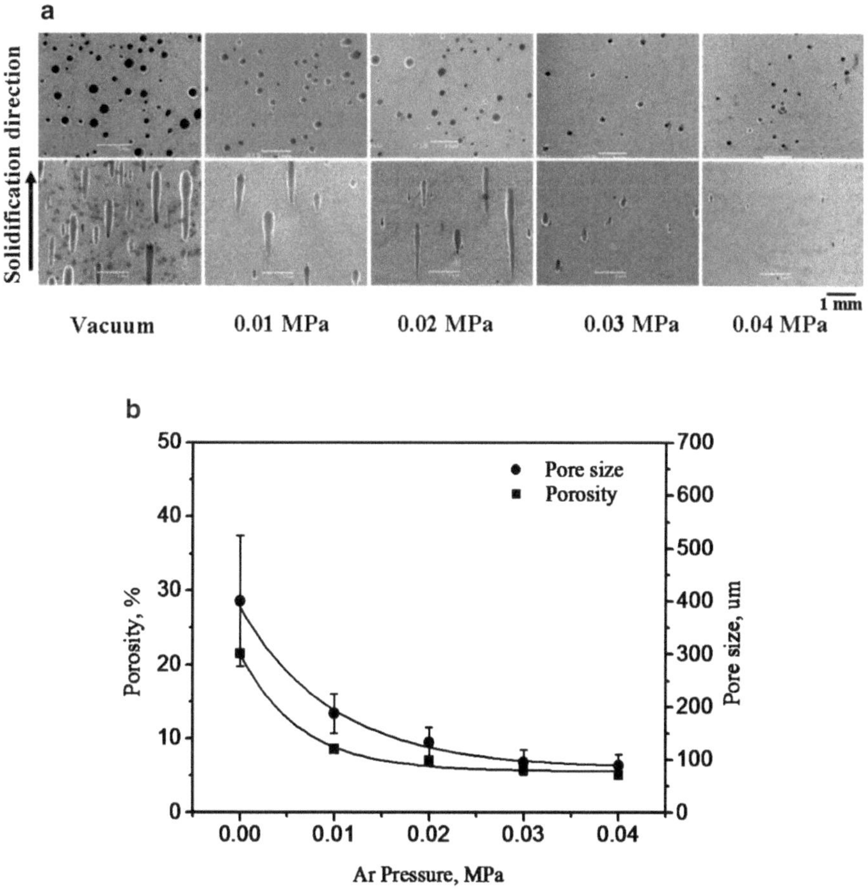

Fig. 2.10 Lotus aluminum fabricated using calcium hydroxide in vacuum or under argon pressure (0.01–0.04 MPa). The amount of calcium hydroxide was kept to be 0.2 g. (**a**) Pore morphology. The *upper* and *lower* micrographs are the cross sections perpendicular and parallel to the solidification direction, respectively. (**b**) Variation of the porosity and pore size as a function of argon pressure. Reproduced from Kim SY, Park JS, Nakajima H 2009 Fabrication of lotus-type porous aluminum through thermal decomposition method. Metall. Mater. Trans. **40A**, 937–942, with permission from Springer

pressure. The aligned pores formed under the pressure less than 0.03 MPa argon; however, spherical pores formed over 0.04 MPa argon. This may indicate that the applied pressure in the chamber reduces the driving force for pore nucleation and growth. Figure 2.10b shows the dependence of the porosity and the average pore size as a function of argon pressure. The effect of external pressure is obvious, and the pore growth is suppressed under higher pressure. Both the porosity and the average pore size decrease with increasing argon pressure. The pore volume v, which is equivalent to the porosity, is inversely proportional to the external argon pressure P, which can be described by the Boyle's law, $v = nRT/P$, where n, R and T are the hydrogen molar number, the gas constant, and the temperature, respectively. Therefore, the pore diameter d can be written as $d \propto P^{-1/3}$. The tendency of the pressure dependence of the porosity and pore size is explained by the law.

2.7 Summary

Lotus metals are fabricated by unidirectional solidification of the molten metals dissolving gas atoms. Three solidification techniques were developed: mold casting technique, continuous zone melting technique and continuous casting technique. The continuous casting technique is the most superior for mass production of lotus metals with uniform pore size and porosity. On the other hand, two different supply methods of gas source into the melt are shown: high-pressure gas method and thermal decomposition method. TDM is superior to the PGM, because PGM uses high pressure hydrogen gas with inflammable and explosive risks and gas pressurization in a high-pressure chamber.

Acknowledgments The author would like to appreciate to Drs. S.K.Hyun, T.Ikeda, S.Suzuki, T.Tane, T.Ide and R.Nakamura of Osaka University.

References

1. Banhart J (2001) Prog Mater Sci 46:559
2. Nakajima H (2007) Prog Mater Sci 52:1091
3. Shapovalov V (1994) MRS Bull XIX:24
4. Nakajima H, Ide T (2008) Metall Mater Trans 39A:390
5. Nakajima H (2010) Proc Jpn Acad, Ser B 86:884
6. Ikeda T, Aoki T, Nakajima H (2005) Metall Mater Trans 36A:77
7. Park JS, Hyun SK, Suzuki S, Nakajima H (2007) Acta Mater 55:5646
8. Kim SY, Park JS, Nakajima H (2009) Metall Mater Trans 40A:937

Chapter 3
Modeling of Arc Welding Process

Yoshinori Hirata

Abstract 3D-numerical model is described, which predicts transport phenomena in the arc plasma and the weld pool associated with the arc welding process. Governing equations and boundary conditions are presented for obtaining time-dependent behavior of both thermal and electromagnetic fluids of gaseous plasma and liquid molten metal. And it is emphasized to take into account temperature dependencies of physical properties of shielding gas and metal used for base material at elevated temperature. The calculation results show that the temperature and the velocity distribution in TIG arc plasma are much influenced by the geometry of base metal and the convection in weld pool is driven by the motive forces: electromagnetic force, surface tension force, and plasma stream shear stress.

Keywords TIG arc • Plasma • Weld pool • Modeling • Heat input distribution • Physical property

3.1 Introduction

The rapid progress of computer technology accelerates and promotes the various advancements in every field of science and technology. The industries involving welding and joining processes have been using computers in order to obtain higher productivities and ensure higher joint qualities in design of products, manufacturing plan, factory automation, and so on. The combination of CAD/CAM systems and welding robots is a typical example of practical use in the welding field. However, welding procedure specifications instructed to welding robots have been almost provided on the basis of data-base accumulated in each factory through qualification

Y. Hirata (✉)
Division of Materials and Manufacturing Science, Graduate School of Engineering, Osaka University, 2-1 Yamada-oka, Suita, Osaka 565-0871, Japan
e-mail: hirata@mapse.eng.osaka-u.ac.jp

T. Kakeshita (ed.), *Progress in Advanced Structural and Functional Materials Design*, DOI 10.1007/978-4-431-54064-9_3,

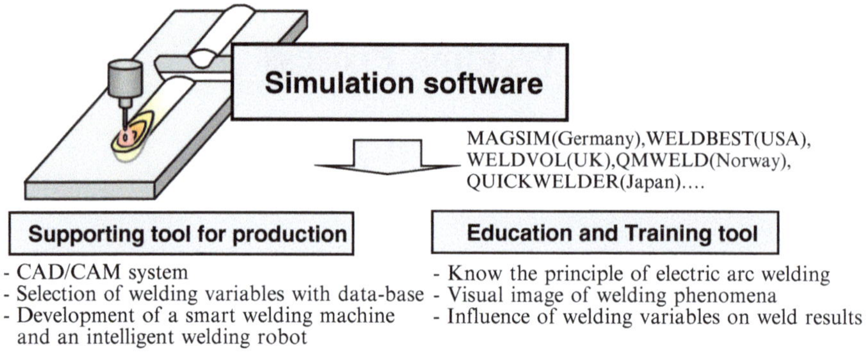

Fig. 3.1 Objects of simulation software for welding process

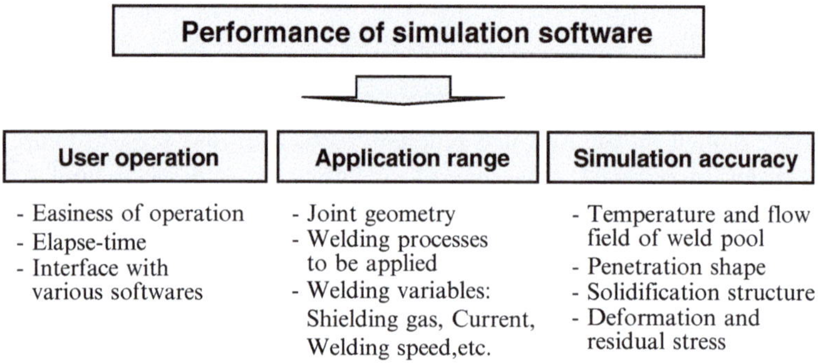

Fig. 3.2 Performance of simulation software

tests performed for many essential variables: kind of material, thickness, groove geometry, welding process, welding position, welding current and so on. Therefore, as for the weld joint not to be experienced in the manufacturing cite, it needs lots of time and cost to carry out the qualification test of the welding procedure in order to ensure the joint performance. Whereas, thermal cycle during welding operation causes the weld deformation and/or the displacement of weld seam line, and also deteriorates the quality of final products. Then, in order to reduce time and expense in the planning stage before fabrication, the developments of simulation software for welding process have been actively carried out in the world [1]. As shown in Fig. 3.1, the simulation software aims at the engineering tool supporting for production such as CAD/CAM, developments of a smart welding machine and an intelligent welding robot, and education/training for welding engineers and welders.

The performance of the simulation software is governed by several factors: the easiness of operation, the scope of application, the accuracy of simulation, etc. As shown in Fig. 3.2, the application range and/or the simulation accuracy are dependent on the numerical model installed into the software. A precise model provides exact solution relevant to the subjects: selection of welding parameters, penetration shape in the welding joint designed, time-dependent temperature field, solidification structure, deformation or residual stress, etc. And it also makes clear the complicated arc welding phenomena. Therefore, numerical models of welding process have been advancing together with spread of high performance personal computer.

3.2 Construction of Numerical Model

Figure 3.3 shows technical issues affecting on welding phenomena, which must be considered in the development of theoretical model. As a matter of course, when the penetration shape and/or the temperature distribution of the work are predicted, temperature at each point corresponding to finite element or mesh in the calculation domain must be acquired by using numerical model. Useful simulation software must enable us to provide temperature distribution of the work relevant to the practical welding having many kinds of joint geometries at various welding positions. And it is necessary to express the features of welding arc as a heat source for calculation. In the case of Tungsten Inert Gas (TIG) welding process, heat input distribution and/or arc pressure distribution must be quantitatively expressed depending on electric current, arc length and so on. In the case of Gas shielded Metal Arc (GMA) welding process, molten metal transfer from electrode wire definitely influences on heat transport and fluid motion in weld pool in addition to

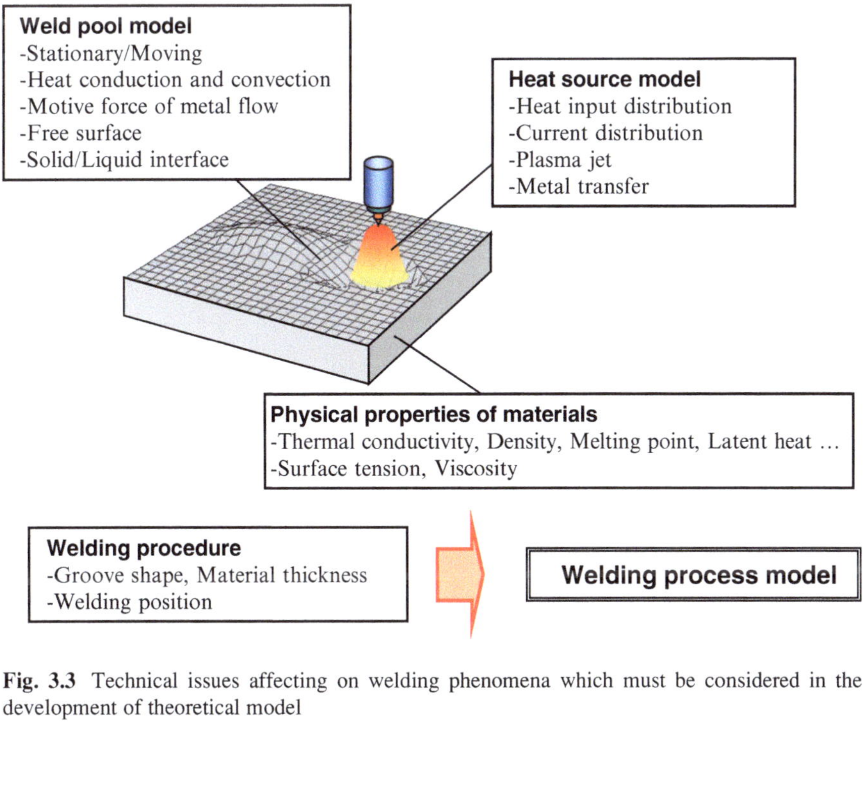

Fig. 3.3 Technical issues affecting on welding phenomena which must be considered in the development of theoretical model

heat and plasma jet from the arc. But from the viewpoint of engineering application, needs for numerical simulation are different depending on the software users: structure-design engineer, production engineer, welding engineer and so on. In other words, it divides into two cases of weld quality prediction requiring simulation accuracy and supporting tool for suitable selection of welding condition. Accordingly, there are lots of needs to reduce calculation time even if the accuracy of the calculation results is rough.

On the other hand, from the scientific viewpoint, the physics of cathode and/or anode, which are interface between arc plasma and liquid/solid metal and dominate characteristics of welding arc discharge, must be deeply understood through development of advanced welding process model. In addition to knowledge concerning the electrode phenomena in the vicinity of the arc discharge, it is necessary to obtain exact and accurate quantities on physical properties of base material and welding wire at elevated temperature.

The arc welding phenomena are associated with heat transfer by high temperature arc plasma and molten metal. Thermal and electromagnetic fluid phenomena are governed by the following equations:

- Mass conservation equation:

$$\nabla \cdot (\rho \vec{v}) + \frac{\partial \rho}{\partial t} = 0 \tag{3.1}$$

- Momentum conservation equation:

$$\frac{\partial}{\partial t}(\rho \vec{v}) + \nabla [\rho \vec{v} \vec{v}] = -\nabla P + \nabla \cdot \tau + \rho \vec{g} + \vec{F} \tag{3.2}$$

here,

$$\tau = \begin{pmatrix} \tau_{xx} & \tau_{xy} & \tau_{xz} \\ \tau_{yx} & \tau_{yy} & \tau_{yz} \\ \tau_{zx} & \tau_{zy} & \tau_{zz} \end{pmatrix} = \begin{pmatrix} 2\eta \frac{\partial u}{\partial x} & \eta\left(\frac{\partial v}{\partial x} + \frac{\partial u}{\partial y}\right) & \eta\left(\frac{\partial u}{\partial z} + \frac{\partial w}{\partial x}\right) \\ \eta\left(\frac{\partial v}{\partial x} + \frac{\partial u}{\partial y}\right) & 2\eta \frac{\partial v}{\partial y} & \eta\left(\frac{\partial w}{\partial y} + \frac{\partial v}{\partial z}\right) \\ \eta\left(\frac{\partial u}{\partial z} + \frac{\partial w}{\partial x}\right) & \eta\left(\frac{\partial w}{\partial y} + \frac{\partial v}{\partial z}\right) & 2\eta \frac{\partial w}{\partial z} \end{pmatrix}$$

- Energy conservation equation:

$$\frac{\partial}{\partial t}(\rho H) + \nabla \cdot (\rho H \vec{v}) = -\nabla \cdot (-\kappa \nabla T) + W - Ra \tag{3.3}$$

here,

$$\rho H = \int \rho c_p dT$$

where ρ: density (kg/m^3), $\vec{v}$: velocity vector (m/s), t: time (s), *P*: pressure (Pa), τ: viscous stress tensor (Pa), $\vec{g}$: gravitational acceleration (m/s^2), $\vec{F}$: external force (N/m^3), η: viscosity (kg/ms), *H*: enthalpy (J/kg), κ: thermal conductivity (J/ms K), *W* is internal heat generation (W/m^3), *Ra* is radiation loss (W/m^3), c_p is specific heat at constant pressure (J/kg K), *u*, *v*, and *w* are the velocity components in the *x*, *y*, and *z* directions, respectively.

When the welding arc is generated, electric current is flowing in the arc plasma and base metal. Therefore, it is necessary to consider electromagnetic force as external force together with Joule's heating as internal heat generation. Here, the electromagnetic force and the Joule's heating are expressed as the following equations:

$$\vec{F} = \vec{j} \times \vec{B} \tag{3.4}$$

$$W = \frac{\vec{j}^2}{\sigma} \tag{3.5}$$

where $\vec{j}$ is current density vector (A/m^2), σ is electrical conductivity (S/m), $\vec{B}$ is magnetic flux density vector (T). The electric current and magnetic field are governed by the following equations:

- Current conservation:

$$\nabla \vec{j} = 0 \tag{3.6}$$

- Ohm's law:

$$\vec{j} = -\sigma \nabla V \tag{3.7}$$

- Magnetic field:

$$\vec{B} = \nabla \times \vec{A} \tag{3.8}$$

- Magnetic vector potential:

$$\nabla^2 \vec{A} = -\mu_0 \vec{j} \tag{3.9}$$

where V: the electrical potential (V), $\vec{A}$: the magnetic vector potential (N/A), and μ_0: the magnetic permeability of free space (H/m).

When the base metal is anode of the arc discharge, the heat input into the base metal is provided by heat conduction and current-carrying electrons from the welding arc plasma. Therefore, the heat input to the anode can be calculated from the following equation:

$$\vec{q} = -\kappa \nabla T + \vec{j} \phi \tag{3.10}$$

where $\vec{q}$: the heat flux (W/m^2), ϕ: the kinetic energy and the condensation energy into the anode metal which are brought by electron in the arc plasma (eV).

Using these governing equations, numerical analyses is carried out using various numerical codes. In this text numerical results are obtained with our own scheme based on the SMAC method [2].

3.3 Modeling of TIG Arc Plasma

3.3.1 Description of TIG Arc Model

Schematic explanations of the 3D numerical model of the TIG arc are shown in Fig. 3.4. Since TIG arc plasma has a wide range of temperatures, the temperature dependence of the physical properties of the shielding gas cannot be ignored [3]. Figure 3.5 shows the physical properties of argon gas [4]. As seen, density, thermal conductivity, electrical conductivity and so on are varied depending on temperature. For example, as for electrical conductivity, at room temperature gas is almost electrical insulator but beyond around 4,000 K it acts as electrical conductor.

In this text the diameter and vertex angle of the electrode are 3.2 mm and 60°, respectively. Shielding gas is argon gas which flows from the gas flow area. The numerical results of arc plasma on the both of flat plate and V-grooved plate are introduced here. For the flat plate, the thickness of the plate is 5 mm. In the case of the grooved plate, the thickness of the plate is 12 mm, the groove depth is 10 mm and its angle is 90°. The kinetic energy and the condensation energy carried by electron in the arc plasma is 4.65 eV for calculation. The definition of the arc length

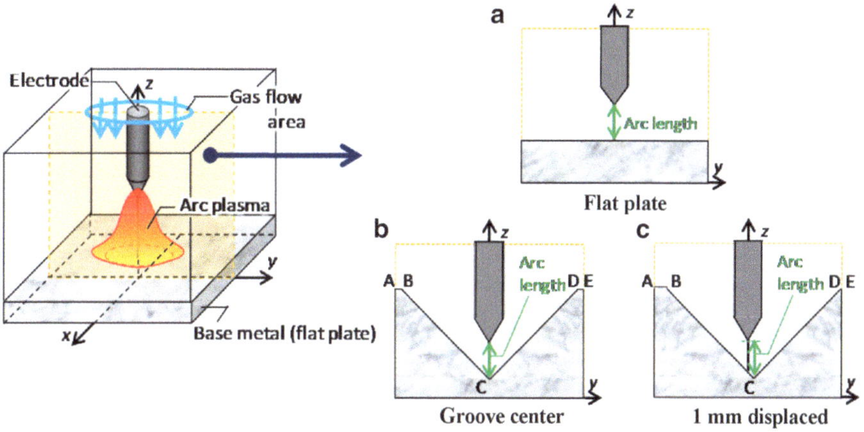

Fig. 3.4 Schematic image of the 3D numerical model of a TIG arc on the flat plate and grooved plate

is shown in Fig. 3.4. In the practical welding, the base metal are melted and deformed by arc heat. Moreover, during practical welding operation, metal vapor generated from weld pool is mixed with the argon plasma, which changes the physical properties of the arc plasma [5]. However, in the present model, in order to avoid these complexities, the anode plate is assumed to be substantially cooled and not to melt nor deformed. In other words, fusion of base metal and metal vapor are ignored, and the calculations are assumed to be pure argon arc plasma. For the V-grooved anode plate, the influence of TIG torch or electrode position on arc plasma is described. As seen in Fig. 3.4b, the electrode tip is set up the just above the groove bottom. In Fig. 3.4c, the electrode tip is displaced 1 mm from the centerline of the groove to left side. The TIG torch is stationary.

Both boundaries of cathode electrode–arc plasma and anode metal surface–arc plasma are taken into account by adjusting the physical properties at the boundary. For the electrical conductivity of the gaseous phase–solid phase boundary, the reciprocal averages of the adjoining grid points are adopted [6]. In the case of non-uniform mesh it can be expressed as follows:

$$\frac{l_G + l_S}{\sigma_B} = \frac{l_G}{\sigma_G} + \frac{l_S}{\sigma_S}, \tag{3.11}$$

where the indices G and S indicate gaseous phase and solid phase, respectively. The symbols, σ_B, σ_G and σ_S are electrical conductivities at the boundary, at the adjoining point of gaseous phase and at the adjoining grid point of solid phase, respectively. The symbols, l_G and l_S are the distance between the boundary and the grid point of gaseous phase, and the distance between the boundary and the grid point of solid phase, respectively. The thermal conductivity of the boundary is calculated using the film temperature.

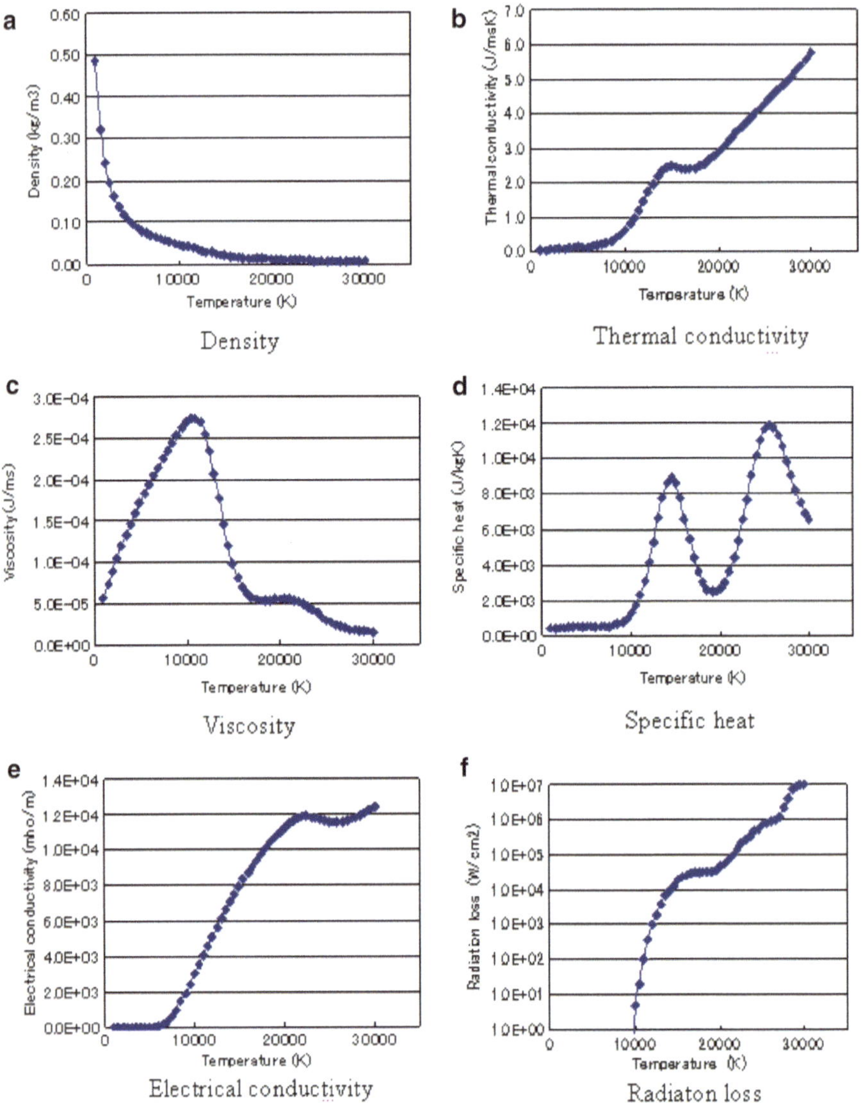

Fig. 3.5 Physical properties of argon gas

3.3.2 Calculation Results

Figure 3.6 shows the temperature and the velocity distribution of the arc plasma [7]. The arc current is 200 A and the arc length is 3 mm. The figure shows the *yz* surface across the electrode tip and the *xy* surface just above the base metal. For the calculation results of just above the grooved plate, shown in Fig. 3.6b(ii), c(ii),

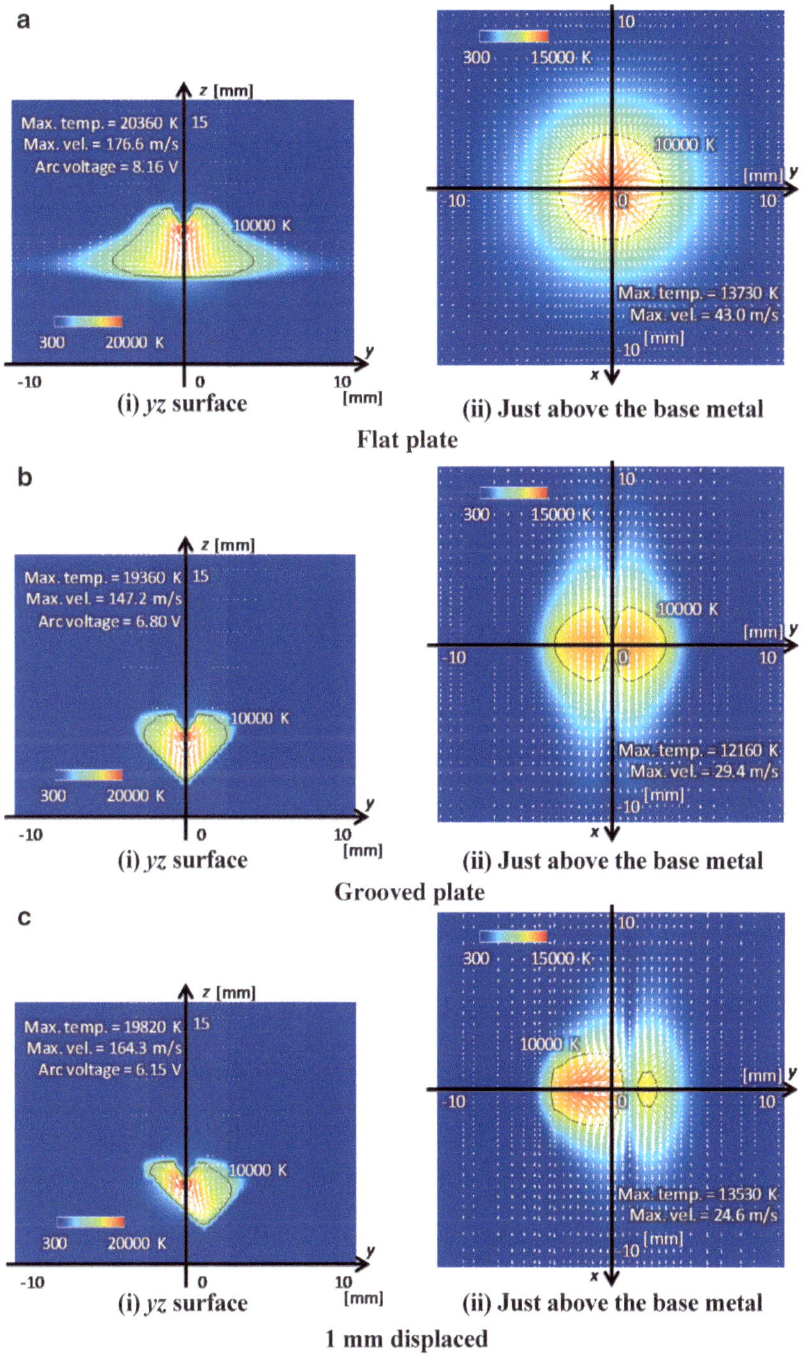

Fig. 3.6 Influence of the base metal shapes on the temperature and the velocity field of an arc plasma

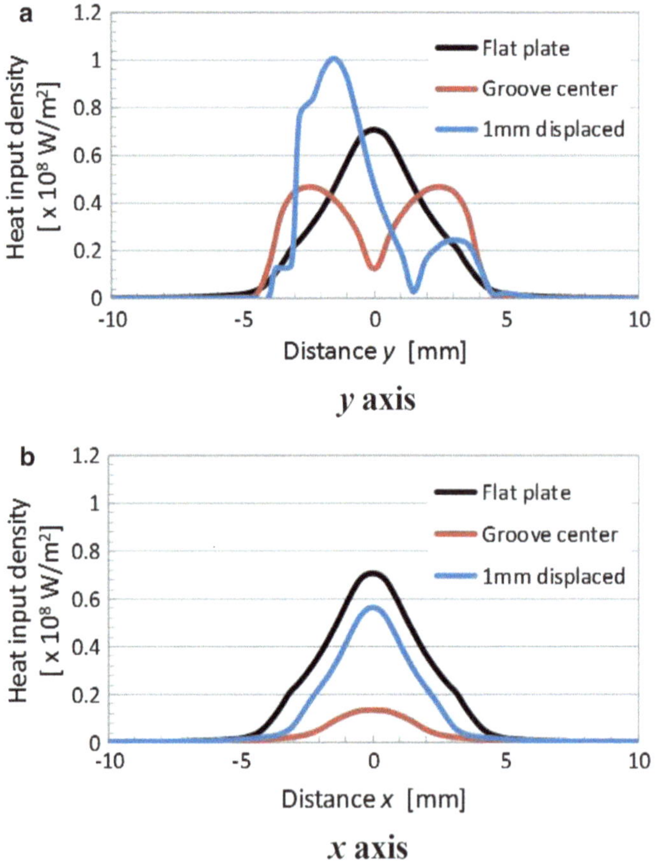

Fig. 3.7 The heat input density distribution on the anode surface for the flat plate and the grooved plate

indicate the surface of along the groove surface that is ABCDE surface shown in Fig. 3.4b, c. In the figure, the isothermal line indicates a temperature of 10,000 K and the white arrows indicate the flow vector. When the flat plate is used, the arc plasma forms a bell shape and its cross section is circular just above the base metal, as shown in Fig. 3.6a. For the grooved plate, shown in Fig. 3.6b, the arc plasma is restricted by the groove wall. And its high-temperature area is located at the groove wall just above the base metal. Moreover, when the TIG torch is displaced to the left direction, the arc plasma shape is deformed from symmetry and its high-temperature area forms at the left side of groove surface, as shown in Fig. 3.6c. Therefore, the arc plasma shape is significantly changed with the base metal shape.

Figure 3.7 shows the heat input density distribution on the anode surface [7]. Figure 3.7a shows the distribution on the *y* axis of Fig. 3.6(ii), which is across the groove. Figure 3.7b shows the distribution on the x axis of Fig. 3.6(ii), which is along to the groove. As seen in Fig. 3.7a, when the flat anode plate is used, the

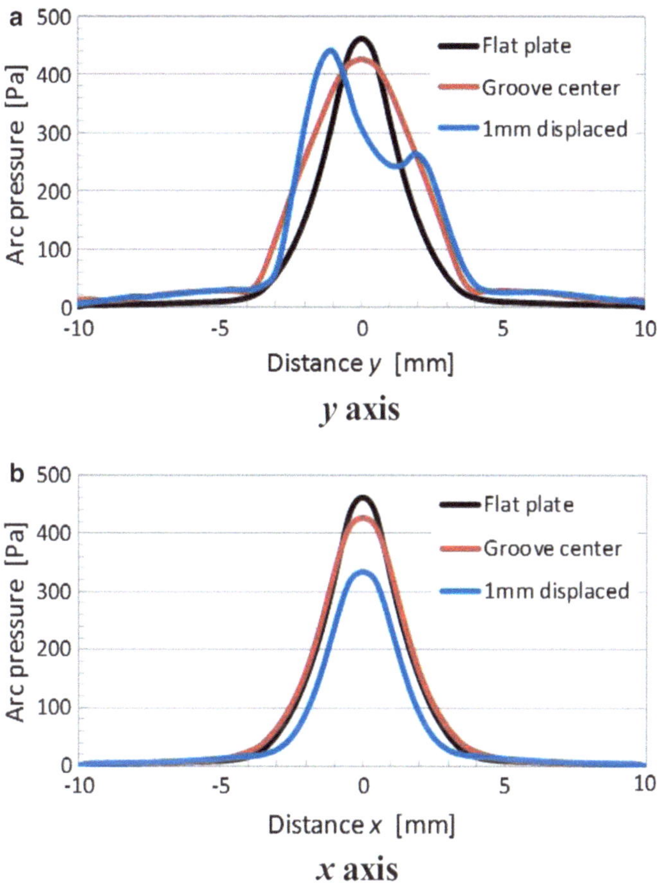

Fig. 3.8 The arc pressure distribution on the anode surface for the flat plate and the grooved plate

maximum heat input from the TIG arc is located at the surface of base metal just below the electrode tip, and its distribution takes like Gaussian distribution. For the grooved plate, the maximum heat input is not located at the bottom of groove just below the electrode. It is located at the groove surface in both sides. When the TIG torch is shifted 1 mm to the left groove surface, heat input from the arc is not symmetry and concentrates on the left groove surface significantly. All of the heat input density distributions on the x axis take like Gaussian distribution and their peaks are located at the just below the electrode as seen in Fig. 3.7b. Figure 3.8 shows the arc pressure distribution of TIG arc on the anode surface [7]. These distributions show the same position as Fig. 3.7. As seen in Fig. 3.8a, when the flat anode plate is used, the maximum pressure of the TIG arc is located at the surface of base metal just below the electrode tip, and its distribution is similar to the heat input, which takes like Gaussian distribution. For the grooved plate, the maximum pressure is also located at just below the electrode, where is the bottom of the groove.

When the TIG torch is shifted 1 mm to the left groove surface, arc pressure distribution is deformed from the symmetry. All of the arc pressure distributions on the x axis take like Gaussian distribution and their peaks are located at the just below the electrode as seen in Fig. 3.8b.

Therefore, the heat source characteristics of arc plasma such as the heat input density distribution and the arc pressure distribution are significantly changed with the base metal shape and the torch position. It is shown that the heat input density distribution changes more dramatically than the arc pressure. The arc pressure of the TIG arc is remarkably affected by the electrode shape [8]. On the other hand, the heat input from the TIG arc strongly depends on the temperature and current density just above the base metal. This causes the difference between the heat input and the arc pressure when the anode plate is changed.

3.4 Modeling of Weld Pool

Recently, most welding experts recognize that variable penetration is associated with the fluid flow pattern in the weld pool, and there are four motive forces generating such flow: electromagnetic force, surface tension force, buoyancy force, and plasma stream shear stress. The problem of cast-to-cast variation of penetration in TIG welding became evident during the 1970s [9]. Especially, minor elements effects on weld penetration shape have been experimentally and theoretically for many years [10, 11]. Considerable works have been done on modeling flow and heat transfer in weld pools during melt-run TIG welding process. Early studies investigated fluid flow due to electromagnetic force in a hemispherical weld pool [12]. An important study on the flow and heat transfer conditions in a stationary TIG weld pool was completed, in which the effect of surface tension gradient on weld pool convection was considered for the first time [13]. Subsequently, the influence of four motive forces on weld penetration of spot TIG welding was investigated [14]. More recently, a unified electrode–arc–weld pool model for a stationary TIG welding was developed [15].

In 1986 the first 3D model, which provides both fields of temperature and flow in the quasi-steady TIG weld pool, was published [16]. A more comprehensive and rigorous model was developed, which considered both a deformable free surface and non-autogenous welds [17]. A correlation between theoretical predictions and experimental results was investigated for time-change of weld pool in TIG welding of type-304 stainless steel [18].

In this section, calculation results of temperature and flow fields in weld pool are shown for melt-run welds of flat plate by TIG arc. The calculation results obtained by TIG arc plasma model mentioned above are used for input conditions to weld pool model. It is required to input the heat input distribution and flow field of TIG arc. In order to make clear the effect of surface tension driven flow in TIG welding of stainless steel, calculations are carried out for two different sulfur contents of

Table 3.1 Physical properties of stainless steel (SUS304) used in the calculation

ρ: density (kg/m^3)	8.0×10^3
mT: melting point	1672.0
K: thermal conductivity of liquid (J/ms K)	28.0
K: thermal conductivity of solid (J/ms K)	1.4×10^{-2} T + 11
c: specific heat (J/kg K)	6.45×10^2
L: latent heat of melting (J/kg)	2.5×10^5
η: kinematic viscosity (m^2/s)	1.0×10^{-6}

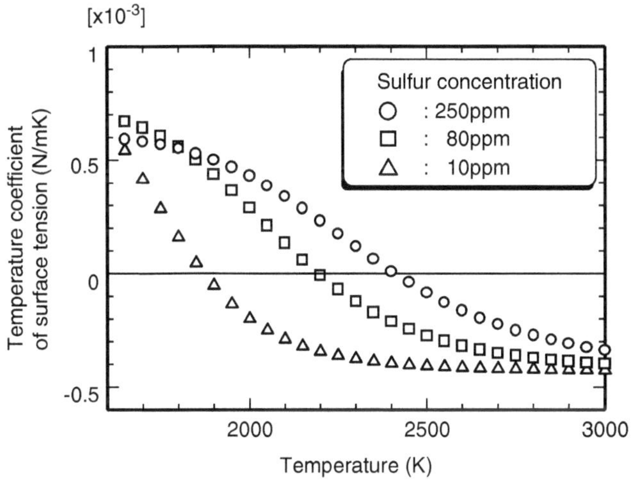

Fig. 3.9 Relationship between temperature and temperature coefficient of surface tension of 18Cr–8Ni–S–Fe alloy

type-304 stainless steel welded by argon gas shielded TIG arc of 150 A. Physical properties of type-304 stainless steel used for calculation are shown in Table 3.1.

Motive force due to surface tension is induced when it is not uniform in the pool. In other words a point having higher surface tension pulls another point having lower surface tension. The surface tension is a function of temperature and chemical composition of the material. Accordingly, when there are temperature differences at the pool surface, surface tension force acts and causes the metal flow. Figure 3.9 shows the temperature coefficient of surface tension of 18Cr–8Ni–S–Fe alloy, used in the calculation [19].

Figure 3.10 shows the calculation results of temperature and flow field of the weld pool in TIG welding of type-304 stainless steel. Arc current is 150 A and welding speed is 12 cm/min. Heat input distribution and shear stress at the pool surface by plasma flow are given from calculation results of TIG arc plasma with current of 150 A. Figure 3.10a shows the calculation result of low sulfur content material (LS: 10 ppm S). As seen, the liquid metal flows from the arc center toward the pool boundary and this convection causes to form the large pool and the shallow penetration. In this case

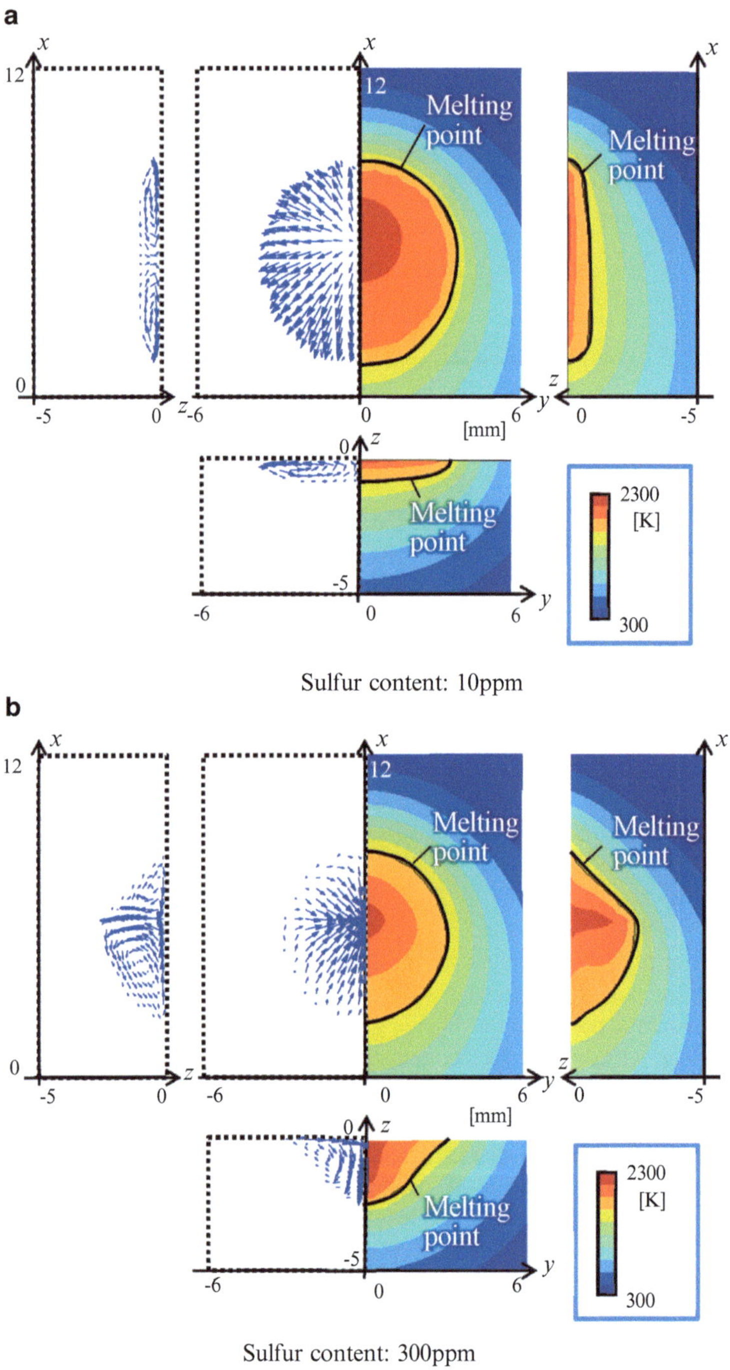

Fig. 3.10 Temperature and flow field of weld pool in TIG welding of type-304 stainless steel (arc current: 150 A, welding speed: 12 cm/min, arc length: 3 mm)

surface temperature gradient is small and the peak temperature is around 2,150 K. While, Fig. 3.10b shows the calculation result of high sulfur content material (HS: 300 ppm S). The weld pool of HS is smaller than that of LS. The peak temperature at the pool surface of HS, 2,200 K is a little higher than that of LS. The molten metal of HS flows from the trailing edge of the pool toward the center of TIG arc. And this flow circulates in the welding direction and contributes to the deep penetration as shown in the longitudinal cross section. As seen in the transverse cross section, inward flow is formed.

3.5 Summary

In order to clarify the behavior of arc plasma and weld pool in the arc welding phenomena, it is necessary to obtain exact and accurate quantities on physical properties of shielding gas and metal used for electrode and/or base material at elevated temperature in addition to knowledge concerning the electrode phenomena in the vicinity of the arc discharge. In the case of GMA welding process which is widely used in various industries all over the world, electrode wire melts due to arc heat and then the molten droplet is formed at the tip of electrode. It detaches from the wire tip and transfers into weld pool in succession. The molten droplet and/or molten pool surface seem to reach considerably high temperature. Accordingly, the metal vapor could be diffused into the plasma, then it greatly affects current path and/or heat input form to base material and electrode wire. Because metal vapor influences on electron density and temperature of the plasma which are directly connected with the electrical conductivity, and then the current path in the arc discharge is governed by the characteristics of arc plasma.

While, it is necessary to establish the measurement technique for temperature and fluid flow of weld pool and molten drop in order to check the accuracy of the numerical results. The verification of the present model enables to develop more advanced model. Then, the prediction based on the refined model is repeatedly compared with the experiment, and it seems to clarify the mechanism of the arc welding phenomena. Consequently, it will be more connected for the development of the high-performance simulation software, and simultaneously, it is expected to develop the new welding process.

References

1. Dilthey U, Bohlmann HC, Willms K, Sudnik W, Mokrov O, Kudinov R (2001) MAGSIM and SPOTSIM—simulation of GMA and spot welding for training and industrial application. In: Proceedings of the 7th international symposium of Japan Welding Society, vol 1, p 143
2. Amsden AA, Harlow FH (1970) The SMAC method: a numerical technique for calculating incompressible fluid flows, Los Alamos Science Laboratory report, LA-4370

3. Capitelli M, Devoto RS (1973) Transport coefficients of high-temperature nitrogen. Phys Fluids 16(11):1835–1841
4. Murphy AB (1995) Transport coefficients of air, argon-air, nitrogen-air, and oxygen-air plasmas. Plasma Chem Plasma Process 15(2):279–307
5. Tanaka M, Yamamoto k, Tashiro S, Nakata K, Yamamoto E, Yamazaki K, Suzuki K, Murphy AB, Lowke JJ (2010) Time-dependent calculations of molten pool formation and thermal plasma with metal vapour in gas tungsten arc welding. J Phys D Appl Phys 43(434009):11 pp
6. Hu J, Guo H, Tsai HL (2008) Weld pool dynamics and the formation of ripples in 3D gas metal arc welding. Int J Heat Mass Transfer 51:2537–2552
7. Ogino Y, Hirata Y, Nomura K (2011) Heat input and pressure distribution of TIG arc on groove surface. Welding in the World 55 (11/12): 107–113
8. Fang D, Ushio M, Matsuda F (1986) Numerical computation of arc pressure distribution. Trans JWRI 1:1–5
9. Lancaster J.F, Mills K.C (1991) Recommendations for the avoidance of variable penetration in gas tungsten arc welding, IIW Doc. 212-796-91
10. Makara AM et al (1977) The effect of refining of the penetration of metal in arc welding. Automatic Welding 30(9):1
11. Heiple CR, Roper JR (1982) Mechanism for minor element effect on GTA fusion zone geometry. Weld J 61(4):97s
12. Sozou C, Pickering WM (1976) Magnetohydrodynamic flow due to the discharge of an electric current in a hemispherical container. J Fluid Mech 76(4):641
13. Oreper GM, Szekely J (1984) Heat and fluid flow phenomena in weld pools. J Fluid Mech 147(10):53
14. Yokoya S, Matsunawa A (1987) Convection in weld pool and its effects on penetration shape, IIW 212-687-87
15. Tanaka K, Tanaka M, Terasaki H, Ushio M, Lowke JJ (2001) Numerical modeling of arc plasma and weld shape in stationary TIG welding. In: Proceedings of the 7th international symposium of Japan Welding Society, vol 1
16. Kou S, Wang YH (1986) Weld pool convection and its effect. Weld J 65(3):63s
17. Zacharia T, Eraslan AH, Aidun DK (1988) Modeling of non-autogenous welding. Weld J 67 (1):18s
18. Zacharia T, David SA, Vitek JM, DebRoy T (1989) Weld pool development during GTA and laser beam welding of type 304 stainless steel, Part II—experimental correlation. Weld J 68(12):510s
19. McNallan MJ, DebRoy T (1991) Effect of temperature and composition on surface tension in Fe-Ni-Cr alloys containing sulfur. Metal Trans B 22B(8):557

Chapter 4
Advanced Materials Design Using Lasers

Tomokazu Sano and Akio Hirose

Abstract The laser, which is one of the greatest inventions of the twentieth century, has opened up new fields of industry as well as science. Femtosecond laser oscillated from the chirped pulse amplifier is a relatively newly-developed system with an extremely short temporal pulse. In this chapter, a state-of-the-art surface treatment method using the femtosecond laser-driven shock wave is described.

Keywords Femtosecond laser • Laser processing • Phase transition • Shock wave

4.1 Introduction

The laser is one of the greatest inventions of the twentieth century [1]. Laser, which is the acronym for "Light Amplification by Stimulated Emission of Radiation," describes a device that produces coherent light of a single wavelength with a single phase. Not only the invention of the laser has opened up new fields of science but the laser has been applied in a variety of industrial areas [2].

Laser processing is used in many applications such as drilling, cutting, welding, joining, cladding, alloying, forming, peening, marking, trimming, scribing, patterning, repairing, cleaning, annealing, etc. [3, 4]. In this Chapter, a state-of-the-art surface treatment method using short laser pulses is described. Synthesis of the metastable phase of carbon and quenching of the high pressure structure of iron are described followed by explanations of the femtosecond laser ablation of solids and the femtosecond laser-driven shock wave in solids.

T. Sano (✉) • A. Hirose
Division of Materials and Manufacturing Science, Graduate School of Engineering, Osaka University, 2-1 Yamadaoka, Suita, Osaka 565-0871, Japan
e-mail: sano@mapse.eng.osaka-u.ac.jp

T. Kakeshita (ed.), *Progress in Advanced Structural and Functional Materials Design*, DOI 10.1007/978-4-431-54064-9_4,

4.2 Femtosecond Laser

A laser with pulse width less than picoseconds order is called an ultrashort pulsed laser or femtosecond laser. Ultrashort pulsed lasers were developed in the middle 1960s. The size of the early systems was large and the pulse was unstable. The ultrashort pulsed laser, however, became smaller in size and highly stable after development of the Kerr lens mode-locked laser using a Ti:Sapphire medium in 1991 [5]. A continuum pumping beam stimulates the Ti:Sapphire medium, and the laser with range of wavelength from infrared to ultraviolet is oscillated and amplified in the oscillator using four mirrors. A slit for mode-locking keeps the laser intensity constant. Scattered light goes back through prisms. The ultrashort pulse is oscillated cyclically through a half-mirror.

A table-top femtosecond pulse above TW was achieved with the development of the chirped pulse amplifier (CPA) [6]. As a result of the irradiation of a low intensity femtosecond pulse into a pair of gratings, the pulse width is stretched (in other words, chirped). This stretched pulse is amplified in an amplifier. The intense femtosecond laser pulse is obtained by compressing the amplified pulse as a result of irradiation into another pair of gratings.

4.2.1 Femtosecond Laser Ablation of Solids

New applications of the intense femtosecond laser have opened in the fields of industry, materials science, medicine, etc., because of the rapid development of the intense femtosecond laser in this decade. Femtosecond laser ablation is one of the important physical phenomena, and is applied to microprocessing, film deposition, new material production, and so on. Distinctive features of the femtosecond laser ablation compared with the nanosecond laser ablation are: highly efficient energy deposition due to no absorption of laser energy into the laser generated plasma because the pulse is over before the expansion of the plasma, direct transition from solid to gas or plasma via no solid–liquid process, and little secondary damage to solids due to thermal conduction. Therefore, the femtosecond laser has the advantage for the applications described above [7].

Nonequilibrium dynamics of the electron gas in metals irradiated by the femtosecond laser has been studied actively in the last 20 years. Direct experimental studies on fundamental processes such as electron–electron scattering and electron–phonon interaction have become possible due to the appearance of the femtosecond pulse laser [8–11]. Theoretical studies on these processes based on the data obtained from experimental studies have also been performed [12–15].

Electron–phonon nonequilibrium is important in the regime of picoseconds order. At first, free electrons in the metal absorb the laser energy as the lattice remains cold. The energy is delivered to all the free electrons by the electron–electron collisions within femtoseconds order, and thermalization of the electron gas occurs. Energy transfer between the electron and the lattice is dominated by electron–phonon collisions. The electron–phonon collision time τ_{ep} is as short as the electron–electron collision time τ_{ee} [16]. The time for energy transfer from hot electrons to the lattice is usually several tens of picoseconds and longer than the thermalization of the electron gas because of the difference in mass between the electron and the phonon. This process was verified experimentally [9–11], and is described by the classical two temperature model [17, 18].

The fundamental mechanism of the ablation process is not yet understood precisely. Pressure wave formation [19], thermodynamic evolution of expanding materials [20], and identification of the collective emission process [7, 14, 15, 20, 21] have to be understood in order to describe the process at the mesoscopic scale. Many mechanisms are thought to play a role in the ablation below the plasma formation threshold: optical dynamic spallation in organic materials [22], heterogeneous nucleations of gas bubbles and phase explosion [14, 20, 22], spinodal decomposition [20, 21], fragmentation [14], and vaporization [7]. The ablation mechanism that follows was suggested using molecular dynamic simulations based on these phenomena [15].

The main response to the absorption of the pulse energy is the expansion to release the storage of the important thermoelastic pressure induced by the heating of the constant volume of the target. The material is, however, relaxed by emitting a strong pressure wave, which plays an important role in the ablation process [22, 23].

Although the tensile component is formed at low fluences below the ablation threshold, it actually disappears with the increment of the fluence due to the thermo-softening of the surface material. Thus, the tensile wave intermediate effect such as spallation is observed only at low fluences. The relaxation of the thermoelastic stress occurs at an early stage by the irradiation of two compressive pressure waves: One goes toward the free surface, and the other goes inside the bulk [19, 22]. The wave irradiated at the free surface reflects and becomes the tensile stress (negative pressure). However, the tensile component is not formed completely before the reflected wave reaches approximately skin depth under the surface. Thus, the resulting acoustic wave has a bipolar profile: the compressive stress and the following tensile stress.

At middle fluences, phase explosion is the main mechanism of the ablation. This mechanism occurs in the region of gradual expansion of the material, and may form the condition that forms Newton's rings.

At high fluences, the pressure profile has a single structure; the tensile component disappears completely. Thus, reflection does not occur because the wave irradiated at the free surface is dissipated at the surface layer. This pressure intensity is proportional to the incident energy. The tensile stress is also formed. This is not induced by the elastic wave but by the development of the melting front. At an early stage, this stress propagates at the sound velocity, and becomes lower later. At high strain rates, a plume is formed by the mechanical fragmentation of the expanded materials. Complete evaporation of the surface layer is also observed. This mechanism can occur at different places under the surface of the target at the same time. Thus, the formation of the pressure wave must be considered in predicting the ablation rate.

4.2.2 Femtosecond Laser-Driven Shock Wave in Solids

The shock wave propagates in metals due to shock loading on the metal surface when an intense femtosecond laser is irradiated on the surface as described in the previous section. In this section, the properties of the femtosecond laser driven shock wave are described.

For many years, the nanosecond laser driven shock wave has been used to study materials at extreme conditions of pressure, density, and temperature [24–29]. The critical difference between the femtosecond and the nanosecond laser ablations is the absorption of the laser energy into the laser induced plume during the laser pulse. For the nanosecond laser, the temporal shock wave profile is relatively long due to the pressure loading from the plume which absorbs the laser energy. The heating effect of the target emitted from the plume is also not negligible. While for the femtosecond laser, the femtosecond laser driven shock wave is characterized only by the femtosecond laser–metal interaction because the ablation occurs after the deposition of the entire laser energy.

The ultrasonic heat wave driven by the heat conduction propagates into the undisturbed target when the thin layer of the target is heated rapidly to 100–1,000 eV. The heat wave slows down when the thickness of the heated material becomes larger. Coincident with this rapid heating is the hydrodynamic expansion of the heated material into the vacuum. The shock front overtakes the heat front when the heat front approaches the velocity of sound. This physical state is the classical problem of the hydrodynamic phenomena [30]. When the intense femtosecond laser is irradiated on the solid surface, the shock pressure of approximately 1 TPa is generated in the laser absorbed region because the lattice is heated long before the thermal expansion occurs. In this situation, the shock front overtakes the heat front after the heat front propagates in the solid through 100–200 nm, which distance depends on the laser intensity [31].

The shock velocity and the particle velocity were measured simultaneously using a frequency domain interferometer with time resolution of sub picoseconds [32] when the femtosecond laser (800 nm, 120 fs, ~10^{14} W/cm^2) was irradiated on the surface of a thin Al film (10–400 nm on fused silica substrate (2 mm)), and the shock pressure was estimated at 100–300 GPa assuming that the shock is along the Hugoniot [33].

Rise times and temporal profile of the femtosecond laser driven shock wave were measured using the frequency domain interferometer [34–36]. The shock wave was driven by the femtosecond laser (800 nm, 130 fs, 0.2–0.5 mJ) which was irradiated on deposited metal thin films (polycrystalline Al and Ni (250–2,000 nm)) through the cover glass for microscope observation. The Gaussian profile of the laser profile of the incident beam is flattened because of the nonlinear absorption of the laser driving the shock wave into the glass substrate that functions as an optical limiter. Therefore, the planar shock wave is generated in the metal [37]. The dynamic behavior of the surface and the reflectivity of the laser from the thin metal film during the generation of the shock wave were measured at the same time using the frequency domain interferometer, and the shock rise time from 10% to 90% was estimated at several picoseconds.

4.3 Synthesis of Hexagonal Diamond from Highly Oriented Pyrolytic Graphite

The stable phase of carbon is graphite in the lower pressure regime and cubic diamond in the higher pressure regime [38]. Cubic diamond is one of the most important materials in the manufacturing industry due to its high hardness and thermal conductivity. Hexagonal diamond was discovered in the Canyon Diablo iron meteorite [39] and is considered the metastable high pressure phase of carbon. Hexagonal diamond is synthesized artificially from graphite using the shock compression method with a catalyst [40] and from cubic diamond without a catalyst [41], using the static compression method [42], and the chemical vapor deposition method [43]. There still exist many unresolved questions about the synthesis mechanism of cubic and hexagonal diamonds. The crystal structure of the femtosecond laser-driven shock-compressed graphite has been analyzed.

4.3.1 Experimental Method

The target used in this study was the highly oriented pyrolytic graphite (HOPG, NT-MDT Co., Russia, 10 mm × 10 mm × *t* 1.5 mm) with ZYA quality, mosaic spread of 0.4–0.7°, and mass density of 2.267 g/cm^3. A femtosecond laser pulse (Spitfire, Spectra-Physics Inc.) with wavelength 800 nm, pulse width 130 fs, and nearly Gaussian spatial energy distribution was first passed through an aperture of 6 mm diameter, and second was focused onto a target surface in air using a plano-convex lens with focal length of 70 mm. The femtosecond laser pulse was irradiated normal to the basal plane of the HOPG target. A single pulse was shot at a point, and the shot to shot interval was 100 μm on the surface. Two kinds of laser pulse energy, 0.7 and 5.5 mJ, were used. The spatially averaged laser intensity was approximately 3×10^{14} and 2×10^{15} W/cm^2 for the laser pulse energies of 0.7 and 5.5 mJ, respectively. The laser spot size was approximately 50 μm. Crystalline structures were analyzed using the grazing incident XRD method at the BL13XU in the SPring-8 [44]. The synchrotron X-ray with wavelength of 1.000 Å was passed through a slit with horizontal width of 410 μm and vertical width of 50 μm, and then was irradiated onto the sample. The incident angle α was fixed and the detector angle δ was varied. A solar slit was located in front of the detector, which is the YAP scintillation counter.

4.3.2 Results and Discussion

The laser irradiated area was explosively removed and a deep crater was created at the laser pulse energy of 5.5 mJ, while no significant crater was created at laser

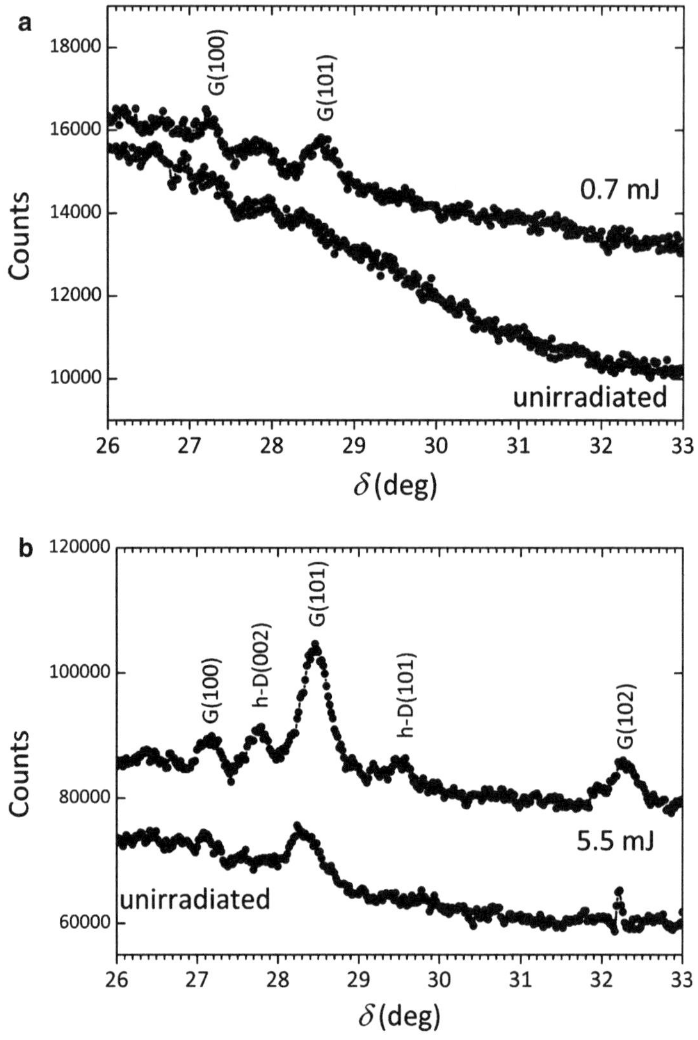

Fig. 4.1 Grazing incidence XRD patterns of the femtosecond laser irradiated HOPG. Laser pulse energy: (**a**) 0.7 and (**b**) 5.5 mJ. *G* Graphite, *h-D* hexagonal diamond

pulse energy of 0.7 mJ. The explosively created deep crater indicates that explosive ablation occurs and that a strong shock wave was driven in the sample.

Grazing incidence XRD patterns for the laser pulse energy of (a) 0.7 and (b) 5.5 mJ are shown in Fig. 4.1. The incident angle of the X-ray to the sample surface was 0.1°, the angular resolution of the detector was 0.02°/step, and the exposure time was 5.0 s/step. The critical angle of carbon for light of wavelength 1.000 Å is 0.13°. Therefore, there is no scattered X-ray if the HOPG surface is perfectly planar. However, the laser irradiated region is roughened so that any

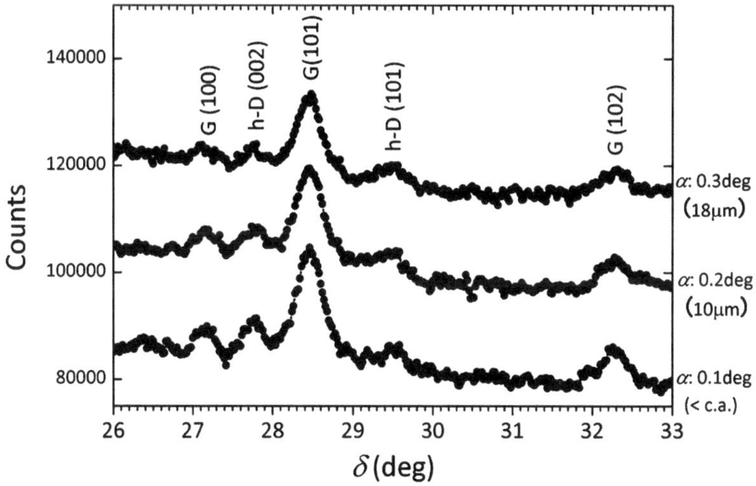

Fig. 4.2 Grazing incidence XRD patterns for incident angles of 0.1°, 0.2°, and 0.3°

X-rays are scattered at the region. Peaks of (100) and (101) planes of the graphite appear after the 0.7 mJ laser pulse irradiation as shown in Fig. 4.2a. This means that the plastic deformation induced by the femtosecond laser-driven shock wave collapsed the orientation in the laser irradiated region. We found peaks of not only (100), (101), and (102) planes of graphite, but (002) and (101) planes of hexagonal diamond after the 5.5 mJ laser pulse irradiation. This means that the 5.5 mJ laser pulse induced a shock wave strong enough to induce the graphite–diamond transition.

Grazing incidence XRD patterns of the HOPG which was irradiated by the 5.5 mJ laser pulse are shown in Fig. 4.2 for incident angles of 0.1°, 0.2°, and 0.3°. The X-ray penetration depth is 10 and 18 μm for incident angles of 0.2° and 0.3°, respectively. The smaller incident angle produces the larger peak of the hexagonal diamond. This means that the induced hexagonal diamond is distributed mainly near the surface.

We calculated the pressure-temperature curve under shock compression (temperature-Hugoniot) using the thermodynamic equation given below [45–47] in order to investigate the synthesis mechanism of hexagonal diamond;

$$C_{VH}\frac{dT_H}{dV_H}+\frac{\gamma_0}{V_0}C_{VH}T_H=\frac{1}{2}\frac{dp_H}{dV_H}(V_0-V_H)+\frac{1}{2}(p_H-p_0), \qquad (4.1)$$

where T is the temperature, p is the pressure, V is the specific volume, C_V is the constant-volume specific heat, γ is the Grüneisen parameter, and subscript 0 indicates an ambient state, and subscript H a shocked state. Constant values

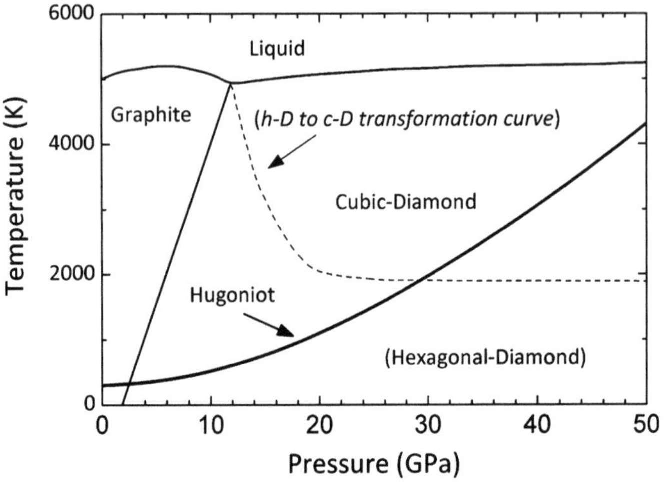

Fig. 4.3 Calculated temperature-Hugoniot described on the carbon phase diagram

such as C_V and γ are taken from Nellis's data [48]. The calculated result is shown on the phase diagram of carbon [38] in Fig. 4.3. The Hugoniot curve passes through the hexagonal diamond to cubic diamond transformation curve at approximately 30 GPa. The femtosecond laser-driven shock pressure, which was estimated at 100–300 GPa for a pulse intensity of around 10^{14} W/cm^2 [33], is strong enough to induce the graphite–hexagonal diamond–cubic diamond transformation. The mechanism of the transformation from graphite to hexagonal diamond is diffusionless, while from hexagonal diamond to cubic diamond it is diffusive. More than a few microseconds are required to induce the diffusive hexagonal to cubic diamond transformation in contrast to the relaxation time of a few picoseconds in the case of the diffusionless graphite–hexagonal diamond transformation. Therefore, the femtosecond laser-driven shock compression with duration of sub-nanoseconds [36] can only induce the graphite→hexagonal diamond transformation. We suggest that the recovery of the hexagonal diamond induced by the femtosecond laser shot is due to the rapid cooling in the shock heated region [49].

4.4 Quenching of High Pressure Phase of Iron

Iron is one of the most important elements in the field of geophysics as well as industry because iron is the principal element in the Earth's core [50]. The phase diagram of iron below 50.2 GPa and 2,000 K is well established [51–53]: the lower pressure and temperature α phase (body-centered cubic lattice: bcc), the lower pressure and higher temperature γ phase (face-centered cubic lattice: fcc) and δ phase (bcc), and the higher pressure ε phase (hexagonal close-packed structure: hcp).

Shock induced α–ε phase transition in iron is one of the most famous high pressure phase transitions. α–ε phase transition in iron was first reported by Minshall [54], and the Hugoniot in the phases were first measured by Bancroft et al. [55]. The temporal profile of the shock wave of approximately 180 ns was required to complete the shock-induced α→ε transition [56]. This phase transition is extremely sluggish compared to the pulse width of the laser-driven shock wave of several nanoseconds. This transition is considered martensitic because this process is athermal and the quantity of the phase varies as a function of the pressure not the time although the mechanism is still an open question [57]. In addition, the shock-induced α–ε phase transition is regarded as a completely reversible process because the quenched high pressure ε phase has never been observed in the material after shock loading.

High power nanosecond laser driven shock induced α↔ε transition in iron was first reported by Romain et al. in 1987 [58]. High density deformation following a characteristic needle-like micro structure due to the occurrence of the α↔ε phase transition was observed in the laser irradiated iron. They suggested the occurrence of the α↔ε phase during the shock wave propagation as the reason for the existence of the needle-like microstructure in the irradiated sample. Existence of the ε phase in the sample has not been reported by other researchers.

4.4.1 Experimental Method

Polycrystalline iron was annealed in vacuum of 10^{-3} Pa at 1,200 K in order to make the grain size larger. The grain size obtained was of millimeter order. The mirror-polished surface was irradiated by the focused femtosecond laser (Spitfire, Spectra-Physics Inc., wavelength: 800 nm, pulse width: 120 fs, intensity: 10^{14} W/cm^2, Gaussian profile of the spatial distribution of the intensity, linear polarization) in an argon atmosphere. The spot size was approximately 50 μm, which is small enough compared to the grain size, so that a femtosecond laser pulse will irradiate a single crystal. The crystalline structure in the irradiated iron was determined using an electron backscatter diffraction (EBSD) method and a synchrotron X-ray diffraction method.

2,000 laser pulses were irradiated at a point on the surface for the EBSD analysis sample. The mirror-finished surface of the vertical cross section was analyzed using EBSD systems (Oxford Instruments plc, TexSEM Laboratories Inc.) equipped with FE-SEMs (JEOL Ltd., JSM-6500F) after the laser irradiated iron was embedded in resin.

A femtosecond laser pulse was irradiated at 50 μm intervals on the mirror-finished surface of iron for XRD analysis. An X-ray diffraction analysis was performed using a six-circle diffractometer at beamline BL13XU for surface and interface structures, SPring-8 [44]. Wavelength 1.000 Å was used in the XRD analysis. The incident angle was fixed at 1.0° so that the incident X-ray could penetrate deeper into the sample and measurements were performed at 0.05°/step and 100 s/step out of the peak angles of α phase.

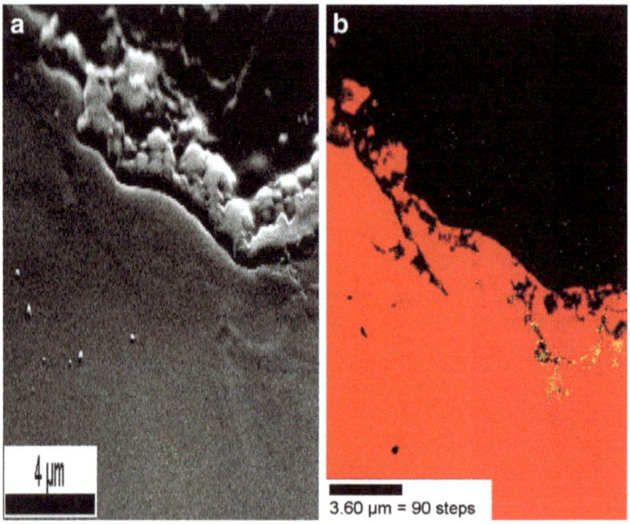

Fig. 4.4 (**a**) SEM image of the area analyzed using the EBSD system, and (**b**) EBSD mapping data of iron sample, where *red*, *yellow*, and *green* colors indicate the α, ε, and γ phases, respectively

4.4.2 Results and Discussion

SEM image of the analyzed region and the EBSD mapping data are shown in Fig. 4.4a, b, respectively. Red, yellow, and green colors indicate α, ε, and γ phases, respectively in Fig. 4.4b. Black region corresponds to an unanalyzable region such as resin. Crystalline grains of the ε phase of several nanometers size scatter around 4 μm deeper from the bottom surface. A small number of crystalline grains of the γ phase also exist in the same area.

XRD pattern of the raw data for the detector angle of 30–34° is shown in Fig. 4.5a and the data, after the background is subtracted is shown in Fig. 4.5b. A peak of ε(101) is found in the pattern.

Experimental results show the existence of the high pressure ε phase which is not quenched using the conventional shock compression methods in the femtosecond laser irradiated iron. A small quantity of the γ phase also exists.

The pulse width of the femtosecond laser used in this study was 120 fs. The shortness of this 120 fs is shown by relating it to the phonon vibrational periods at the Debye temperature. The Debye temperature of the ε phase at high pressures is approximately 700 K [59]. The phonon vibrational periods at this temperature of 70 fs and 120 fs, which correspond to two vibrations of the phonon, are not long enough to drive the structural transition. This is evidence that the femtosecond laser pulse itself does not synthesize the ε phase. Therefore, the ε phase is considered to be induced by the shock wave.

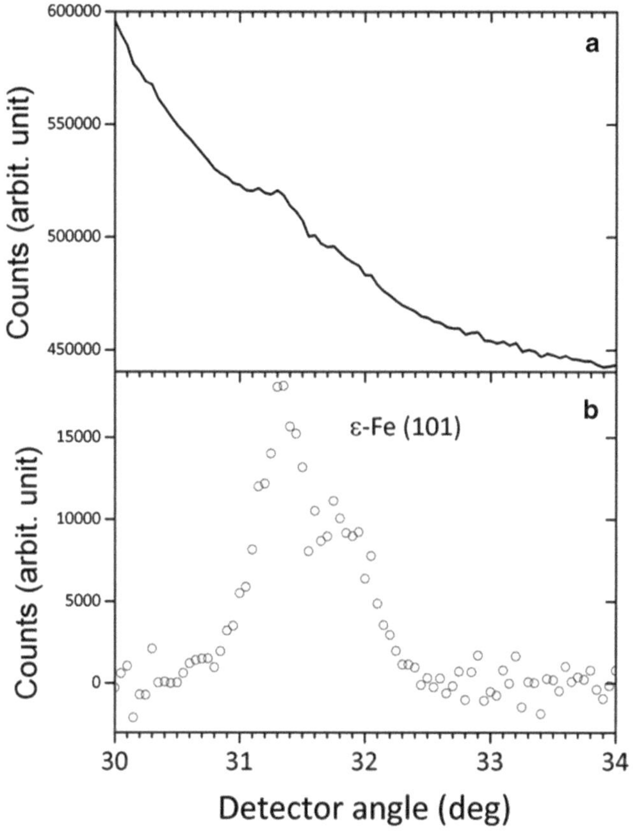

Fig. 4.5 Synchrotron X-ray diffraction pattern of the femtosecond laser irradiated iron. (**a**) Pattern of the raw data for the detector angle of 30–34°. (**b**) Data with the background subtracted

Result of EBSD analysis shows that the ε phase exists around 4 μm deeper from the bottom surface. On the other hand, the depth of the heat affected zone due to the femtosecond laser irradiation is 100–200 nm [31]. Therefore, the region where the ε phase exists is not affected by the heat due to the femtosecond laser irradiation itself but influenced by the femtosecond laser driven shock wave. The thermodynamic state inside the shock front has to be known in order to investigate the mechanism of the transition because the shock induced phase transition occurs inside the shock front. Thus, the temperature inside the shock front is estimated as a function of the pressure using the inside temperature method implicitly, including the heat transport [46, 47]. The thermodynamic state inside the shock front, where there is local thermal equilibrium [30, 46, 47, 59], is expressed by the following equation:

$$C_V \frac{dT}{dV} + \frac{\gamma}{V} C_V T = -(p - p_E), \tag{4.2}$$

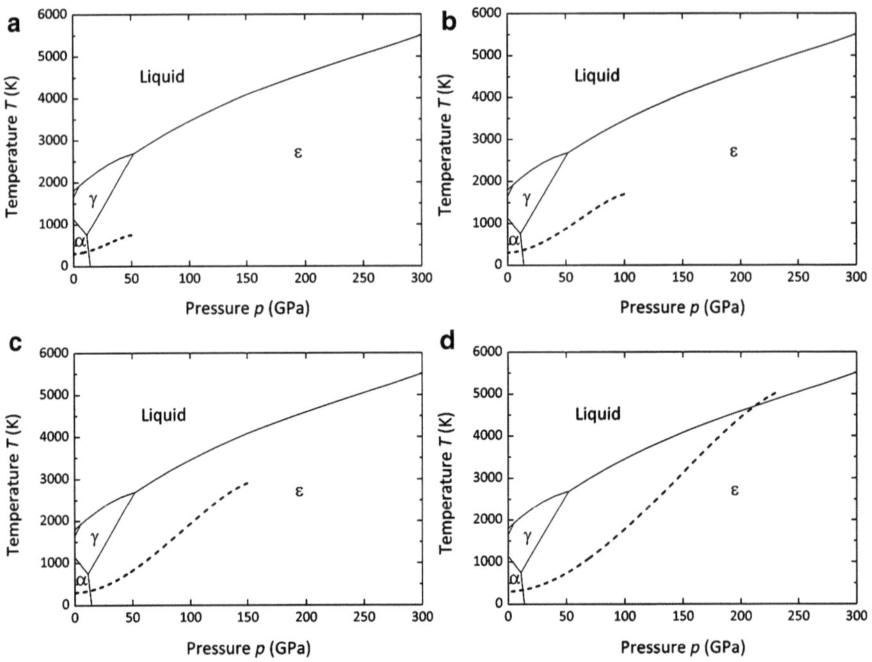

Fig. 4.6 Calculated temperatures inside the overdriven shock wave (*bold dashed curves*) for the shock amplitude of (**a**) 50, (**b**) 100, (**c**) 150, and (**d**) 230 GPa

where C_V is the constant-volume specific heat on the Rayleigh line, and T is the temperature, V is the constant volume, γ is the Grüneisen parameter, p is the pressure, and p_E is the thermoelastic component of the pressure p. These parameters indicate the state inside the shock front. The following equation was used for the constant-volume specific heat [60],

$$C_V = 3Nk_B + \Gamma_0 \left(\frac{V}{V_0}\right)^g T, \tag{4.3}$$

where N is the number of atoms per unit mass, k_B is the Boltzmann constant, V_0 is the constant volume in an ambient state, $\Gamma_0 = 0.091$ J/kgK^2, and $g = 1.34$. Revised shock data from Brown et al. [61] was applied to the known Hugoniot function. Calculations were performed below 230 GPa, which is the Hugoniot melting point and is considered to be achieved by the femtosecond laser driven shock wave.

The thermodynamic state inside the shock front can be drawn on the phase diagram because the state inside the shock front is locally in thermal equilibrium [30, 46, 47, 59]. Estimated temperatures inside the shock front are shown in Fig. 4.6 as a function of the pressure for the shock amplitude (a) 50, (b) 100, (c) 150, and (d) 230 GPa, where we apply the data of Bundy [52] to the α–γ–ε triple point and the data of Anderson and Isaak [62] to the γ–ε-liquid triple point and the melting curve.

The inside temperatures above 50 GPa are in the region where the ε phase is stable and are always below the transition point to the γ phase. Therefore, the femtosecond laser driven shock itself induces the ε phase directly, but not the γ phase.

The amplitude and the rise time were reported as 100–300 GPa [33] and several picoseconds [34, 35], respectively, for the femtosecond laser driven shock in the thin Al film under similar conditions to this study. On the other hand, the relaxation time of the shock induced α→ε phase transition is approximately 180 ns [56]. Pulse width of the femtosecond laser driven shock is thought to be shorter than the several ten nanoseconds of the nanosecond laser driven shock although it has never been measured. Therefore, the pulse width of the femtosecond laser driven shock is shorter than the relaxation time of the shock induced α→ε phase transition.

Bcc–hcp transition of iron is martensitic. A three step model that includes the fcc structure as the intermediate phase is considered valid as the transition model [57]. The fcc structure may be metastable due to the lattice matching of the bcc and the fcc phases after a small quantity of the bcc-fcc transition. Thus, the next step of the transition does not proceed without additional pressure or a long waiting time. Therefore, the fcc structure remains because a part of the fcc does not transform to the hcp structure when the additional pressure is insufficient or there is not sufficient time. The femtosecond laser driven shock formed in this study has enough amplitude to drive the α→ε phase transition, whereas not only the ε phase that is induced by the α→ε transition process but the γ phase that is the intermediate structure during the α→ε transition are induced due to the shortness of the pulse width. The ε and γ phases once induced may be quenched during the incomplete ε→α and γ→α transitions due to the same reason.

References

1. Schawlow AL, Townes CH (1958) Infrared and optical masers. Phys Rev 112:1940
2. Slusher RE (1999) Laser technology. Rev Mod Phys 71:S471
3. Steen WM, Mazumder J (2010) Laser material processing. Springer, London
4. Spence DE, Kean PN, Sibbett W (1991) 60-fsec pulse generation from a self-mode-locked Ti: sapphire laser. Opt Lett 16:42
5. Stricland D, Mourou G (1985) Compression of amplified chirped optical pulses. Opt Commun 56:219
6. Chichkov BN, Momma C, Nolte S, von Alvensleben F, Tünnermann A (1996) Femtosecond, picosecond and nanosecond laser ablation of solids. Appl Phys A 63:109
7. Eesley GL (1983) Observation of nonequilibrium electron heating in copper. Phys Rev Lett 51:2140
8. Fujimoto JG, Liu JM, Ippen EP, Bloembergen N (1984) Femtosecond laser interaction with metallic tungsten and nonequilibrium electron and lattice temperatures. Phys Rev Lett 53:1837
9. Eesley GL (1986) Generation of nonequilibrium electron and lattice temperatures in copper by picosecond laser pulses. Phys Rev B 33:2144
10. Schoenlein RW, Lin WZ, Fujimoto JG, Eesley GL (1987) Femtosecond studies of nonequilibrium electronic processes in metals. Phys Rev Lett 58:1680

11. Kanavin AP, Smetanin IV, Isakov VA, Afanasiev YV, Chichkov BN, Wellegehausen B, Nolte S, Momma C, Tünnermann A (1998) Heat transport in metals irradiated by ultrashort laser pulses. Phys Rev B 57:14698
12. Rethfeld B, Kaiser A, Vicanek M, Simon G (2002) Ultrafast dynamics of nonequilibrium electrons in metals under femtosecond laser irradiation. Phys Rev B 65:214303
13. Perez D, Lewis LJ (2002) Ablation of solids under femtosecond laser pulses. Phys Rev Lett 89:255504
14. Perez D, Lewis LJ (2003) Molecular-dynamics study of ablation of solids under femtosecond laser pulses. Phys Rev B 67:184102
15. Bejan D, Raseev G (1997) Nonequilibrium electron distribution in metals. Phys Rev B 55:4250
16. Kaganov MI, Lifshitz IM, Tanatarov LV (1957) Relaxation between electrons and crystalline lattice. Sov Phys JETP 4:173
17. Allen PB (1987) Theory of thermal relaxation of electrons in metals. Phys Rev Lett 59:1460
18. Etcheverry JI, Mesaros M (1999) Molecular dynamics simulation of the production of acoustic waves by pulsed laser irradiation. Phys Rev B 60:9430
19. Sokolowski-Tinten K, Bialkowski J, Cavalleri A, von der Linde D, Oparin A, Meyer-ter-Vehn J, Anisimov SI (1998) Transient states of matter during short pulse laser ablation. Phys Rev Lett 81:224
20. Vidal F, Johnston T, Laville S, Bathélemy O, Chaker M, Drogoff BL, Margot J, Sabsabi M (2001) Critical-point phase separation in laser ablation of conductors. Phys Rev Lett 86:2573
21. Zhigilei LV, Garrison BJ (2000) Microscopic mechanisms of laser ablation of organic solids in the thermal and stress confinement irradiation regimes. J Appl Phys 88:1281–1298
22. Schafer C, Urbassek HM, Zhigilei LV (2002) Metal ablation by picosecond laser pulses: a hybrid simulation. Phys Rev B 66:115404
23. Veeser LR, Solem JC (1978) Studies of laser-driven shock waves in aluminum. Phys Rev Lett 40:1391
24. Trainor RJ, Shaner JW, Auerbach JM, Holmes NC (1979) Ultrahigh pressure laser-driven shock-wave experiments in aluminum. Phys Rev Lett 42:1154
25. Koenig M, Faral B, Boudenne JM, Batani D, Benuzzi A, Bossi S, Rémond C, Perrine JP, Temporal M, Atzeni S (1995) Relative consistency of equations of state by laser driven shock waves. Phys Rev Lett 74:2260
26. Kodama R, Norreys PA, Mima K, Dangor AE, Evans RG, Fujita H, Kitagawa Y, Krushelnick K, Miyakoshi T, Miyanaga N, Norimatsu T, Rose SJ, Shozaki T, Shigemori K, Sunahara A, Tampo M, Tanaka KA, Toyama Y, Yamanaka T, Zepf M (2001) Fast heating of ultrahigh-density plasma as a step towards laser fusion ignition. Nature 412:798
27. Ozaki N, Tanaka KA, Ono T, Shigemori K, Nakai M, Azechi H, Yamanaka T, Wakabayashi K, Yoshida M, Nagao H, Kondo K (2004) GEKKO/HIPER-driven shock waves and equation-of-state measurements at ultrahigh pressures. Phys Plasmas 11:1600
28. Glenzer SH, MacGowan BJ, Michel P, Meezan NB, Suter LJ, Dixit SN, Kline JL, Kyrala GA, Bradley DK, Callahan DA, Dewald EL, Divol L, Dzenitis E, Edwards MJ, Hamza AV, Haynam CA, Hinkel DE, Kalantar DH, Kilkenny JD, Landen OL, Lindl JD, LePape S, Moody JD, Nikroo A, Parham T, Schneider MB, Town RPJ, Wegner P, Widmann K, Whitman P, Young BKF, Van Wonterghem B, Atherton LJ, Moses EI (2010) Symmetric inertial confinement fusion implosions at ultra-high laser energies. Science 327:1228
29. Pakula R, Sigel R (1985) Self-similar expansion of dense matter due to heat transfer by nonlinear conduction. Phys Fluids 28:232
30. Ng A, Forsman A, Celliers P (1995) Heat front propagation in femtosecond laser-heated solids. Phys Rev E 51:5208
31. Tokunaga E, Terasaki A, Kobayashi T (1992) Frequency-domain interferometer for femtosecond time-resolved phase spectroscopy. Opt Lett 17:1131
32. Evans R, Badger AD, Falliès F, Mahdieh M, Hall TA, Audebert P, Geindre J-P, Gautheier J-C, Mysyrowicz A, Grillon G, Antonetti A (1996) Time- and space-resolved optical probing of femtosecond laser-driven shock waves in aluminum. Phys Rev Lett 77:3359

33. Gahagan KT, Moore DS, Funk DJ, Rabie RL, Buelow SJ, Nicholson JW (2000) Measurement of shock wave rise times in metal thin films. Phys Rev Lett 85:3205
34. Funk DJ, Moore DS, Gahagan KT, Buelow SJ, Reho JH, Fisher GL, Rabie RL (2001) Ultrafast measurement of the optical properties of aluminum during shock-wave breakout. Phys Rev B 64:115114
35. McGrane SD, Moore DS, Funk DJ, Rabie RL (2002) Spectrally modified chirped pulse generation of sustained shock waves. Appl Phys Lett 80:3919
36. Moore DS, Gahagan KT, Reho JH, Funk DJ, Buelow SJ, Rabie RL (2001) Ultrafast nonlinear optical method for generation of planar shocks. Appl Phys Lett 78:40
37. Bundy FP, Bassett WA, Weathers MS, Hemley RJ, Mao HK, Voncharov AF (1996) The pressure-temperature phase and transformation diagram for carbon; updated through 1994. Carbon 34:141
38. Frondel C, Marvin UB (1967) Lonsdaleite, a hexagonal polymorph of diamond. Nature 214:587
39. Trueb LF (1968) An electron-microscope study of shock-synthesized diamond. J Appl Phys 39:4707
40. He H, Sekine T, Kobayashi T (2002) Direct transformation of cubic diamond to hexagonal diamond. Appl Phys Lett 81:610
41. Bundy FP, Kasper JS (1967) Hexagonal diamond—a new form of carbon. J Chem Phys 46:3437
42. Misra A, Tyagi PK, Yadav BS, Rai P, Misra DS, Pancholi V, Samajdar ID (2006) Hexagonal diamond synthesis on h-GaN strained films. Appl Phys Lett 89:071911
43. Sakata O, Furukawa Y, Goto S, Mochizuki T, Uruga T, Takeshita K, Ohashi H, Ohata T, Matsushita T, Takahashi S, Tajiri H, Ishikawa T, Nakamura M, Ito M, Sumitani K, Takahashi T, Shimura T, Saito A, Takahasi M (2003) Beamline for surface and interface structures at SPring-8. Surf Rev Lett 10:543
44. Walsh JM, Christian RH (1955) Equation of state of metals from shock wave measurements. Phys Rev 97:1544
45. Sano T, Sano Y (2001) Equilibrium thermodynamic theory for the evaluation of temperature distributions in overdriven steady-plane wave fronts. J Appl Phys 90:3754
46. Sano T, Sano Y (2001) Equilibrium thermodynamic theory explicitly including heat transport for evaluation of temperature distributions in steady plane-wave fronts. J Appl Phys 90:5576
47. Nellis WJ, Mitchell AC, McMahon AK (2001) Carbon at pressures in the range 0.1–1 TPa (10 Mbar). J Appl Phys 90:696
48. Colombier JP, Combis P, Stoian R, Audouard E (2007) High shock release in ultrafast laser irradiated metals: scenario for material ejection. Phys Rev B 75:104105
49. Birch F (1952) Elasticity and constitution of the Earth's interior. J Geophys Res 57:227
50. Strong HM (1959) The experimental fusion curve of iron to 96,000 atmospheres. J Geophys Res 64:653
51. Bundy FP (1965) Pressure-temperature phase diagram of iron to 200 kbar, 900 °C. J Appl Phys 36:616
52. Boehler R (1986) The phase diagram of iron to 430 kbar. Geophys Res Lett 13:1153
53. Minshall S (1955) Investigation of a polymorphic transition in iron at 130-kb. Phys Rev 98:271
54. Bancroft D, Peterson EL, Minshall S (1956) Polymorphism of iron at high pressure. J Appl Phys 27:291
55. Barker LM, Hollenbach RE (1974) Shock wave study of the $\alpha \rightleftarrows \varepsilon$ phase transition in iron. J Appl Phys 45:4872
56. Wang FM, Ingalls R (1998) Iron bcc-hcp transition: local structure from x-ray-absorption fine structure. Phys Rev B 57:5647
57. Romain JP, Hallouin M, Gerland M, Cottet F, Marty L (1988) In: Schmidt SC, Holmes NC (eds) Shock waves in condensed matter – 1987. Elsevier Science Publishers B.V., Amsterdam, p 787

58. Trainor RJ, Lee YT (1982) Analytic models for design of laser-generated shock-wave experiments. Phys Fluids 25:1898
59. Brown JM, McQueen RG (1986) Phase transitions, Grüneisen parameter, and elasticity for shocked iron between 77 GPa and 400 GPa. J Geophys Res 91:7485
60. Brown JM, Fritz JN, Hixon RS (2000) Hugoniot data for iron. J Appl Phys 88:5496
61. Anderson OL, Isaak DG (2000) Calculated melting curves for phases of iron. Am Mineral 85:376
62. Burgers WG (1934) On the process of transition of the cubic-body-centered modification into the hexagonal-close-packed modification of zirconium. Physica 1:561

Chapter 5
Advanced Material Designs Using Friction Stir Welding Technique

Hidetoshi Fujii

Abstract A variety of material designs using FSW (Friction Stir Welding) and FSP (Friction Stir Processing) are demonstrated. The FSW and FSP are solid state processing techniques, which can be used for many processes such as welding, surface modification and fabrication of partial composites. In particular, this method is very useful for the material design of steel. When the FSW is performed below the A_{C1} point, the optimal microstructure consisting of very fine ferrite and globular cementite is obtained, regardless of the carbon content. A combination of FSW and a laser allows both grains and carbides to be refined to about 100 nm. FSPP (Friction Stir Powder Processing) is also introduced as a new technique for the material designs. It is the Friction Stir Processing over a gap which is filled with a powder. Using this method, the modification and alloying can freely be carried out, depending on the purposes.

Keywords FSW • Recrystallization • Severe deformation • Steel • Transformation

5.1 Friction Stir Welding

During FSW (Friction Stir Welding), unlike conventional welding, the materials are maintained in the solid state [1]. Accordingly, this new method has a variety of excellent advantages, that have already been used for various industrial applications such as trains, ships, automobiles, and civil engineering structures for Al alloys [2–9], although it is a relatively new technique which was invented about 20 years ago.

H. Fujii (✉)
Joining and Welding Research Institute, Osaka University, 11-1 Mihogaoka,
Ibaraki, Osaka 567-0047, Japan
e-mail: fujii@jwri.osaka-u.ac.jp

T. Kakeshita (ed.), *Progress in Advanced Structural and Functional Materials Design*,
DOI 10.1007/978-4-431-54064-9_5,

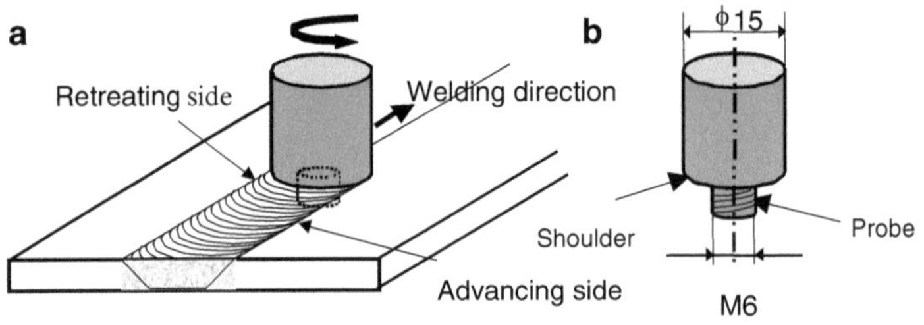

Fig. 5.1 Principles of FSW and tool shape

In FSW, an about ϕ10–20 cylindrical tool rotating at a high speed is brought into contact with the materials which generates a frictional heat, as shown in Fig. 5.1a, thus, the two materials are welded using the frictional heat [3, 4]. As shown in Fig. 5.1b, the tool consists of a large diameter part (Shoulder) and a small tip part (Probe). While only the probe is inserted into the materials, the tool is moved along the butt interface. At this time, the materials are fixed onto a backing plate, and welded through a plastic flow caused by the tool.

The maximum temperature is below the melting point, which indicates that the welding is performed in the solid state, accordingly the reduction in the joint strength is low. In some cases, the joint strength is higher than the base metal. Especially in the case of steel, the heat-affected zone is not generally softened, thus a 100% joint efficiency can easily be obtained [10–17], except for some special steel, such as high strength steel [18].

However, most practical structures welded using the FSW are made of Al alloys. Thus, it is desired to establish an FSW technology for relatively high melting point materials such as steel. When joining aluminum alloys, an SK or SKD tool steel, such as SKD61, is widely used. For the FSW of steels, on the other hand, high strength, toughness wear resistance and non-reactive properties at high temperature are required for the tool materials. In the initial study, a W alloy [10, 11] and Mo alloy [11] have been used for the tool materials, and, subsequently, ceramic materials, such as polycrystalline cubic boron nitride (PCBN) tools [19, 20] and coated Si_3N_4 [21], and tungsten carbide [13–15, 17] are used. Recently, a high-strength and long-life Co alloy tool (http://www.tohoku.ac.jp/japanese/newimg/pressimg/20100326_01.pdf) and Ir alloy tool [22, 23] have also been developed in Japan, which made – significant progress towards commercialization.

While the tungsten carbide tool is not suitable for welding over 1,000°C, it is suitable for FSW at low temperatures of about 650–850°C, which enables the FSW below the A_{C1} point [13–15]. Thus, it is desirable to select the proper tool, depending on the welding temperature and the material properties.

Due to these efforts, FSW is getting closer to practical applications even for steel. For example, its practical use for pipelines in North America has been significantly examined, because the FSW of 12 mm thick steels has become possible [24]. Also, the high-speed FSW of stainless steel over 1 m per minute

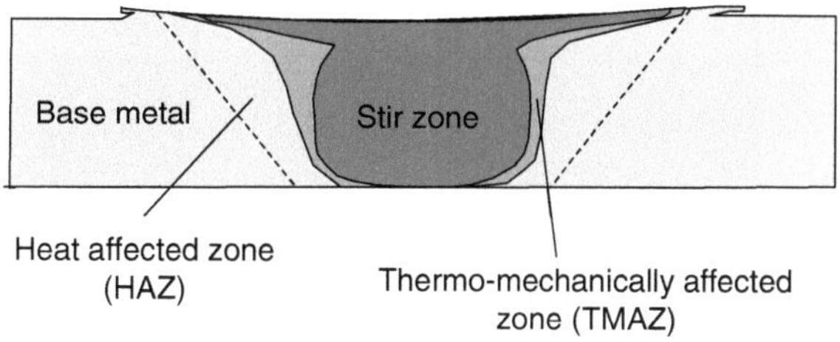

Fig. 5.2 Schematic illustration of a joint

has been reported [25]. The hurdle for the FSW of steels has become much lower, because the FSW of Mo with a melting point of 2,620°C, which is 1,000°C higher than that of steel, was successful [26].

5.2 Features of the FSW

Unlike the conventional welding methods, FSW is an asymmetric welding method. As shown in Fig. 5.1, the side where the movement and rotational directions of the tool are the same is called the advancing side, and the side where the movement and rotational directions are opposite is called the retreating side [3, 4].

Figure 5.2 shows a schematic illustration of a joint and Fig. 5.3 shows actual microstructures of an 1,080 aluminum alloy joint on a cross section [4, 27]. An equiaxial and recrystallized structure of several microns are formed at the center of the joint, and this area is called the stir zone (SZ). Outside of the stir zone, a thermo-mechanically affected zone (TMAZ) is formed, where elongated grains are formed due to the plastic deformation by the tool. Outside the TMAZ, a heat affected zone (HAZ) is present, which is not affected by plastic deformation, but affected by the heat.

Figure 5.4 [28] shows TEM bright field images of the stir zones of Al, pure iron (IF steel) and pure Ti. The stir zones consist of very fine recrystallized grain structures for all the materials. The Al alloys, which have an fcc structure, but a high stacking fault energy, and ferrous materials having a bcc structure prone to recovery during cooling after the FSW, accordingly a recrystallized structure with fewer dislocations is obtained in the stir zone. A recrystallized structure with a high density of dislocations is obtained in the Ti stir zone, which indicates that the welding is completed due to the dynamic recrystallization during the FSW [28].

5.3 Advanced Material Designs of Carbon Steel

Since Thomas et al. succeeded in the FSW of 12% Cr steels and low carbon steel and showed the potential for the FSW of steel in 1999 [29], several papers have been published on the FSW of steel such as carbon steel, [10–17, 24, 30], pure iron, steel IF (low carbon steel) [13, 31–33], and stainless steel [25, 34–38].

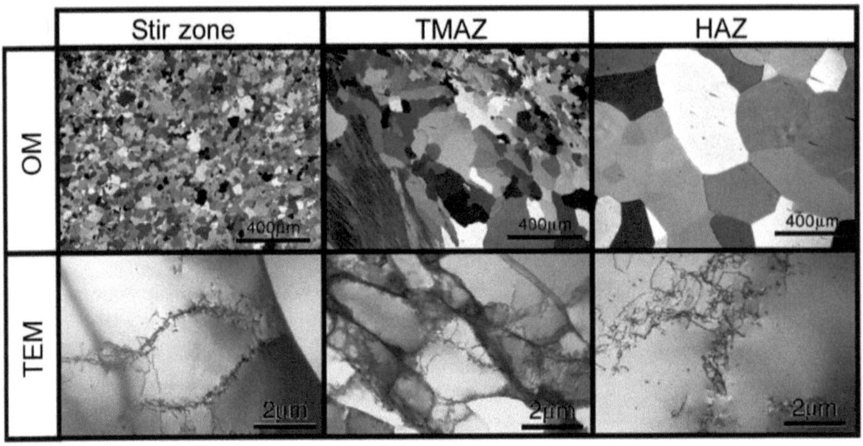

Fig. 5.3 Microstructures of a 1,080 aluminum alloy joint [27]. (**a**) Macrostructure, (**b**) optical microscope and TEM observations

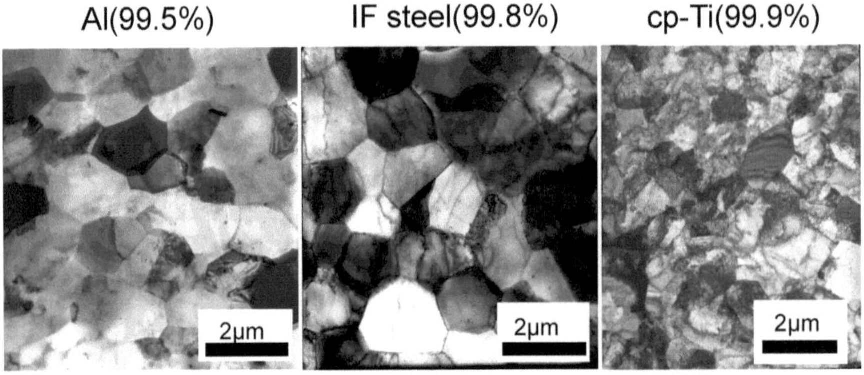

Fig. 5.4 TEM bright field images of the stir zones of pure Al, pure iron (IF steel) and pure Ti [28]

However, unlike the FSW of aluminum alloys or austenitic stainless steels, the FSW of carbon steel is accompanied by a transformation. Thus, by controlling the transformation during the FSW, the joint strength is significantly changed, and various different phenomena can also be observed, which never occur in the Al alloys [13–15, 30, 31].

Figure 5.5 [14] shows the change in the microstructure of a high carbon steel, S70C (0.70% C), which is close to the eutectoid composition. When normal fusion welding is used for such a material, the joint is very brittle and thus the welding is very difficult, because martensite is formed in the entire joint. The welding speed is reduced from the right to left side in Fig. 5.5, thereby reducing the cooling rate. As a result, under the 400 rpm to 25 mm/min conditions, a pearlite and about 16 vol.% martensite structure is formed, while almost 100% martensite is formed under

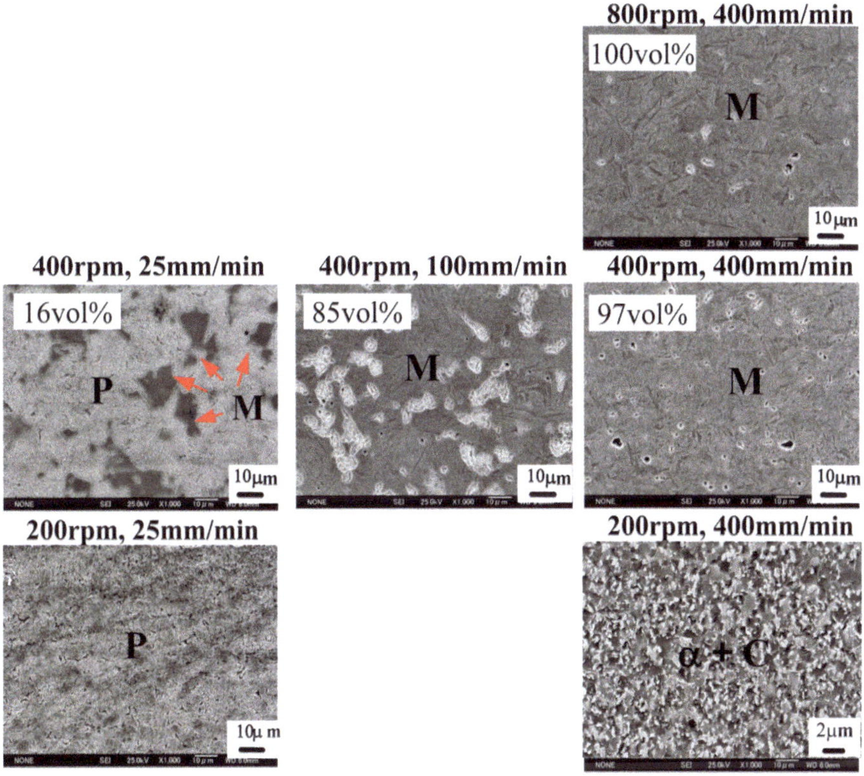

Fig. 5.5 Relationship between welding conditions and the microstructure of a high carbon steel, S70C (0.70 % C) [14]. *P* perlite, *M* martensite, *α* ferrite, *C* globular cementite

the 400 rpm to 400 mm/min conditions. Thus, the amount of martensite can be controlled by the welding conditions. Under the 400 rpm to 25 mm/min conditions, the mechanical properties with a 1,432 MPa tensile strength and 11% elongation are obtained. By decreasing the rotation speed to 200 rpm to further decrease the cooling rate, a complete pearlite structure is obtained. In this case, the elongation is significant improved.

By reducing the rotational speed (changing from the top to bottom in Fig. 5.5), on the other hand, the peak temperature can be decreased. Under the 200 rpm to 400 mm/min welding conditions, the peak temperature is below the A_{C1} point (723°C), indicating that the welding can be performed without any transformation. In this case, the resulting microstructure consists of a very refined ferrite and globular cementite, which is the ideal microstructure with both a good strength and ductility. As shown in Fig. 5.6, when the rotation speed is 400 or 600 rpm, the peak temperature exceeds the A_{C1} point, thus a very hard and brittle microstructure is formed, while at 200 rpm, the hardness is slightly increased from the base material, and the joint ensures a sufficient strength and elongation.

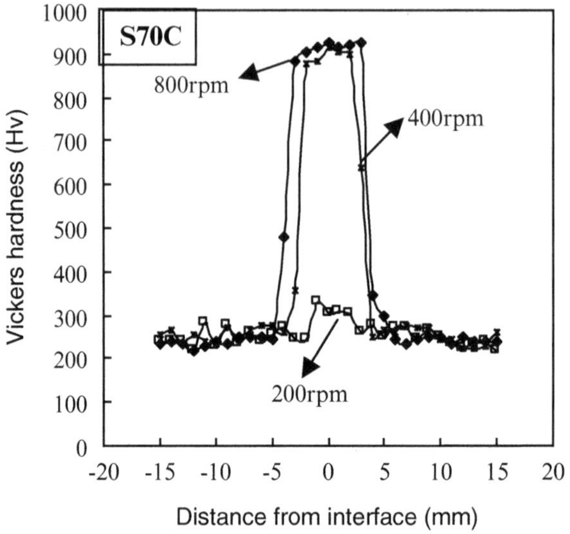

Fig. 5.6 Effect of rotation speed on hardness of S70C (400 mm/min) [14]

Because this method can be performed, regardless of the carbon content of steel, it may induce a significant change in the design and welding method of various structures in the future. By performing welding at a low temperature of about 700–900°C, which was not possible before, a flexible strength design becomes possible in response to the user's requests. A tungsten carbide (WC) tool is very effective for this purpose.

Of course, this method can be used for hypereutectoid steels. Figure 5.7 [39, 40] shows the Charpy absorbed energy of SK85 (0.85% C) joints. When the peak temperature is below the A_{C1} point, the absorbed energy is increased by about three times when compared to the joint obtained above the A_{C1} point. The fracture surfaces are also significantly changed.

5.4 Advanced Materials Design by Combination of Laser and FSW

Figure 5.8 [41] shows an example of the microstructure control by the combination of a laser and FSW. In this case, as a surface modification method instead of welding, FSW (or FSP) has been applied to tool steel, i.e., SKD11 (C: 1.48%).

In general, the FSP (Friction Stir Processing) only allows the grain size to be decreased, but it does not very effectively decrease the carbide size. To solve this problem, the tool steel was first melted by the laser, then solidified to segregate the carbides at the grain boundaries [41]. When the FSP is performed after this process, a very fine microstructure is obtained. In this case, both the grains and carbides are

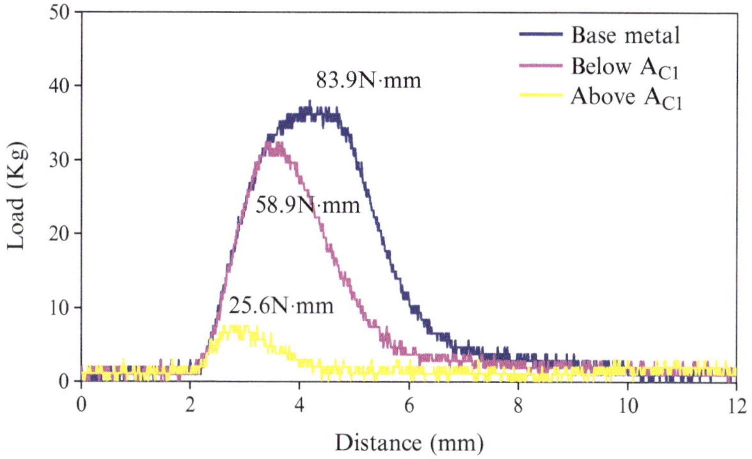

Fig. 5.7 Effect of peak temperature on Charpy absorbed energy of SK85 (0.85% C) joints [39]

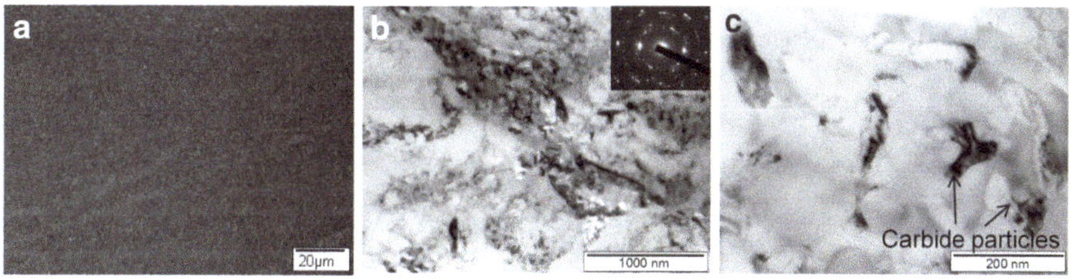

Fig. 5.8 Microstructure of SKD11 after laser+FSP [41]. (**a**) Optical microscope, (**b** and **c**) TEM bright field images

significantly refined to about 100 nm, as shown in Fig. 5.8 [41], and the obtained microstructure is the ideal microstructure for a knife. A good sharpness and significant small missing teeth have been proven [41].

5.5 Friction Stir Powder Processing (FSPP)

Friction stir powder processing (FSPP) is a method of FSP over a gap which is filled with a powder [42], as shown in Fig. 5.9. Using this method, modification and alloying can freely be carried out, depending on the applications [42, 43].

Figure 5.10 shows the Vickers hardness distribution on a cross section of a pure Al plate (AA1050) with pure Cu powder perpendicular to the processing direction. The horizontal axis is the distance from the interface. Because the Al–Cu alloy is a typical precipitation strengthening system, the strength can be increased by

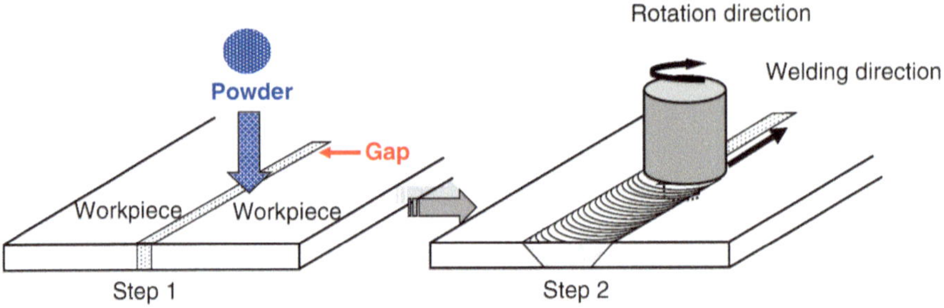

Fig. 5.9 Friction stir powder processing (FSPP) [42]

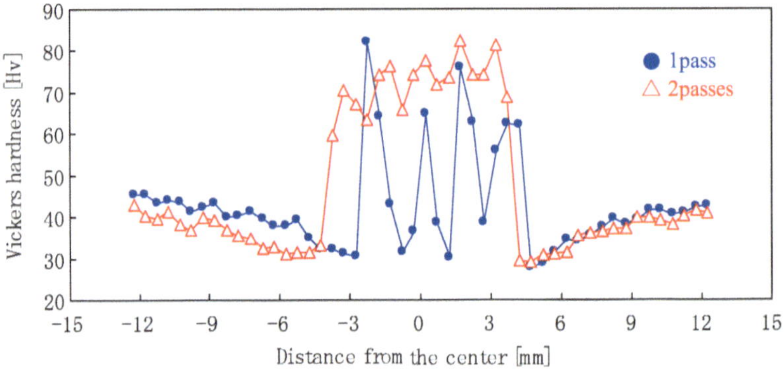

Fig. 5.10 Hardness distribution on a cross section of a pure Al plate (AA1050) with pure Cu (1,500 rpm to 100 mm/min) [42]

dispersing fine precipitates in the matrix after the Cu is once dissolved in pure Al by the FSPP. Whereas the Vickers hardness in the base material is about 40 Hv, it increased to about 80 Hv in the stir zone after the FSPP [42]. In particular, the hardness is uniformly distributed to be twice value throughout the stir zone after the second pass.

Figure 5.11 is a TEM bright field image of the stir zone obtained under the conditions of 1,500 rpm - 100 mm/min-two passes, under which the hardness is significantly increased. Many fine intermetallic compounds caused by the precipitation are observed. Focusing on the size and shape of the precipitates, about 150 nm bulk-shaped and about 10 nm plate-shaped precipitates are observed. This result indicates that both the dynamic recrystallization and precipitation occur during the FSPP, and the precipitation is affected by the recrystallization behavior. Moreover, it is very interesting that a similar result is obtained even when using Fe powder with a limited solid solubility in Al [43]. These results are important as a unique phenomenon of the FSW (FSPP), in which heating and severe deformation are simultaneously given by the rotating tool.

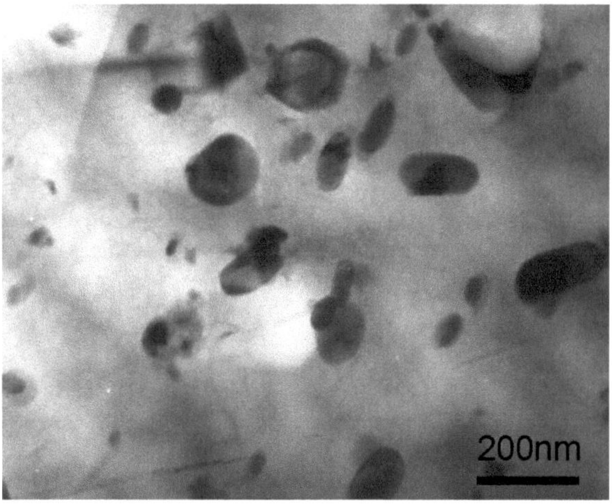

Fig. 5.11 TEM bright field image of the stir zone after FSPP of a pure Al plate (AA1050) with pure Cu (1,500 rpm - 100 mm/min-two passes) [42]

5.6 Summary

FSW has a variety of possibilities for material designs, because it is a solid state processing. It was initially used only as a welding method, but, some other applications, such as surface modification and fabrication of partial composites have been proposed. Even now, new technologies have been continuously developed, and further development is also expected in the future.

In particular, the surface modification of steel, such as knives, has already been commercialized, and much research is being performed on the FSW of steel. In addition to this, the FSW without transformation or a combination of FSW and a laser to obtain about 100 nm grains and carbides are very useful for practical use, as shown in this chapter. Also, the FSW of stainless steel over 1 m/min and 3,000 spots or more using one cheap tool for the spot FSW of steel seems to be linked to future technologies.

FSPP is also introduced as a new technique for material designs. Using this method, the modification and alloying can be freely carried out. Accordingly, a large structure is first constructed using deformable materials and the structure can then be partially strengthened after the construction, depending on users' purposes.

References

1. Thomas WM, Nicholas ED, Needhan JC, Murch MG, Temple-Smith P, Dawes CJ (1991) International Patent Application PCT/GB92/02203 and GB Patent Application 9125978.8. UK Patent Office, London, 6 December 1991
2. Nandan R, DebRoy T, Bhadeshia HKDH (2008) Prog Mater Sci 53:980–1023
3. Mishra RS, Ma ZY (2005) Mater Sci Eng R 50:1–78
4. Friction Stir Welding (2006) Japan, Welding Society, Sampo Shuppan

5. Okamura H, Aota K, Ezumi M (2000) J Jpn Inst Light Met 50:166–171
6. Campbell G, Stotler T (1999) Weld J 78:45–47
7. Johnsen MR (1999) Weld J 78:35–39
8. Knipstron KE, Pekkari B (1997) Weld J 76:55–57
9. Dawes CJ, Thomas WM (1996) Weld J 75:41–45
10. Lienert TJ, Stellwag WL Jr, Grimmett BB, Warke RW (2003) Weld J 82:1S–9S
11. Reynolds AP, Tang W, Posada M, DeLoach J (2003) Sci Technol Weld Join 8:455
12. Ozekcin A, Jin HW, Koo JY, Bangaru NV, Ayer R (2004) Int J Offshore Polar Eng 14:284
13. Fujii H, Cui L, Tsuji N, Maeda M, Nakata K, Nogi K (2006) Mater Sci Eng A 429:50–57
14. Cui L, Fujii H, Tsuji N, Nogi K (2007) Scr Mater 56:637–640
15. Cui L, Fujii H, Tsuji N, Nakata K, Nogi K, Ikeda R, Matsushita M (2007) ISIJ Int 47(2):299–306
16. Sato YS, Yamanoi H, Kokawa H, Furuhara T (2008) ISIJ Int 48:71–76
17. Saeid T, Abdollah-zadeh A, Assadi H, Malek Ghaini F (2008) Mater Sci Eng A 496:262–268
18. Matsushita M, Kitani Y, Ikeda R, Ono M, Fujii H, Chung YD (2011) Sci Technol Weld Join 16:181
19. Sorensen CD, Nelson TW, Packer SM (2001) Proceedings of 3rd international symposium on FSW, TWI, Kobe, Japan, CD-ROM
20. Collier M, Steel R, Nelson TW, Sorensen C, Packer S (2003) Mater Sci Forum 426:3011
21. Ohashi R, Fujimoto M, Koga S, Ikeda R, Ono M (2008) Proceedings of 7th international FSW symposium, Awaji, Japan, CD-ROM, 2-2, 20–22 May 2008
22. Miyazawa T, Iwamoto Y, Maruko T, Fujii H (2011) Sci Technol Weld Join 16:188–192
23. Miyazawa T, Iwamoto Y, Maruko T, Fujii H (2012) Sci Technol Weld Join 17:207–212
24. Ayer R, Fairchild DP, Ford SJ, Nissley NE, Ozekcin A (2008) Proceedings of 7th international FSW symposium, Awaji, Japan, CD-ROM, 9B-1, 20–22 May 2008
25. Ishikawa T, Fujii H, Genchi K, Iwaki S, Matsuoka S, Nogi K (2009) ISIJ Int 49:897–901
26. Fujii H, Sun YS, Kato H (2011) Scr Mater 64:657–660
27. Sato YS, Park SHC, Kokawa H (2001) Metall Mater Trans 32A:3033
28. Fujii H, Sun YF, Kato H, Nakata K (2010) Mater Sci Eng A 527:3386–3391
29. Thomas WM, Threadgill PL, Nicholas ED (1999) Sci Technol Weld Join 4:365–371
30. Ueji R, Fujii H, Cui L, Nishioka A, Kunishige K, Nogi K (2006) Mater Sci Eng A 423:324–330
31. Fujii H, Ueji R, Takada Y, Kitahara H, Tsuji N, Nakata K, Nogi K (2006) Mater Trans 47:239–242
32. Mironov S, Sato YS, Kokawa H (2008) Acta Mater 56:2602–2614
33. Mehranfara M, Dehghanib K (2011) Mater Sci Eng A 528:3404–3408
34. Park SHC, Sato YS, Kokawa H, Okamoto K, Hirano S, Inagaki M (2003) Scr Mater 49:1175
35. Reynolds AP, Tang W, Gnaupel-Herold T, Prask H (2003) Scr Mater 48:1289
36. Sato YS, Nelson TW, Sterling CJ (2005) Acta Mater 53:637
37. Zhu XK, Chao YJ (2004) J Mater Process Technol 146:263
38. Chabok A, Dehghani K (2010) Mater Sci Eng A 528:309–313
39. Chung YD, Fujii H, Ueji R, Tsuji N (2010) Scr Mater 63:223–226
40. Chung YD, Fujii H, Ueji R, Nogi K (2009) Sci Eng Weld Join 14:233–238
41. Morisada Y, Fujii H, Mizuno M, Abe G, Nagaoka T, Fukuzumi M (2009) Mater Sci Eng A505:157–162
42. Inada K, Fujii H, Ji YS, Sun YF, Morisada Y (2010) Sci Tech Weld Join 15:131–136
43. Fujii H, Sun YF, Inada K, Yokoyama Y, Kimura H, Inoue A (2011) Mater Trans 52:1634–1640

Chapter 6
Advanced Analysis of Surface Films Formed on Passive Metals and Alloys Using X-ray Photoelectron Spectroscopy

Shinji Fujimoto

Abstract Most of high corrosion resistance advanced structural and functional metals and alloys are protected by passive films, that is oxide and/or hydroxide films of few nm in thickness. In this chapter, properties of oxide/hydroxide film formed on metals and alloys are briefly summarized, then the procedure of quantitative analysis of passive film using X-ray photoelectron spectroscopy is described in detail as a one of characterization technique. Passive films on Cr containing high corrosion alloys, such as stainless steels, high nickel alloys, Co–Cr alloys, consist of highly Cr enriched oxide layer and covering hydroxide layer. Assuming the duplex model, the thickness and the content including chemical states in both layers, are quantitatively estimated from deconvoluted XPS spectra acquired without any sputtering technique.

Keywords Fe-Cr • Staintess steel • Cr enrichement • Corrosion • Chemical shift

6.1 Introduction

Properties of surface oxide and/or hydroxide films on metals and alloys are important for understanding their corrosion property, because corrosion resistance of metals and alloys are usually derived from surface oxide films. Therefore, many kinds of surface characterization techniques, such as, ellipsometry [1–3], Raman spectroscopy [4, 5], electrochemical impedance spectroscopy [6], modulated UV–vis reflectometry [7, 8], photoelectrochemical response spectroscopy [9, 10], Auger electron spectroscopy [11, 12], and X-ray photoelectron spectroscopy [13–15] are developed in order to discuss corrosion behaviour. In this chapter, role of oxide/hydroxide films on metal and alloys are explained mainly for passive

S. Fujimoto (✉)
Division of Materials and Manufacturing Science, Graduate School of Engineering,
Osaka University, 2-1 Yamadaoka, Suita, Osaka 565-0871, Japan
e-mail: fujimoto@mat.eng.osaka-u.ac.jp

T. Kakeshita (ed.), *Progress in Advanced Structural and Functional Materials Design*,
DOI 10.1007/978-4-431-54064-9_6, © Springer Japan 2013

films on high corrosion materials. Then, quantitative X-ray photoelectron spectroscopy (XPS) will be described in detail.

6.2 Surface Oxide and/or Hydroxide Films on Metals and Alloys

Metals and alloys are usually covered with oxide and/or hydroxide films that are formed by reaction of substrate metal or alloy with surrounding environment. Oxide or hydroxide layers formed on metals and alloys are generally classified in to three categories; thick rust layers, anodizing films and passive films.

Thick rust layer is often observed; red rust on iron and steel [16], patinated copper and brass, for instance. Such rust layers are formed as accumulation of colloidal deposit. Metallic ions released into water excess solubility in water, then precipitate as colloid particle of hydroxide or oxide. Such colloidal deposits are accumulated on the surface, and dehydrated to be deposited layer. Rust layer is usually water and ions permeable, therefore basically not protective. The rust layers formed on weathering steels [17] and bronze exceptionally exhibit high corrosion resistance.

Anodizing oxide films [18, 19] are formed by anodic polarization of Al, Ti, Mg, etc. Anodizing oxide is usually dense and insulating, therefore protective for substrate metal. Anodizing oxide film is able to grow proportionally depending on applied potential, occasionally reaches to few μm. Most of structural materials made of Al alloys are used with anodizing oxide films. Al, Ta, Nb covered with insulating anodized oxide films are applied for electric capacitor.

Passive films [20–22] are very thin oxide and/or hydroxide formed naturally on metals and alloys. For example, passive film on iron is formed in aqueous solution containing some oxidant without harmful anion such as Cl^- and SO_4^{2-}. Passive films are formed on most of metals and alloys, usually 1–5 nm in thickness and protective for corrosion. Figure 6.1 [23] shows variation of the thickness of passive film on pure iron as a function of applied potential. As shown in this figure, the thickness of passive film on iron is in the range from 1 to 4 nm. In the ordinary environment, potential is controlled by oxidant, such as dissolved oxygen and H^+ ions and is in the range of horizontal axis of this Figure. Above a critical potential, Fe is more oxidized into soluble FeO_4^{2-} ions. Similar behavior is observed for Ni [24, 25], Cr [12], Co [26], etc.

6.3 Passive Films on Stainless Steels

High corrosion resistant alloys containing Cr as alloying elements, such as stainless steels, high nickel alloys and Co–Cr alloys are protected by Cr enriched passive films. Figure 6.2 [27] shows Cr cation fraction in the passive film and Cr content of substrate alloy underneath the passive film measured by X-ray photo electron

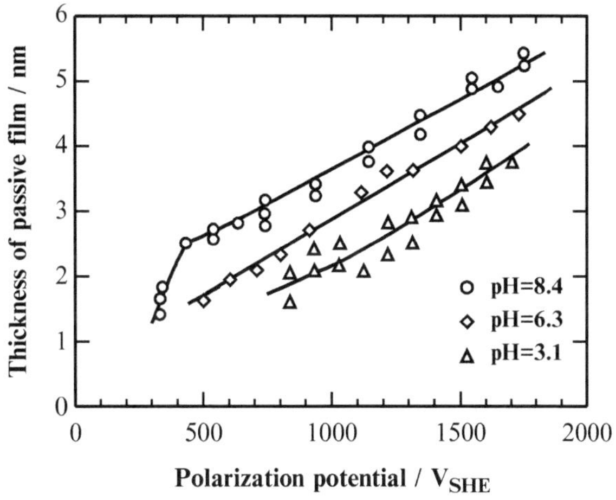

Fig. 6.1 Thickness of passive film on Fe formed at various applied potentials [23]

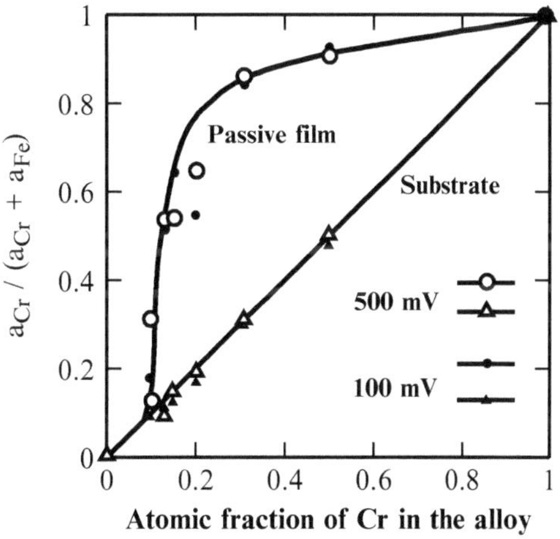

Fig. 6.2 Changes in composition of passive film and substrate alloy beneath passive film on Fe–Cr alloys polarized at 500 and 100 mV (SCE) in 1 M H_2SO_4 as a function of Cr faction in substrate alloy [27]

spectroscopy as a function of Cr content in Fe–Cr alloys. Cr content in passive film abruptly increases with increasing Cr content in the alloy above 12% Cr, then reaches around 80% at 20% Cr in the alloy. On the other hand Cr content underneath passive film is the same with alloy composition. Therefore, it is concluded that Cr enrichment is due to selective dissolution of Fe into aqueous solution and preferential oxide/hydroxide formation of Cr. Similar enrichment of Cr is observed for Ni–Cr alloys [28–30] and Co–Cr alloys [31, 32]. Properties of passive film, especially Cr content, depend on the aqueous environment and affects corrosion resistance, therefore characterization of passive film is important for considering corrosion behavior.

6.4 Principle and Characteristics of X-ray Photoelectron Spectroscopy (XPS)

Photoelectron is yielded from occupied electron orbitals around atoms by X-ray adsorption. The kinetic energy, E_k, of photoelectron emitted is described as follows:

$$E_k = h\nu - E_b - e\Phi \tag{6.1}$$

where $h\nu$ is photon energy of irradiated X-ray, E_b binding energy of electron in a specific orbital of an atom and Φ work function of a photoelectron analyser. The binding energy of electron in the core levels slightly shifts depending on the chemical state of the atom. Therefore, XPS is also called Electron Spectroscopy for Chemical Analysis (ESCA). Photoelectron emitted from the most surface of a solid is captured by an analyser. However, photoelectron from inside of solid is inelastically scattered to be back ground noise. In another words, the electron generated inside of material is attenuated before emitted from the surface. The attenuation length, λ, which depends on kinetic energy and materials, is defined as the length in a material after passes through which the intensity of photoelectron without inelastic scattering becomes 1/e. Typical attenuation length for photoelectron generated by commonly used X-ray source, such as AlKα and MgKα, is few nm. Therefore, XPS is very surface sensitive characterization technique. XPS is widely utilized for surface characterization in research areas such as metallurgy, catalyst, corrosion, and surface treatment etc. In the following, the procedure of quantitative analysis of passive films on corrosion resistant metals and alloys will be described.

6.5 Procedure of Quantitative Analysis of Layered Surface

Intensity of photoelectron, $i_{z,0}$, yielded from atoms, z, existing inside an infinitesimal volume, dv, is given by:

$$i_{z,0} = XC_z\sigma_z \mathrm{dv} \tag{6.2}$$

where X is intensity of irradiated X-ray, C_z mol concentration of the element, z, for an unit volume, and σ_z photoionization cross section which is the sensitivity factor to yield photoelectron. When dv is located inside of some solid, s, at a depth of y, as shown in Fig. 6.3(a), the intensity of photoelectron of z which emitted from the surface of the solid is described as;

$$i_z = i_{z,0}\exp(-y/\lambda_z^s) \tag{6.3}$$

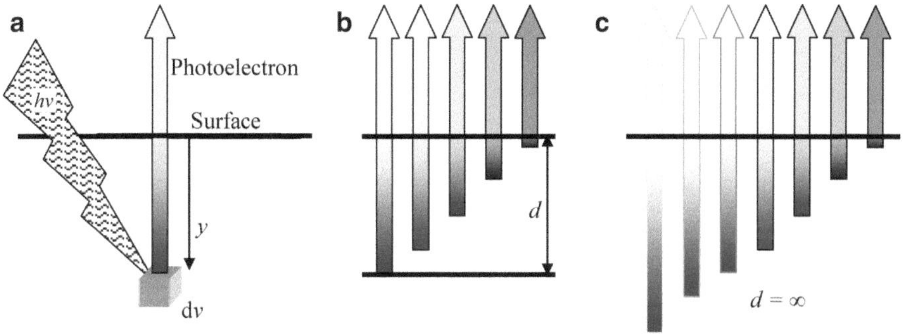

Fig. 6.3 Generation of Photoelectron: (**a**) yielded at infinitesimal volume, dv, which is located inside of solid of y in depth, (**b**) generated from a layer of thickness d, (**c**) generated from bulk solid (thickness is infinite)

where λ_z^s is the attenuation length of photoelectron of the atom, z, in the solid, s. As shown in Fig. 6.3(b), when z is distributed homogeneously in the solid s, the photo electron emitted from a unit area (v = 1 × 1 × y) and thickness of d is a summation of i_z:

$$I_{z,0} = \int_0^d i_{z,0}\exp\left(\frac{-y}{\lambda_z^s}\right)dy = i_{z,0}\lambda_z^s(1 - \exp(-d/\lambda_z^s)) \tag{6.4}$$

If photo electron is emitted from bulk solid, that is $d = \infty$, as shown in Fig. 6.3(c),

$$I_{z,0} = \int_0^\infty i_{z,0}\exp\left(\frac{-y}{\lambda_z^s}\right)dy = i_{z,0}\lambda_z^s. \tag{6.5}$$

The counts of photoelectron of z yielded in a bulk solid and detected by an analyzer is described as:

$$I_z = \Psi I_{z,0}\cos\theta = \Psi I_{z,0} = \Psi X C_z \sigma_z \lambda_z^s \quad \text{(infinite thickness)} \tag{6.6}$$

where Ψ is an acquisition constant which is specific to apparatus and usually changes with E_K. If photo electron is emitted from a thin layer of thickness d,

$$I_z = \Psi X C_z \sigma_z \lambda_z^s(1 - \exp(-\mathrm{d}/\lambda_z^s\cos\theta) \text{ (a layer with thickness } d) \tag{6.7}$$

where θ is photoelectron take off angle measured from normal to surface as shown in Fig. 6.4. The term cosθ is applied, because the path inside the solid where photoelectron passes through increases by a factor of 1/cosθ as described in Fig. 6.4.

If the infinite or limited thickness layer is covered with another solid sc with thickness of t, the photoelectron is attenuated during passing through the covering layer by a factor of $\exp(-t/\lambda_z^{sc})$, where λ_z^{sc} is the attenuation length of photoelectron of z through the solid sc.

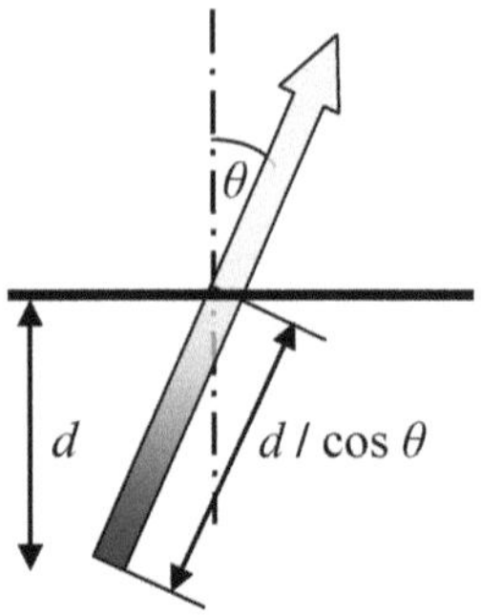

Fig. 6.4 Change in the length of path inside solid with detection angle, θ, of photoelectron

Quantitative analysis of XPS spectra is proceeded using above equations. If subjected material, s, consists of a single layer, Eq. (6.6) or (6.7) directly provides concentration and thickness, d_s, as described in the following. When a solid, s, consists of components, z1–zn, Eq. (6.7) is applicable for all components, including various chemical states;

$$I_{z1} = \Psi X C_{z1} \sigma_{z1} \lambda_{z1}^{s} (1 - \exp(-d_s / \lambda_{z1}^{s} \cos\theta) \quad (6.8)$$

$$I_{z2} = \Psi X C_{z2} \sigma_{z1} \lambda_{z2}^{s} (1 - \exp(-d_s / \lambda_{z2}^{s} \cos\theta) \quad (6.9)$$

$$I_{zn} = \Psi X C_{zn} \sigma_{zn} \lambda_{zn}^{s} (1 - \exp(-d_s / \lambda_{zn}^{s} \cos\theta) \quad (6.10)$$

For the layer of s which consists of z1, z2, ... zn, the following equation is obtained:

$$C_{z1} M_{z1} + C_{z2} M_{z2} + \cdots + C_{zn} M_{zn} = \rho_s d_s \quad (6.11)$$

Where M_{z1}, M_{z2}, ... M_{zn} are atomic weight of element z1, z2, ... zn, respectively, ρ_s is density of the layer of s. C_{z1}, C_{z2}, ... C_{zn} in Eq. (6.11) are substituted by Eqs. (6.8)–(6.10). As a result, only d_s becomes unknown variable in Eq. (6.11). Therefore, thickness d of the layer s and concentration of each elements (states) C_{zn} are obtained.

On the other hand, if a sample consists of multi layers, some structural model is to be assumed. Therefore, an appropriate procedure for quantitative analysis should be developed for each subject. In the following, the quantitative analysis on passive films formed on high corrosion alloys is described in detail.

6.6 Procedure of the Quantitative Analysis of Passive Films

As mentioned before, passive films on stainless steels formed in aqueous environment consist of oxide layer and covering hydroxide layer. Therefore, passive films are assumed to be composed of two layers [33, 34]. Actually, specimens exposed to atmosphere must be covered with contaminant hydrocarbon layer.

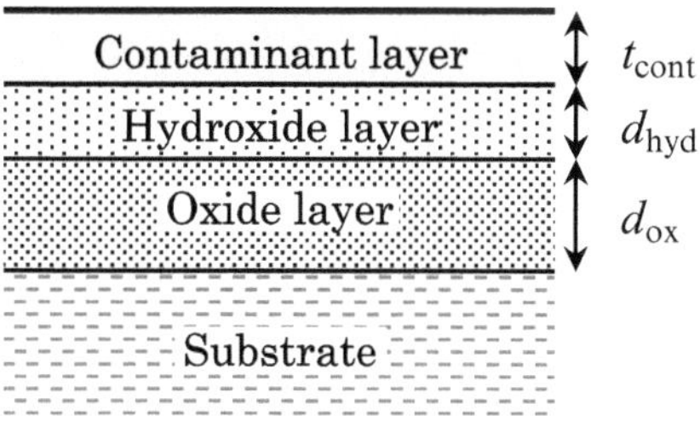

Fig. 6.5 Multi-layered model for passive films

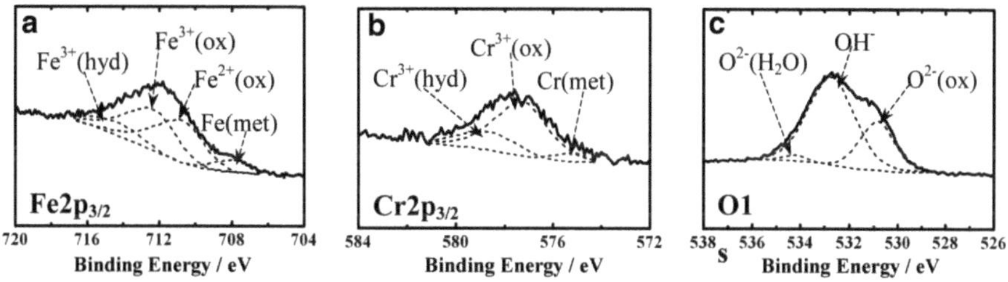

Fig. 6.6 (XPS spectra of Fe2p3/2, Cr2p3/2 and O1s detected for the passive films formed on Type 304 stainless steel under humid atmosphere of 90% at (a) 30°C)

Moreover, the substrate alloy beneath the passive films occasionally changes the composition because of dealloying. Therefore a multi-layers model which is composed of contaminant/hydroxide/oxide/substrate alloy is assumed as shown in Fig. 6.5.

In order to analyse passive films on stainless steel, photoelectron spectra of Fe2d, Cr2d, Ni2d, O1s, and C1s orbitals are measured. If minor element like Mo is required to be analysed, spectra of such elements are also measured.

Typical spectra obtained for passive film on Type304 stainless steel are shown in Fig. 6.6 Spectra of contaminant carbon are integrated to an area $I_{C,con}$. Eq. (6.7) is applied for contaminant carbon, C_{con}:

$$I_{C,con} = \Psi_C X_{con} C_{con} \sigma_C \lambda_C{}^{con} (1 - \exp(-t_{con}/\lambda_C^{con} \cos\theta)) \tag{6.12}$$

$$I_{C,gra} = \Psi_C X_{gra} C_{gra} \sigma_C \lambda_C{}^{gra}, \tag{6.13}$$

where $I_{C,gra}$ is area of C1s spectrum measured for pure Carbon, for example graphite. $\lambda_C{}^{gra}$ is escape length of photoelectron yielded from carbon through graphite. These equations are modified into:

$$\frac{I_{C,con}}{I_{C,gra}} = \frac{X_{con}}{X_{gra}} \cdot \frac{C_{con}}{C_{gra}} \cdot \frac{\lambda_C^{con}}{\lambda_C^{gra}} \cdot (1 - \exp(-t_{con}/\lambda_C^{con} \cos\theta)) \tag{6.14}$$

$$t_{\mathrm{con}} = -\lambda_{\mathrm{C}}^{\mathrm{con}} \ln\left(1 - \frac{X_{\mathrm{gra}}}{X_{\mathrm{con}}} \cdot \frac{C_{\mathrm{gra}}}{C_{\mathrm{con}}} \cdot \frac{\lambda_{\mathrm{C}}^{\mathrm{gra}}}{\lambda_{\mathrm{C}}^{\mathrm{con}} \cos\theta} \cdot \frac{I_{\mathrm{C,con}}}{I_{\mathrm{C,gra}}}\right) \tag{6.15}$$

As shown above, thickness of contaminant hydrocarbon layer is estimated.

Spectrum of Fe is deconvoluted into metallic: $\mathrm{Fe}^{\mathrm{met}}$, ferrous oxide: $\mathrm{Fe}^{2+,\mathrm{ox}}$, ferrous oxide: $\mathrm{Fe}^{3+,\mathrm{ox}}$, and hydroxide: $\mathrm{Fe}^{\mathrm{hyd}}$ states as shown in Fig. 6.6(a). Similarly, spectra of Cr, Ni and other metallic elements are also deconvoluted into metallic, oxide and hydroxide. Intensities, that are area of spectrum of each element and state in hydroxide layer are described as:

$$I_{\mathrm{Fe,hyd}} = \Psi_{\mathrm{Fe}} X_{\mathrm{Fe}} C_{\mathrm{Fe}} \sigma_{\mathrm{Fe}} \lambda_{\mathrm{Fe}}{}^{\mathrm{hyd}} \left(1 - \exp\left(-d_{\mathrm{hyd}}/\lambda_{\mathrm{Fe}}^{\mathrm{hyd}} \cos\theta\right)\right) \exp(-t_{\mathrm{con}}/\lambda_{\mathrm{Fe}}{}^{\mathrm{con}} \cos\theta) \tag{6.16}$$

$$I_{\mathrm{Cr,hyd}} = \Psi_{\mathrm{Cr}} X_{\mathrm{Cr}} C_{\mathrm{Cr}} \sigma_{\mathrm{Cr}} \lambda_{\mathrm{Fe}}{}^{\mathrm{hyd}} \left(1 - \exp\left(-d_{\mathrm{hyd}}/\lambda_{\mathrm{Cr}}^{\mathrm{hyd}} \cos\theta\right)\right) \exp(-t_{\mathrm{con}}/\lambda_{\mathrm{Cr}}{}^{\mathrm{con}} \cos\theta) \tag{6.17}$$

$$I_{\mathrm{Ni,hyd}} = \Psi_{\mathrm{Ni}} X_{\mathrm{Ni}} C_{\mathrm{Ni}} \sigma_{\mathrm{Ni}} \lambda_{\mathrm{Ni}}{}^{\mathrm{hyd}} \left(1 - \exp\left(-d_{\mathrm{hyd}}/\lambda_{\mathrm{Ni}}^{\mathrm{hyd}} \cos\theta\right)\right) \exp(-t_{\mathrm{con}}/\lambda_{\mathrm{Ni}}{}^{\mathrm{con}} \cos\theta) \tag{6.18}$$

$$I_{\mathrm{O,hyd}} = \Psi_{\mathrm{O}} X_{\mathrm{O}} C_{\mathrm{O}} \sigma_{\mathrm{O}} \lambda_{\mathrm{O}}{}^{\mathrm{hyd}} \left(1 - \exp\left(-d_{\mathrm{hyd}}/\lambda_{\mathrm{O}}^{\mathrm{hyd}} \cos\theta\right)\right) \exp(-t_{\mathrm{con}}/\lambda_{\mathrm{O}}{}^{\mathrm{con}} \cos\theta) \tag{6.19}$$

$$C_{\mathrm{Fe,hyd}} M_{\mathrm{Fe}} + C_{\mathrm{Cr,hyd}} M_{\mathrm{Cr}} + C_{\mathrm{Ni,hyd}} M_{\mathrm{Ni}} + C_{\mathrm{O,hyd}} M_{\mathrm{O}} = \rho_{\mathrm{hyd}} d_{\mathrm{hyd}} \tag{6.20}$$

The last term in Eqs. (6.16)–(6.19) refers to attenuation of photo electron during passing through the contaminant layer which covers hydroxide layer. $C_{\mathrm{Fe,hyd}}$, $C_{\mathrm{Cr,hyd}}$, $C_{\mathrm{Ni,hyd}}$, and $C_{\mathrm{O,hyd}}$ in Eq. (6.20) are replaced by Eqs. (6.16)–(6.19). Accordingly,

$$\begin{aligned}
& I_{\mathrm{Fe,hyd}} M_{\mathrm{Fe}} / \left\{ \Psi_{\mathrm{Fe}} X_{\mathrm{Fe}} \sigma_{\mathrm{Fe}} \lambda_{\mathrm{Fe}}{}^{\mathrm{hyd}} \left(1 - \exp\left(-d_{\mathrm{hyd}}/\lambda_{\mathrm{Fe}}^{\mathrm{hyd}} \cos\theta\right)\right) \exp(-t_{\mathrm{con}}/\lambda_{\mathrm{Fe}}{}^{\mathrm{con}} \cos\theta) \right\} \\
& + I_{\mathrm{Cr,hyd}} M_{\mathrm{Cr}} / \left\{ \Psi_{\mathrm{Cr}} X_{\mathrm{Cr}} \sigma_{\mathrm{Cr}} \lambda_{\mathrm{Cr}}{}^{\mathrm{hyd}} \left(1 - \exp\left(-d_{\mathrm{hyd}}/\lambda_{\mathrm{Cr}}^{\mathrm{hyd}} \cos\theta\right)\right) \exp(-t_{\mathrm{con}}/\lambda_{\mathrm{Cr}}{}^{\mathrm{con}} \cos\theta) \right\} \\
& + I_{\mathrm{Ni,hyd}} M_{\mathrm{Ni}} / \left\{ \Psi_{\mathrm{Ni}} X_{\mathrm{Ni}} \sigma_{\mathrm{Ni}} \lambda_{\mathrm{Ni}}{}^{\mathrm{hyd}} \left(1 - \exp\left(-d_{\mathrm{hyd}}/\lambda_{\mathrm{Ni}}^{\mathrm{hyd}} \cos\theta\right)\right) \exp(-t_{\mathrm{con}}/\lambda_{\mathrm{Ni}}{}^{\mathrm{con}} \cos\theta) \right\} \\
& + I_{\mathrm{O,hyd}} M_{\mathrm{O}} / \left\{ \Psi_{\mathrm{O}} X_{\mathrm{O}} \sigma_{\mathrm{O}} \lambda_{\mathrm{O}}{}^{\mathrm{hyd}} \left(1 - \exp\left(-d_{\mathrm{hyd}}/\lambda_{\mathrm{O}}^{\mathrm{hyd}} \cos\theta\right)\right) \exp(-t_{\mathrm{con}}/\lambda_{\mathrm{O}}{}^{\mathrm{con}} \cos\theta) \right\} \\
& = \rho_{\mathrm{hyd}} d_{\mathrm{hyd}}
\end{aligned} \tag{6.21}$$

The thickness of d_{hyd} is thus obtained, because d_{hyd} is only unknown variable in Eq. (6.22). Then, substituting d_{hyd} in Eqs. (6.16)–(6.19) gives values of concentration of each element, C_z, in the hydroxide layer.

A similar relation can be applied for the oxide layer:

$$
\begin{aligned}
& I_{\mathrm{Fe2+,ox}} M_{\mathrm{Fe}} / \{\Psi_{\mathrm{Fe}} X_{\mathrm{Fe}} \sigma_{\mathrm{Fe}} \lambda_{\mathrm{Fe}}{}^{\mathrm{ox}} (1 - \exp(-d_{ox}/\lambda_{\mathrm{Fe}}^{\mathrm{ox}} \cos\theta)) \exp(-t_{\mathrm{con}}/\lambda_{\mathrm{Fe}}{}^{\mathrm{con}} \cos\theta) \\
& \cdot \exp(-t_{\mathrm{con}}/\lambda_{\mathrm{Fe}}{}^{\mathrm{hyd}} \cos\theta)\} + I_{\mathrm{Fe3+,ox}} M_{\mathrm{Fe}} / \{\Psi_{\mathrm{Fe}} X_{\mathrm{Fe}} \sigma_{\mathrm{Fe}} \lambda_{\mathrm{Fe}}{}^{\mathrm{ox}} \\
& (1 - \exp(-d_{ox}/\lambda_{\mathrm{Fe}}^{\mathrm{ox}} \cos\theta)) \exp(-t_{\mathrm{con}}/\lambda_{\mathrm{Fe}}{}^{\mathrm{con}} \cos\theta) \cdot \exp(-t_{\mathrm{con}}/\lambda_{\mathrm{Fe}}{}^{\mathrm{hyd}} \cos\theta)\} \\
& + I_{\mathrm{Cr,ox}} M_{\mathrm{Cr}} / \{\Psi_{\mathrm{Cr}} X_{\mathrm{Cr}} \sigma_{\mathrm{Cr}} \lambda_{\mathrm{Fe}}{}^{\mathrm{ox}} (1 - \exp(-d_{\mathrm{ox}}/\lambda_{\mathrm{Cr}}^{\mathrm{ox}} \cos\theta)) \exp(-t_{\mathrm{con}}/\lambda_{\mathrm{Cr}}{}^{\mathrm{con}} \cos\theta)\} \\
& \cdot \exp(-t_{\mathrm{con}}/\lambda_{\mathrm{Cr}}{}^{\mathrm{hyd}} \cos\theta)\} + I_{\mathrm{Ni,ox}} M_{\mathrm{Ni}} / \{\Psi_{\mathrm{Ni}} X_{\mathrm{Ni}} \sigma_{\mathrm{Ni}} \lambda_{\mathrm{Ni}}{}^{\mathrm{ox}} (1 - \exp(-d_{\mathrm{ox}}/\lambda_{\mathrm{Ni}}^{\mathrm{ox}} \cos\theta)) \\
& \exp(-t_{\mathrm{con}}/\lambda_{\mathrm{Ni}}{}^{\mathrm{con}} \cos\theta)\} \cdot \exp(-t_{\mathrm{con}}/\lambda_{\mathrm{Ni}}{}^{\mathrm{hyd}} \cos\theta)\} \\
& + I_{\mathrm{O,ox}} M_{\mathrm{O}} / \{\Psi_{\mathrm{O}} X_{\mathrm{O}} \sigma_{\mathrm{O}} \lambda_{\mathrm{O}}{}^{\mathrm{ox}} (1 - \exp(-d_{\mathrm{ox}}/\lambda_{\mathrm{O}}^{\mathrm{ox}} \cos\theta)) \exp(-t_{\mathrm{con}}/\lambda_{\mathrm{O}}{}^{\mathrm{con}} \cos\theta)\} \\
& \cdot \exp(-t/\lambda_{\mathrm{o}}{}^{\mathrm{hyd}} \cos\theta)\} = \rho_{\mathrm{ox}} d_{\mathrm{ox}}
\end{aligned}
\tag{6.22}
$$

From Eq. (6.22) the thickness of oxide layer, d_{ox}, is calculated. With same procedure as hydroxide layer, concentrations of each element, C_z, in the oxide layer are obtained.

When the thickness of passive film is fairly thin for detection of photoelectron yielded from the substrate steel, spectra of metallic states are detected and their intensities are described as:

$$
\begin{aligned}
I_{\mathrm{Fe,met}} = {} & \Psi_{\mathrm{Fe}} X_{\mathrm{Fe}} C_{\mathrm{Fe}} \sigma_{\mathrm{Fe}} \lambda_{\mathrm{Fe}}{}^{\mathrm{met}} \exp(-t_{\mathrm{con}}/\lambda_{\mathrm{Fe}}{}^{\mathrm{con}} \cos\theta) \\
& \cdot \exp(-d_{\mathrm{hyd}}/\lambda_{\mathrm{Fe}}{}^{\mathrm{hyd}} \cos\theta)\} \cdot \exp(-d_{\mathrm{ox}}/\lambda_{\mathrm{Fe}}{}^{\mathrm{ox}} \cos\theta)\}
\end{aligned}
\tag{6.23}
$$

$$
\begin{aligned}
I_{\mathrm{Cr,met}} = {} & \Psi_{\mathrm{Cr}} X_{\mathrm{Cr}} C_{\mathrm{Cr}} \sigma_{\mathrm{Cr}} \lambda_{\mathrm{Cr}}{}^{\mathrm{met}} \exp(-t_{\mathrm{con}}/\lambda_{\mathrm{Cr}}{}^{\mathrm{con}} \cos\theta) \\
& \cdot \exp(-d_{\mathrm{hyd}}/\lambda_{\mathrm{Cr}}{}^{\mathrm{hyd}} \cos\theta)\} \cdot \exp(-d_{\mathrm{ox}}/\lambda_{\mathrm{Cr}}{}^{\mathrm{ox}} \cos\theta)\}
\end{aligned}
\tag{6.24}
$$

$$
\begin{aligned}
I_{\mathrm{Ni,met}} = {} & \Psi_{\mathrm{Ni}} X_{\mathrm{Ni}} C_{\mathrm{Ni}} \sigma_{\mathrm{Ni}} \lambda_{\mathrm{Ni}}{}^{\mathrm{met}} \exp(-t/\lambda_{\mathrm{Ni}}{}^{\mathrm{con}} \cos\theta) \\
& \cdot \exp(-d_{\mathrm{hyd}}/\lambda_{\mathrm{Ni}}{}^{\mathrm{hyd}} \cos\theta)\} \cdot \exp(-d_{\mathrm{ox}}/\lambda_{\mathrm{Ni}}{}^{\mathrm{ox}} \cos\theta)\}
\end{aligned}
\tag{6.25}
$$

These equations provide concentration of each element, C_z.

6.7 Parameters Adopted for Quantitative Analysis

In the previous section, process of calculation to provide the chemical composition and thickness of passive film is described in detail. In the process, many parameters that are specific to elements and substances are required.

6.7.1 Photoionization Cross Section

Sensitivity parameter for yielding photo electron of an element, z, is usually termed photoionization cross section, σ_z. Theoretically calculated values are available in the literature [35]. However, such value is not necessarily applicable for quantitative analysis. Therefore, σ_z is estimated from the intensity of photoelectron, I_z, measured for some standard specimen. The process to obtain σ_z from I_z is described later.

σ_z of metallic element is measured for Ar^+ ion sputtered specimen. For example, σ_z of elements consisting a stainless steel is obtained using the sputtered stainless steel, the chemical composition of which is known. Value of σ_z is regarded as proportional to atomic concentration. Therefore, usage of alloy is convenient, because σ_z of several elements is obtained for a specimen with same measurement conditions that are intensity of X-ray, sensitivity of photoelectron detector and etc. Since σ_z may change depending on the photon energy of irradiated X-ray, it is recommended to measure σ_z using the same X-ray source which is used for measurement of unknown specimen.

Photoionization cross section of carbon, σ_C, is usually necessary, because most of specimen is covered with contaminant hydrocarbon layer of few nm in thickness. σ_C is usually measured using graphite.

Determination of photoionization cross section of oxygen, σ_O, is most difficult but crucial for quantitative analysis of passive films with high reliability. Since pure material of oxygen is not available, standard specimen of some compound with exact stoichiometry is required. Thermally oxidized pure metals could be candidates for such purpose. SiO_2, Cr_2O_3, Al_2O_3 etc. are used as standard. On the other hand, Asami et al. reported that they adopted oxides and hydroxide of metal, M, with several valences that are commercially available as high purity chemicals for standard. They measured intensity of photoelectron of them to obtain averaged ratio of σ_O/σ_M [36–38]. Reliable empirically obtained sensitivity parameters as a form of $\sigma_z \lambda_z$ are reported [39].

As already described, the photoelectron intensity of the elements z in a substance s is measured as

$$I_z = \Psi_z C_z X \sigma_z \lambda_z^s \quad \text{(infinite thickness)} \tag{6.6}$$

Therefore, the value λ_Z^S is necessary in order to determine σ_z. Ψ, acquisition constant of analyzer is usually provided by vendor of apparatus. Otherwise, $\Psi\sigma_z$ is used as a parameter, because Ψ depends not on material examined but only on the kinetic energy of photoelectron. It is to be noted that intensity of irradiated X-ray, X is, also required. Some standard specimen, such as Au, Ag which easily provides pure elemental surface without any compounds could be used as the reference to calibrate intensity of X-ray and kinetic energy of spectrometer. The values of σ_z of elements may be summarized as values with respect to that of the reference element.

6.7.2 Attenuation Length

Attenuation length, λ_Z^S, is probably most difficult parameter to obtain for quantitative analysis of XPS spectra. The value of λ_Z^S depends on kinetic energy and the substance in which photoelectron passes through. Recently, values of inelastic mean free path, IMFP, calculated based on the first principal evaluation are available [40–45]. Such data are useful for some specific purposes. It is also mentioned that attenuation length is smaller than inelastic mean free path [40, 46]. According to the author's experience, the values available in the literature, most of them might be determined empirically, are more reliable than that obtained by first principal calculation for passivity study. It is empirically recognized that attenuation length of photoelectron is roughly described is roughly described as

$$\lambda^s = 0.050\sqrt{E_k}(\mathrm{nm}) \tag{6.26}$$

with binding energy in the range of 70–1,500 eV independent of substance [38]. Therefore, λ_z^S is substituted by attenuation length of oxygen which is always contained in passive films, λ_O^S, as follows.

$$\frac{\lambda_z^s}{\lambda_O^s} = \left(\frac{E_{k,z}}{E_{k,O}}\right)^{0.5}, \tag{6.27}$$

where $E_{k,z}$ and $E_{k,O}$ are kinetic energy of photoelectron yielded in an metallic element, z, and oxygen, respectively, that are known values. If Eq. (6.27) is introduced in Eqs. (6.21)–(6.23), concentration of each component is able to be determined without absolute value of escape depth.

6.7.3 Chemical Shift

Extensive data for binding energy, E_b, of elements are easily available and usually reliable, especially for metallic elements. However, binding energy of compounds is usually empirically obtained and termed as chemical shift. For the passivity study, chemical shifts as oxide and hydroxide of metallic elements and also of oxygen are necessary. Although chemical shift of oxygen as oxide and hydroxide may depend on metallic cation and pH of solution in which passive film is formed, values of chemical shifts available in the literature [13–15, 27–29, 32, 34, 36–38, 47–53] should be adopted with a careful consideration.

6.8 Summary

The procedure of the quantitative analysis of XPS spectra for passive films formed on stainless steel is described concretely in detail. This approach is also applicable for any kind of thin surface films with thickness of up to few nm. In order to conduct quantitative analysis, as mentioned in the Sects. 6.6 and 6.7, many parameters specific for each element and substance are necessary. However, no appropriate date base is established for the passivity study. Therefore, photoionization cross section and attenuation length should be carefully collected and selected with careful consideration.

References

1. Szklarska-Smialovska Z, Kozowski Z (1983) In: Froment M (ed) Passivity of metals and semiconductors. Elsevier, Amsterdam, p 89
2. Ohtsuka T (1992) Denkikagaku 60:1123
3. Kirchheim R (1994) In: Marcus P, Baroux B, Keddam M (eds) The institute of metals., p 102
4. Boucherit N, Hugot-Le Goff A, Joiret S (1989) Thin Solid Films 174:111
5. Gui J, Devine TM (1994) Corros Sci 36:441
6. Azumi K, Ohtsuka T, Sato N (1987) J Electrochem Soc 134:1352
7. Hara N, Sugimoto K (1991) J Electrochem Soc 138:1594
8. Hara N, Sugimoto K (1990) Corros Sci 31(197)
9. Tsuchiya H, Fujimoto S, Shibata T (2004) J Electrochem Soc 151:B39
10. Fujimoto S (2005) In: Waseda Y, Suzuki S (eds) Characterization of corrosion products on steel surfaces. Springer, Benlin, p 33
11. Lumsden JB, Staehle RW (1972) Scr Metall 6:1205
12. Seo M, Saito R, Sato N (1980) J Electrochem Soc 127:1909
13. Asami K, Hashimoto K, Shimodaira S (1977) Corros Sci 17(713)
14. Marcus P, Olefjord I (1982) Surf Interface Anal 4:29
15. Asami K, Ohnuma S, Masumoto T (1998) Surf Interface Anal 26:659
16. Suzuki S (2005) In: Waseda Y, Suzuki S (eds) Characterization of corrosion products on steel surfaces. Springer, Benlin, p 131
17. Asami K (2005) In: Waseda Y, Suzuki S (eds) Characterization of corrosion products on steel surfaces. Springer, p 159
18. Despic A, Parkhutik V (1989) Modern aspects of electrochemistry, vol 20. Plenum, New York, p 401
19. Habazaki H, Shimizu K, Skeldon P, Thompson GE, Wood GC (1998) J Surf Sci Soc Jpn 19:772
20. Marcus P, Maurice V (eds) (2006) Passivity of metals and semiconductors, and properties of thin oxide layers. Elsevier, Amsterdam
21. Ohtsuka T (1995) Mater Jpn 34:1037
22. Fujimoto S, Shibata T (1998) J Surf Sci Soc Jpn 19:812
23. Azumi K, Ohtsuka T, Sato N (1983) In: Froment M (ed) Passivity of metals and semiconductor. Elsevier, Amsterdam, p 199
24. Chao CY, Szklarska-Smialowska Z (1980) Surf Sci 96:426
25. Hoppe HW, Strehblow HH (1990) Corros Sci 31:167
26. Ohtsuka T, Sato N (1983) J Electroanal Chem 147:167
27. Asami K, Hashimoto K, Shimodaira S (1978) Corros Sci 18:151
28. Asami K, Hashimoto K (1979) Corros Sci 19:427
29. Kawashima A, Asami K, Hashimoto K (1985) Corros Sci 25:1103
30. McIntyre MS, Zetaruk DG, Owen D (1979) J Electrochem Soc 126:750
31. Hanawa T, Hiromoto S, Asami K (2001) Appl Surf Sci 183:68
32. Milosev I, Strehblow HH (2003) Electrochim Acta 48:2767
33. Olefjord I, Wegrelius L (1990) Corros Sci 31:89
34. Yang WP, Costa D, Marcus P (1994) J Electrochem Soc 141:2669

35. Scofield JH (1976) J Electron Spectros Relat Phenom 8:129
36. Asami K, Hashimoto K, Shimodaira S (1977) Corros Sci 17:713
37. Asami K, Hashimoto K (1984) Corros Sci 84:83
38. Hashimoto K, Asami K (1977) Boshoku Gijyutsu 26:375
39. Wagner CD, Davis LE, Zeller MV, Taylor JA, Raymound RH, Gale LH (1981) Surf Interface Anal 3:211
40. Tanuma S, Powell CJ, Penn DR (1988) Surf lnferface Anal 11:577
41. Tanuma S, Powell CJ, Penn DR (1991) Surf lnferface Anal 17:911
42. Tanuma S, Powell CJ, Penn DR (1991) Surf lnferface Anal 17:927
43. Tanuma S, Powell CJ, Penn DR (1993) Surf lnferface Anal 20:77
44. Tanuma S, Powell CJ, Penn DR (1993) Surf Interface Anal 21:165
45. Gries WG (1996) Surf Interface Anal 24:38
46. Olefjord I (1991) In: Proceedings of the symposium on the application of surface analytical methods to environmental/material interactions, PV 91–7, The Electrochemical Society, p 22
47. Marcus P, Olefjord I (1988) Corros Sci 28:589
48. De Vito E, Marcus P (1992) Surf lnferface Anal 19:403
49. Yang WP, Costa D, Marcus P (1994) J Electrochem Soc 141:111
50. Maurice V, Yang WP, Marcus P (1998) J Electrochem Soc 145:909
51. Tossi A, Elsener B (1995) Mater Sci Forum 185/188:337
52. Fujimoto S, Yamada T, Shibata T (1998) J Electrochem Soc 145:L79
53. Fujimoto S, Shibata T, Yamada T (1998) J Jpn Soc Mater 62:527

Chapter 7
Advanced Numerical Simulations of Micro-, Macro-, and Mega-Scale Structurization

Masahito Mochizuki

Abstract Materials structurization is the final step for manufacturing science and engineering, and welding is one of the essential technology for it. Welding residual stress generates when materials are structurized and residual stress causes fatigue, stress-corrosion cracking, reduction of structural strength, brittle fracture, buckling, and other failures in various components. A computational method as well as a direct measurement method is useful for evaluating weld residual stress and distortion. This paper introduces recently developed methods for innovative numerical simulations of the weld residual stress for materials structurization on various scales and in structures with various welds. Many applications of these analysis methods are expected in the near future.

Keywords Macro-to-micro analysis • Multi-scale computation • Residual stress • Welded structures

7.1 Introduction

Structuralization of materials is done by using a lot of processes. Welding is one of the important manufacturing processes for metal structures. Residual stress by welding generates when materials are structurized, and various effects of weld residual stress on structures and materials have been detailed in books specializing in fatigue strength, stress-corrosion cracking (SCC), and brittle fracture. However, when it comes to methods for the accurate calculation of residual stress, which is the driving force of damage, no acceptable methods have been completely established, despite the persevering and continuous efforts of researchers, neither measurement methods nor analysis methods are satisfactory. Thus, a lot of research and development are still in progress.

M. Mochizuki (✉)
Division of Materials and Manufacturing Science, Graduate School of Engineering,
Osaka University, 2-1 Yamadaoka, Suita, Osaka 565-0871, Japan
e-mail: mmochi@mapse.eng.osaka-u.ac.jp

T. Kakeshita (ed.), *Progress in Advanced Structural and Functional Materials Design*,
DOI 10.1007/978-4-431-54064-9_7,

As a numerical analysis method, the finite element method has rapidly advanced in the field of structural analysis. The method was applied to thermal elastic–plastic analysis approximately 40 years ago. Since then, the analytical research of weld residual stress has rapidly advanced. As an example, the thermal elastic–plastic finite element method, which considers the temperature dependence of material properties, has been formulated [1–4]. This method has for example clarified the generation mechanism of weld residual stress and applied the combination with material phase transformation or arc physics [5–11]. With the subsequent advancement of computers, very large-scale numerical analyses are possible.

Special consideration is however necessary for convergence because of the complexity of the phenomenon and the very strong nonlinearity in dynamics. When it comes to weld residual stress, the areas of application of numerical simulation have not been extensive compared with those of other fields. Nevertheless these boundary conditions, several numerical analysis methods has been newly developed by the authors, and the essence of these numerical analysis methods and analysis examples for problems of various scales are reported in this paper.

7.2 Fundamentals of Thermal Elastic–Plastic Analysis

In the thermal elastic–plastic analysis, the governing equations are as follows. The equation of the strain–displacement relation is

$$\{\varepsilon\} = [A]\{U\}$$

where $\{\varepsilon\}$ and $\{U\}$ are the tensor of strain and the displacement, respectively, and $[A]$ is the matrix that includes the differential operator.

The constitutive equation is

$$\{\sigma\} = [D^e]\{\varepsilon^e\} = [D^e](\{\varepsilon\} - \{\varepsilon^t\})$$

where $\{\sigma\}$ is the tensor of stress, and $\{\varepsilon^e\}$ and $\{\varepsilon^t\}$ are the tensors of elastic strain and thermal strain, respectively. $[D^e]$ is the elastic stress–strain matrix.

The virtual work principle, shown in the following, can substitute for the equation of equilibrium:

$$\int_V \delta\{\varepsilon\}^T\{\sigma\}dV - \int_V \delta\{U\}^T\{\overline{F}\}dV - \int_{S_\sigma} \delta\{U\}^T\{\overline{T}\}dS = 0$$

where $\{\overline{F}\}$ is the tensor of body force per unit volume, and $\{\overline{T}\}$ is the tensor of surface force per unit area. V is the volume of the body and S_σ is the area for which the boundary conditions are given. $\delta\{\ \}$ is the amount of virtual change, $\{\ \}^T$ is the transposed tensor.

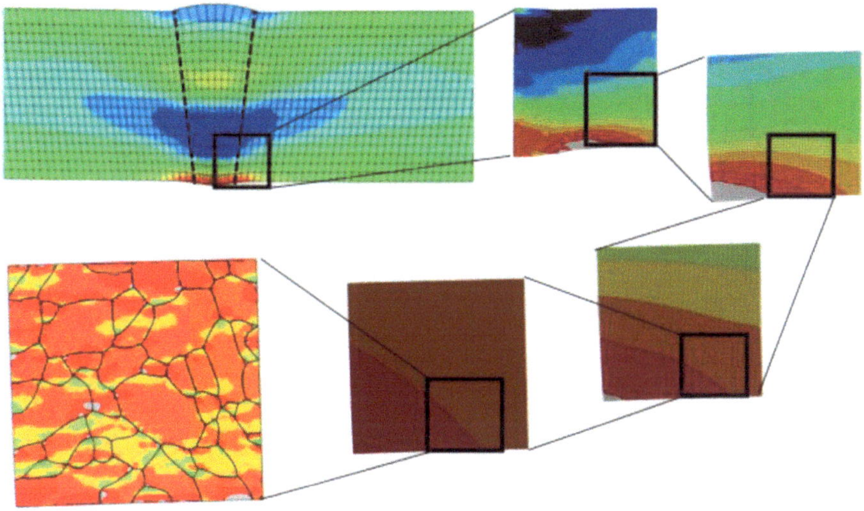

Fig. 7.1 An example of a multi-scale analysis of weld residual stress

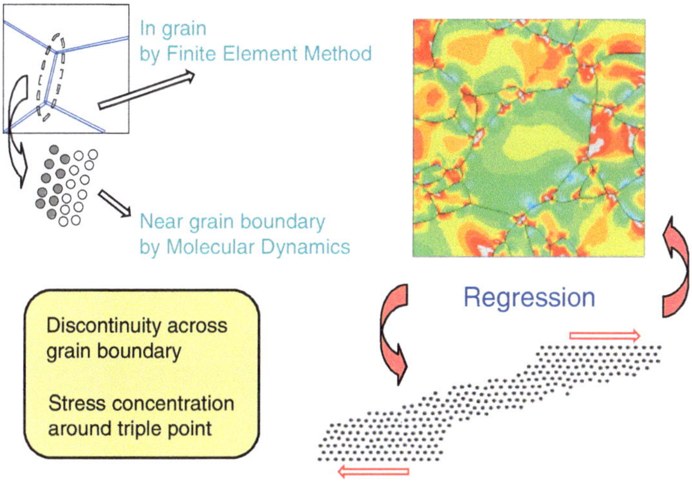

Fig. 7.2 Conceptual diagram for the modeling of crystal grains and crystal grain boundaries

7.3 Multi-scale Analysis of Weld Residual Stress

Weld residual stress has various effects on structures and materials. Thus, the numerical simulation technology of various scales, from large structures such as a pressure vessel structurization to crystal grains for SCC, is necessary. The setting of

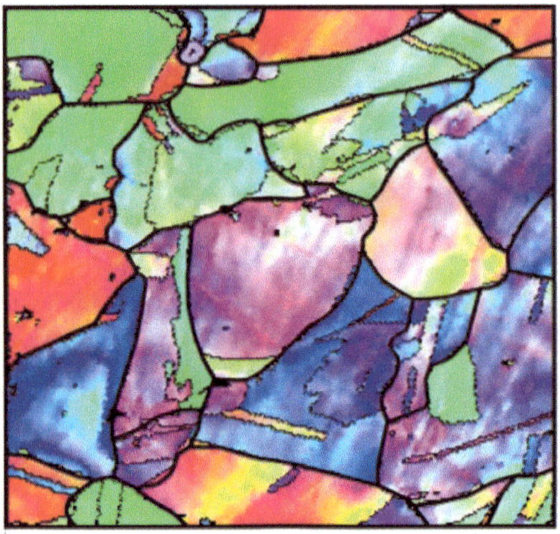

Fig. 7.3 Crystal orientation measured by EBSP-OIM

boundary conditions is extremely important. A heat and stress coupled multi-scale analysis method is developed in order to express realistic boundary conditions in numerical analysis [12–15].

Figure 7.1 shows an example of a millimeter-scale welded joint model coupled with a micron-scale crystal grain model. A similar multi-scale analysis is possible for a mega-scale structure by using the same procedure.

7.4 Example of Numerical Analysis of Weld Residual Stress

7.4.1 Prediction Simulation of SCC by Considering Inhomogeneity and Crystal Plasticity at the Grain Boundaries

In a microscopic phenomenon such as SCC, it is important to understand the residual stress at the crystal grain level and investigate its effect. Thus, an analysis method has been developed in which microscopic residual stress can be determined under the condition of crystal plasticity. This is achieved by measuring the crystal orientation of each crystal grain by electron backscattered pattern-orientation imaging microscopy (EBSP-OIM) and inputting the obtained value into each crystal grain. As shown in Fig. 7.2, discontinuous distortion in the vicinity of the grain boundary can also be simulated by combining the finite element method and molecular dynamics.

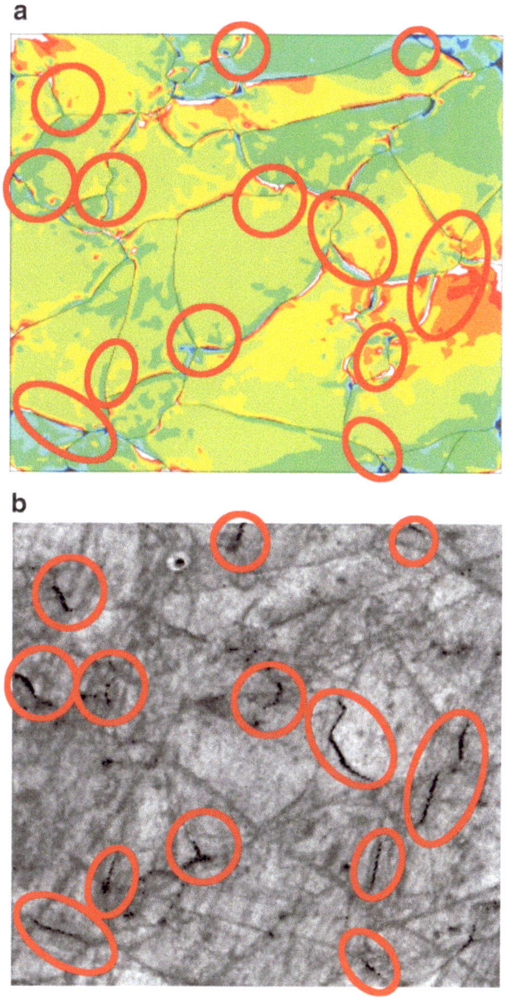

Fig. 7.4 Numerical analysis for the prediction of SCC by considering crystal plasticity (**a**) Locations of high-stress regions based on the results of numerical analysis. (**b**) Locations of SCC by real operating-condition simulated testing

The analysis results for the prediction of SCC for nickel-based alloy type 600 are shown as an example. The crystal orientation of each crystal grain was firstly measured by the EBSP-OIM method, as shown in Fig. 7.3. A numerical calculation was carried out by using the measured value as the input data and considering the crystal plasticity of the polycrystalline body [14, 15]. The calculated high-stress locations, which do not correlate with the direction of the main macroscopic stress, in the vicinity of the grain boundary match the cracking locations in actual SCC testing, as shown in Fig. 7.4. By using such an analysis method, the effect of microscopic residual stress on SCC and its relationship with the progression of SCC can be examined.

a

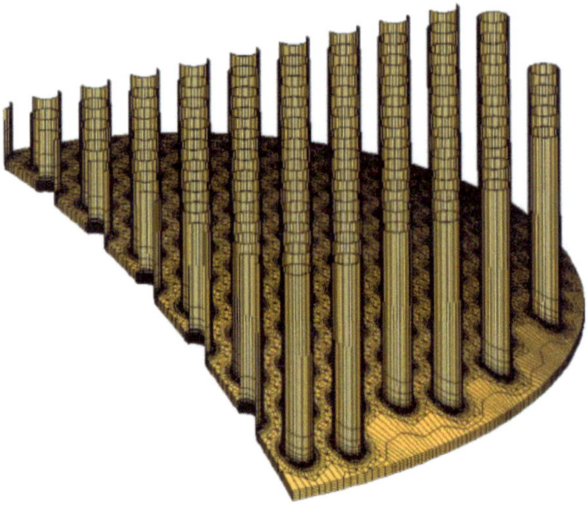

b

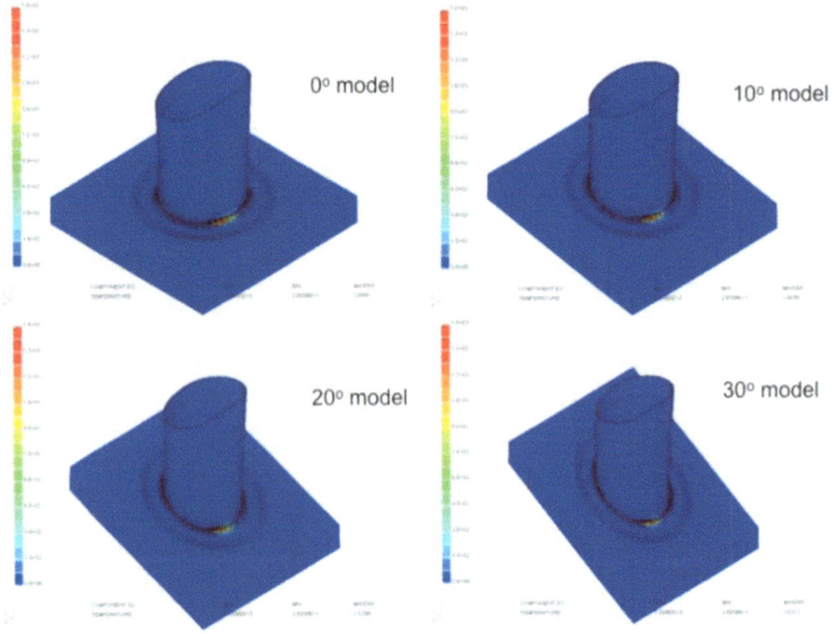

Fig. 7.5 (continued)

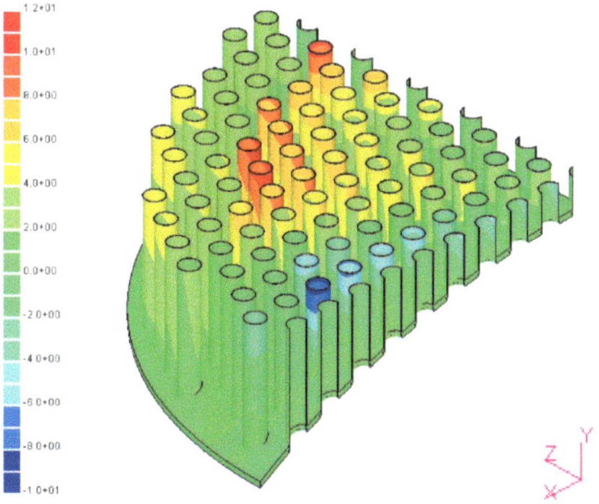

Fig. 7.5 Residual stress analysis for a structure having numerous welds. (**a**) Fillet weld structure of head plate and numerous pipes. (**b**) Example of numerical analysis for various tilt angles models. (**c**) Example of analysis results for residual stress along the direction of the pipe axis

7.4.2 Simulation of Welding Distortion and Residual Stress of Core Internals Having Numerous Welds

Among welded structures, many intricately shaped structures have numerous welds in the neighboring region. For core internals in the pressure vessel of nuclear power plants, meticulous attention is necessary to prevent welding distortion for installation precision and to control the residual stress for structural soundness. Such intricately shaped devices were prepared based on the intuition and experience of skilled workers in the past, and numerical calculations are helping to realize fast computing analyses by the newly developed iterative substructure method. A large-scale computational simulation with one-million finite-element order becomes possible by a normal personal computer such as Windows PC or Macintosh [16]. As an example, the residual stress analysis for a structure having numerous pipe welds on the head plate is shown in Fig. 7.5.

7.4.3 Simulation of Assembling of a Large Structure

Even for a much larger welded structure on the scale of tens of meters, the numerical simulation for welding distortion and residual stress is becoming possible. A numerical simulation example for the assembly of a large structure with a side approximately 20 m in length is shown in Fig. 7.6. At the time of assembly at a plant or setting and mounting on-site, the selection of welding order and the method of installing the restraining jig are very important. The suitable welding conditions

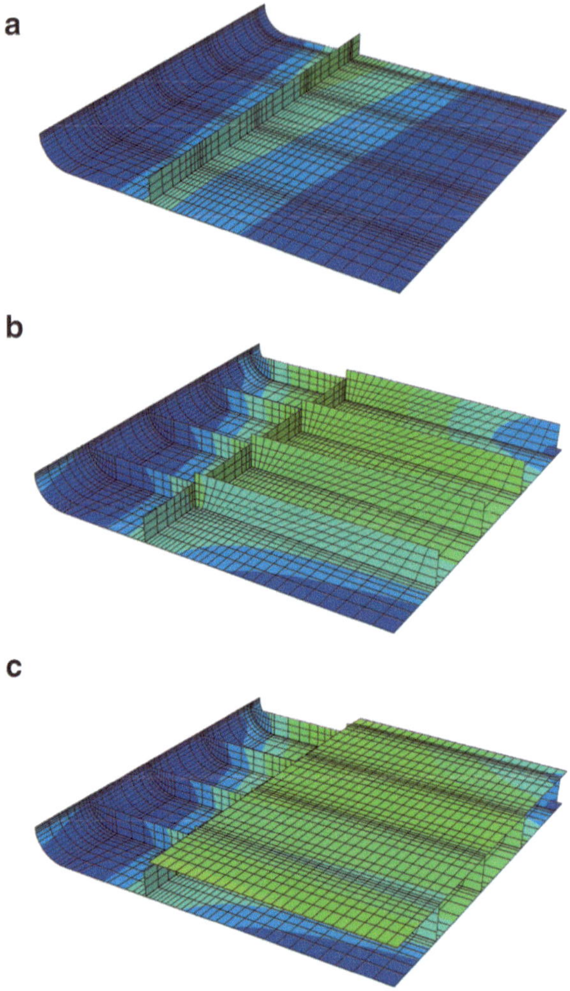

Fig. 7.6 Analysis examples of the weld residual stress of a large structure. (**a**) Assembly order no. 1. (**b**) Assembly order no. 2. (**c**) Assembly order no. 3

can be determined analytically when the appropriate numerical analysis method is applied. That is, high precision of the products can be achieved by pre-examination, and high reliability can also be achieved by the investigation of low residual stress structures.

7.5 Summary

Fundamental theory and an innovative analysis technology are introduced, which have been developed by the authors, for weld residual stress in mega-structures to micro-structures. Presently, it is possible to carry out very detailed modeling by combining a material model, a process physical model, and a dynamic/structural model. It is considered thus that the application of the technology to various fields will be possible.

Acknowledgments This study was supported by Priority Assistance for the Formation of Worldwide Renowned Centers of Research – The Global COE Program (Project: Centre of Excellence for Advanced Structural and Functional Materials Design), from the Ministry of Education, Culture, Sports, Science and Technology (MEXT), Japan.

References

1. Ueda Y, Yamakawa T (1971) Trans Jpn Weld Soc 2:90–100
2. Muraki T, Bryan JJ, Masubuchi K (1975) Trans ASME J Eng Mater Tech 97:81–84
3. Friedman E (1975) Trans ASME J Press Vessel Technol 97:206–212
4. Rybicki EF, Schmueser DW, Stonesifer RW, Groom JJ, Mishler HW (1978) Trans ASME J Press Vessel Technol 100:256–262
5. Mochizuki M (2006) Sci Technol Weld Join 11:496–501
6. Mochizuki M, Toyoda M (2007) Trans ASME J Press Vessel Technol 129:619–629
7. Mochizuki M (2007) Nucl Eng Des 237:107–123
8. Mikami Y, Morikage Y, Mochizuki M, Toyoda M (2009) Sci Technol Weld Join 14:97–105
9. Mochizuki M, An GB, Toyoda M (2009) Trans ASME J Press Vessel Technol. 131:031202-1–031202-11. doi:10.1115/1.3027477
10. Yamamoto J, Hiraoka K, Mochizuki M (2010) Sci Technol Weld Join 15:104–110
11. Mochizuki M, Toyoda M (2011) Trans ASME J Press Vessel Technol 133:031401-1-031401-8. doi:10.1115/1.4002670
12. Okano S, Tanaka M, Mochizuki M (2012) Sci Technol Weld Join 17:264–268
13. Mochizuki M, Mikami Y, Okano S, Itoh S (2009) J Phys Conf Ser 165:012014-1–012014-6
14. Mochizuki M, Mikami Y (2010) In: Proceedings of ASME pressure vessel piping conference, Seattle, PVP2010-25899
15. Mikami Y, Uraguchi R, Sogabe K, Mochizuki M (2011) In: Cerjak H (ed) Mathematical 144 modelling of weld phenomena, vol 9. TU Graz Publishing, Graz : 699–713
16. Itoh S, Shibahara M, Mochizuki M, Murakawa H (2009) Proceedings of 12th international conference pressure vessel technology, Jeju, ICPVT12-0275

Chapter 8
Advanced Analysis of Solidification by X-ray Imaging

Hideyuki Yasuda and Tomoya Nagira

Abstract To observe the solidification of metallic alloys in situ is desired to help understand solidification phenomena, build physical models and validate theories/ models. X-ray imaging using a monochromatized X-ray in a third-generation synchrotron radiation facility has allowed us to observe metallic alloy solidification in situ. In this chapter, the observation technique is briefly explained. Some observations such as dendrite coarsening, transformation from δ phase (bcc) to γ phase (fcc) during solidification and shear deformation of semisolid in Fe alloys are also discussed to highlight the advantages of in situ observation for analyzing solidification phenomena.

Keywords Solidification • In-situ observation • Synchrotron radiation

8.1 Introduction

To observe a phenomenon of interest in situ is a first step toward understanding it. However, it is often difficult to achieve in situ observation. A typical example is solidification of metallic alloys, which are optically opaque. Even though most materials are produced through casting and solidification processing, there have been ambiguities in understanding how microstructures evolve and related defects form during solidification. One possible solution to this problem is X-ray imaging using a monochromatized X-ray at a third generation synchrotron radiation facility.

In third generation facilities such as SPring-8 [1], a hard monochromatized X-ray (10–100 keV), which can penetrate though metallic alloys, is available for X-ray imaging. There are several advantages to imaging in this way. One is

H. Yasuda (✉) • T. Nagira
Department of Adaptive Machine Systems, Graduate School of Engineering, Osaka University, 2-1 Yamadaoka, Suita, Osaka 565-0871, Japan
e-mail: yasuda@ams.eng.osaka-u.ac.jp

T. Kakeshita (ed.), *Progress in Advanced Structural and Functional Materials Design*,
DOI 10.1007/978-4-431-54064-9_8,

the monochromatic light, which can enhance the contrast in transmission images. Another is high coherency, which results in high spatial resolution. A third is the intensity of the light, which improves time resolution. These advantages enable us to observe solidification of metallic alloys in situ by X-ray imaging.

X-ray imaging has been developed to observe solidification of Sn, Zn and Al alloys [1–19]. Microstructure evolution during dendritic solidification (dendrite arm fragmentation, the columnar/equiaxed transition and development of segregation) has been observed in situ. In addition, melt flow in and ahead of the mushy region (solid + liquid present) in Ga–In alloys was also measured by analysis of X-ray transmission images using a conventional X-ray source [20].

Observation of solidification in Cu, Ni and Fe alloys has been limited because of difficulties such as their high melting temperature and reactivity, although knowledge of the solidification process in these alloys is important from the viewpoint of practical application. The first observation of steel solidification was performed by X-ray topography [21]. The planar solid/liquid interface and transition from the planar to the columnar interface in Fe-3mass%Si alloys were detected. However, this technique did not allow dendrite growth to be probed. Recently, X-ray transmission imaging using synchrotron radiation X-rays has allowed dendritic growth in Fe–Si–Al alloys [22] and in Fe–C alloys [23] to be observed. New findings have been realized. For example, the δ/γ transformation observed differed significantly from the expected peritectic reaction (δ: bcc phase and γ: fcc phase) [24]. In addition, shear deformation of semisolids in a Fe–C system was also reported [25]. The observation clearly showed collision and rearrangement of solid grains and provided insight into the deformation mechanism. In this chapter, the technique of X-ray imaging and some examples that provide understanding of solidification of Fe alloys are summarized.

8.2 X-ray Imaging

8.2.1 Requirements for In Situ Observation

Time-resolved X-ray transmission imaging for Fe–C alloys is briefly explained in this section. The intensity of the transmission X-ray, I, is expressed by

$$I = I_0 \exp[-\mu t] \tag{8.1}$$

Here, I_0 is the intensity of the incident beam and t is thickness. The linear X-ray absorption coefficient of the Fe–C specimen, μ, is given by

$$\mu = \rho_{avr}\left[\left(\frac{\mu}{\rho}\right)_{Fe}(1 - w_C) + \left(\frac{\mu}{\rho}\right)_{C} w_C\right], \tag{8.2}$$

where (μ/ρ) and ρ are the mass X-ray absorption coefficient and mass density, respectively. The suffix indicates constituent element, ρ_{avr} is the average density, and

w is the mass fraction. The mass X-ray absorption coefficient, (μ/ρ), which is a function of photon energy, is uniquely defined by the element. The mass X-ray absorption coefficients of Fe and C are 2.57 and 0.044 m^2/kg at 20 keV, respectively [26]. Because the mass fraction of C is less than 0.01 in conventional carbon steels, the mass X-ray absorption coefficient and the density of Fe determine the linear X-ray absorption coefficient of the Fe–C sample.

The X-ray absorption coefficient of Fe–C alloys suggests that the essential requirement for observing the solid/liquid interface is to detect the contrast caused by the difference in density between solid and liquid phases (4.2% for pure Fe).

8.2.2 *Influence of Photon Energy*

The linear X-ray absorption coefficients of solid and liquid phases of pure Fe are expressed as

$$\mu_{\text{Liquid}} = \left(\frac{\mu}{\rho}\right)_{Fe} \rho_{\text{Fe,Liquid}}, \quad \text{and} \quad \mu_{Solid} = \left(\frac{\mu}{\rho}\right)_{\text{Fe}} \rho_{\text{Fe,Solid}} \tag{8.3}$$

Time-resolved observation of a solid/liquid interface simultaneously requires a sufficient photon flux to a detector and an appropriate contrast in a transmission image to be attained. The normalized intensity, τ, and the contrast of solid phase to liquid phase, χ, are defined by the following equations:

$$\tau = \frac{I_{\text{Liquid}}}{I_0} = \exp\left[-\mu_{\text{Fe,Liquid}} t\right], \tag{8.4}$$

$$\chi = \frac{I_{\text{Liquid}} - I_{\text{Solid}}}{I_{\text{Liquid}}} = 1 - \exp\left[-\left(\frac{\mu}{\rho}\right)_{\text{Fe}} \left(\rho_{\text{Fe,Solid}} - \rho_{\text{Fe,Liquid}}\right) t\right] \tag{8.5}$$

Figure 8.1 shows τ and χ as a function of sample thickness and photon energy for pure Fe with a thickness of 100 μm. The normalized intensity of 0.1% is too small to allow time-resolved imaging using the present setup. Because a normalized intensity of at least several % is required, an X-ray beam with a photon energy exceeding 15 keV should be used.

If the contrast is less than 1%, it is difficult to detect a solid/liquid interface. As shown in Fig. 8.1b, the contrast decreases with increasing photon energy. Thus, the intensity and contrast in transmission images have a trade-off relationship. In the case of a sample with a thickness of 100–200 μm, an X-ray with a photon energy ranging from 15 to 30 keV is suitable for in situ observation [23]. X-rays of such energy are available at third generation synchrotron radiation facilities.

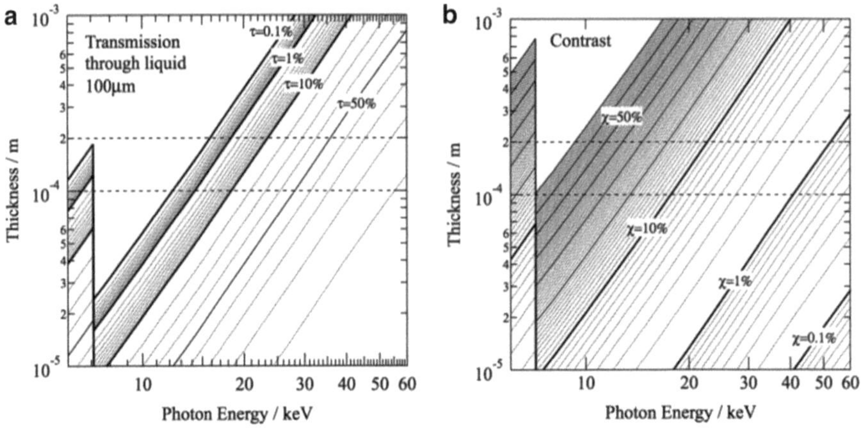

Fig. 8.1 (**a**) Normalized transmission X-ray intensity through the liquid phase, and (**b**) contrast between liquid and solid phases [23]

8.2.3 Setup of Observation Apparatus

Observation experiments were performed using the BL20B2 beamline at SPring-8, Japan. A bending magnet was used as an X-ray source, and the radiation was monochromatized with a Si double crystal monochromator (36.8 m from the X-ray source point). Both an absorption contrast caused by the difference in absorption and a phase contrast induced by the difference in density, which improves the observation of phase boundaries in a sample, are obtained in X-ray transmission images [27, 28].

Figure 8.2 shows a typical setup for observing solidification of pure Fe [23]. An ion chamber, vacuum chamber for heating the sample and an X-ray detector are placed along an X-ray beam. An X-ray direct-sensing pickup tube, SATICON [29], was used to observe transmitted X-ray images. The image signals were stored in frame memory with a format of 1,024 $\times$ 1,024 pixels and 10-bit resolution. In the present setup, the spatial resolution was approximately 10 μm.

8.3 Observations

8.3.1 Solid/Liquid Interface of Pure Fe

Figure 8.3a shows static observation of a solid/liquid interface in pure Fe at 20 keV [23]. The exposure time needed to obtain the transmission images was 4 s. The upper part of the image is the liquid phase and the lower part is the solid

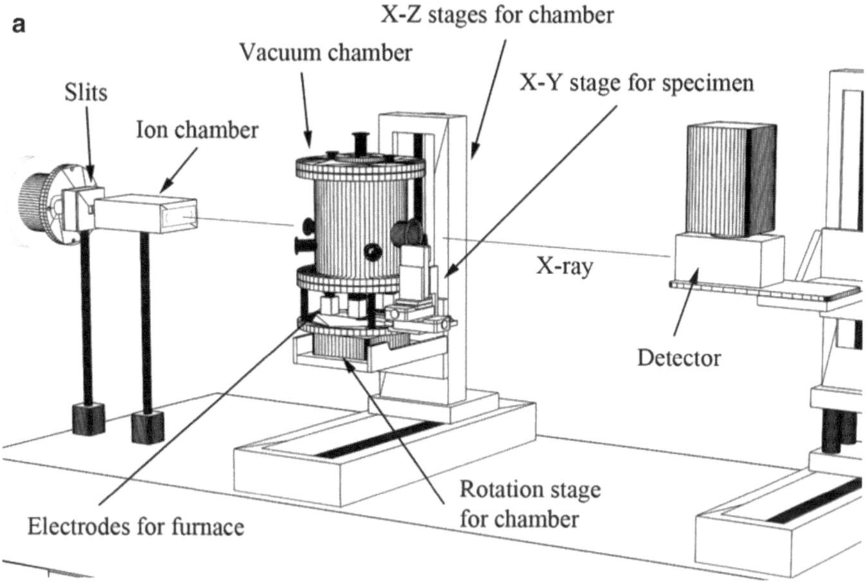

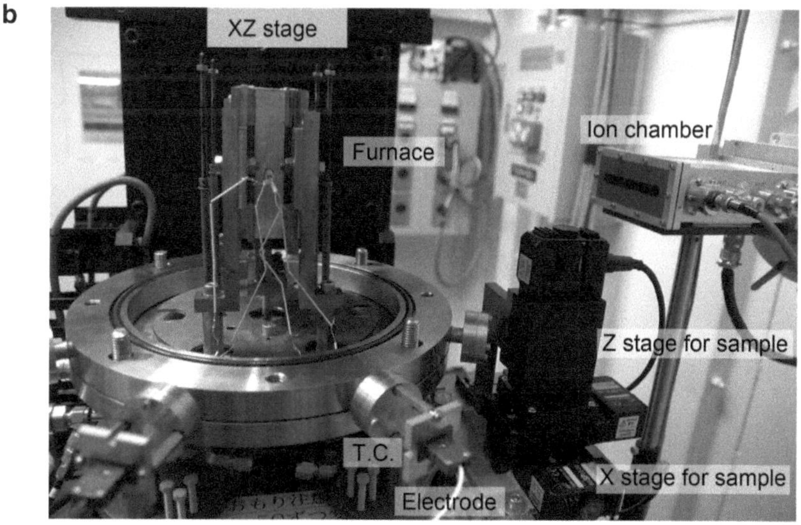

Fig. 8.2 Setup of equipment used for in situ observation of Fe alloys [23]. (**a**) Configuration of X-ray optics, and (**b**) furnace in the vacuum chamber

phase. This solid/liquid interface in pure Fe was clearly detected at photon energies ranging from 16 to 28 keV. As shown in Fig. 8.3b, the phase contrast, which originated from interference of the X-ray beam with high coherency, showed a couple of white and black fringes in the vicinity of the interface. Because the

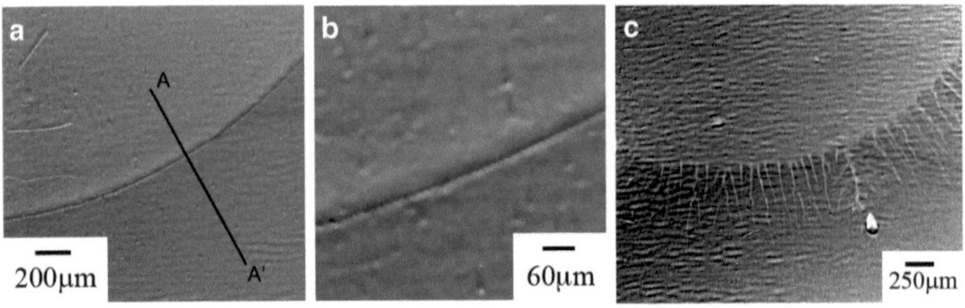

Fig. 8.3 Photographs of the solid/liquid interface in pure Fe [23, 30]. (**a**) 20 keV, (**b**) close-up view at 20 keV, and (**c**) growing interface at a cooling rate of 0.33 K/s

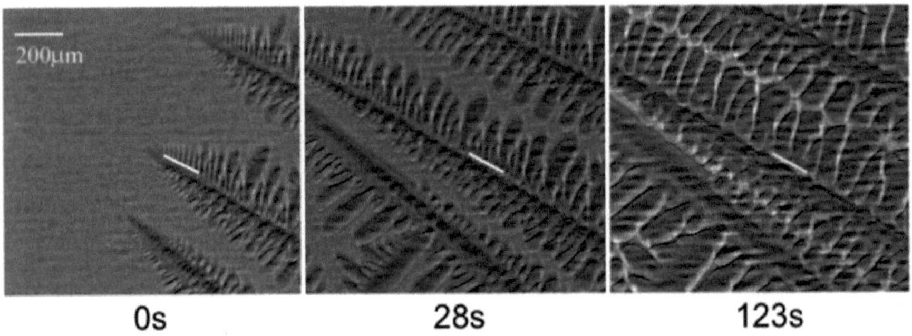

Fig. 8.4 Coarsening of secondary arms in Fe-0.3mass%C alloy at a cooling rate of 0.17 K/s [30]

solid/liquid interface was smooth enough and not parallel to the X-ray beam, reflection of the X-ray beam at the solid/liquid interface was also observed.

8.3.2 Coarsening of Secondary Arms in Fe-0.3mass%C Alloys

Secondary arm spacing is often used to characterize solidification structure. The spacing is used to evaluate the cooling rate in castings and is closely related to mechanical properties. Thus, it is of interest to know how the dendrite arms coarsen during solidification. Figure 8.4 shows the dendrite solidification of Fe-0.3mass%C alloys at a cooling rate of 0.17 K/s [30]. Relatively fine secondary arms with a spacing of 20 μm or less were formed just behind the dendrite tips and then coarsened in the mushy region as indicated by a white line. Coarsening was classified into three stages. In stage I ($t < 150$ s), some arms were selected through competitive growth between the initial arms. The coarsening caused liquid channels to form between the secondary arms. In stage II, the depth of the liquid channel decreased and consequently the coarsened arms coalesced (150–170 s). In stage III,

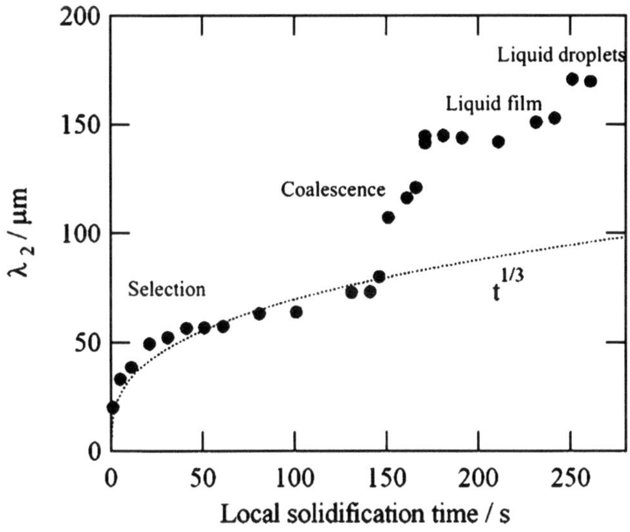

Fig. 8.5 Change of dendrite arm spacing during solidification [30]. Stage I: selection of arms ($0 < t < 140$ s), stage II: coalescence of coarsened arms ($150 < t < 160$ s), and stage III: formation of a liquid film and droplets

the liquid phase was isolated by solid, leading to a liquid film between the primary arms or liquid droplet.

The relationship between the secondary arm spacing and local solidification is shown in Fig. 8.5. The spacing was roughly proportional to $t_f^{1/3}$ (t_f: local solidification time) in stage I. Thus, the coarsening in stage I is well described by the conventional coarsening model [31]. The arm spacing at 150 s (beginning of stage II) was 60 μm. In stage II, the arm spacing deviated from the $t_f^{1/3}$ law and rapidly increased. The liquid channel between the secondary arms controlled the coalescence. Because the change of the liquid channel is controlled not by selection but by the curvature effect, the secondary arm coarsening in stage II differs from that in stage I. To know the transitions from stage I to II and from stage II to III is useful to determine the permeability of the melt in the mushy region, and to help understand the mechanical properties of the solidifying shell.

8.3.3 Transformation of δ Phase to γ Phase

It has generally been accepted that the peritectic reaction occurs during or after solidification in Fe–C alloys (<0.5mass%). Because the transformation from δ phase to γ phase causes volume shrinkage of 1%, the transformation can influence casting defects such as deformations, cracks and unevenness of the solidifying

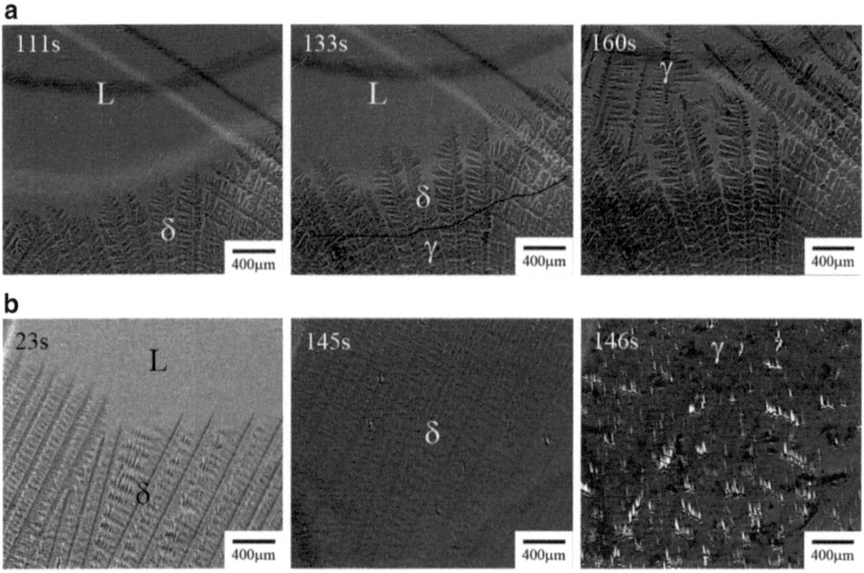

Fig. 8.6 Peritectic transformation modes observed in Fe—0.45mass%C alloy by X-ray imaging [24, 30]. (**a**) Peritectic-like mode at 0.167 K/s, and (**b**) massive-like mode at 0.83 K/s

shell. Thus, it is of interest to know how the γ phase is produced during or after solidification in Fe–C alloys.

The solidification and phase transformation of Fe-0.45C-0.6Mn-0.3Si alloys (mass%) were observed [24]. The observed transformation differed significantly from the peritectic reaction. Figure 8.6a shows the δ/γ transformation during solidification at a cooling rate of 0.17 K/s. δ dendrites grew from the bottom to the top (111 s). The transformation from the δ to the γ phase proceeded from the root to the tip of δ dendrites (133 s). When the γ phase reached the tips of δ dendrites, γ dendrites grew ahead of δ dendrite tips (160 s). Because the crystallographic orientation of the γ phase differed from that of the δ phase, the γ dendrites changed the growth direction. The transformation occurred in the mushy region. Thus, the observed transformation was classified into the peritectic transformation. However, this mode was hardly observed in Fe–C alloys even at a cooling rate of 0.17 K/s.

The massive-like transformation was observed at higher cooling rates. Figure 8.6b shows δ dendrite and γ phase transformed by the massive-like transformation at a cooling rate of 0.83 K/s. δ dendrites grew in advance (23 s), and the sample solidified without γ phase formation (145 s). When the temperature was more than 100 K below the liquid temperature, the δ phase directly transformed into the γ phase within 1 s (145–146 s). Because the volume shrinkage caused by the δ/γ transformation was not completely compensated for by melt flow, grooves were produced (white region). Many dark spots were also observed, indicating relatively large strain in the γ phase. The large undercooling for the δ/γ transformation implied that γ nucleation was difficult in the semisolid containing δ phase and liquid, as well as in the δ phase.

In the massive-like transformation, the volume shrinkage caused by the δ/γ transformation is not compensated for by melt flow. Thus, a relatively large strain is induced. In addition, the strain rate in the massive-like transformation will be higher than that in the peritectic reaction. As a result, observation by X-ray imaging can provide valuable information on the microstructure evolution and defect formation in alloys.

8.3.4 Shear Deformation of a Semisolid

Semisolid processing (SSP) is a promising solidification method, in which a mixture of solid and liquid is poured into a mold. The potential advantages include lower processing pressure, smaller machines, and the ability to realize rather complex shapes compared with conventional forging. SSP can also reduce porosity compared to traditional casting methods. There have been significant developments in SSP of steels [32–39].

It is well known that semisolids exhibit various mechanical phenomena. For example, thixotropic properties [40, 41], agglomeration/disagglomeration [40], deformation of solid globules [42], and dilatancy during crystal rearrangement [43–45] have been realized. It is therefore valuable to observe the deformation of semisolids in situ [25, 44].

High carbon steel (Fe-2mass%C-1mass%Mn-0.5mass%Si), which has a relatively wide freezing range and is a candidate for SSP, was used as the sample [35]. Semisolid microstructure was generated by partially remelting the as-cast alloy. The average grain size in the sample was 310 μm.

Figure 8.7 shows the deformation of a semisolid with solid fraction of 0.65 [25]. An Al_2O_3 plate inserted into the sample cell was moved at a rate of 40 μm/s (strain rate: 10^{-3}/s, push-plate motion: 2d increment, where d is grain size). Rearrangement of solid grains, induced by the motion of the plate, produced a liquid-filled space between globules, as shown in Fig. 8.7a, b. Figure 8.7c clearly shows that the liquid-filled spaces enlarge during rearrangement. An example of the dilation was demonstrated by highlighting five globules (a–e). First, a moved upwards into b and c. The displacement of c and arrangement of contacts between c/e and c/d push e to the left and d upwards, opening up a space between d, e and c. Thus, dilation of the globule assembly was observed.

The time-resolved sequences showed that direct shear was accommodated by globule rearrangement and that the semisolid deformed as a largely cohesionless granular material. A loose assembly of solid grains in mechanical contact is consistent with recent work on Al and Mg alloys [43–45]. The in situ observation proved that the rearrangement of solid grains plays an important role in the dilation of a sample.

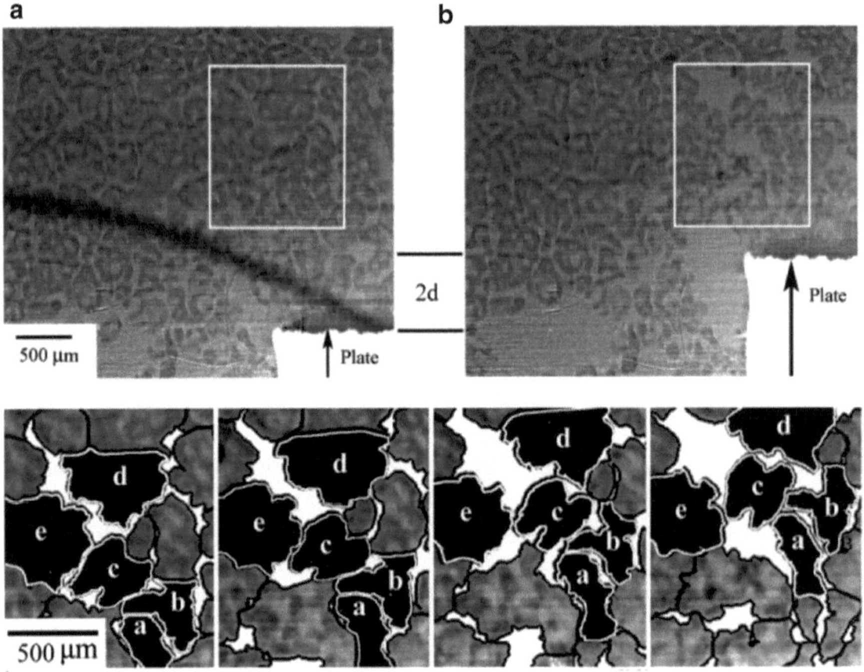

Fig. 8.7 Deformation of a steel semisolid (grain size: 310 μm) [25]. (**a**) Before, and (**b**) after a 2d increment of push-plate motion. (**c**) Close-up view of the dilation observed during the 2d increment

8.4 Summary

Time-resolved absorption imaging using synchrotron radiation X-rays has been developed for metallic alloys with high melting temperatures. The observation of solidification in pure Fe proved that this technique is suitable for studying various metallic alloy systems.

Coarsening of the secondary arms in Fe-0.3mass%C alloys was classified into three stages: I Secondary arms were selected, II coalescence occurred, leading to a rapid increase of arm spacing, and III the liquid phase becomes isolated by solid. The arm spacing followed the $t_f^{-1/3}$ law in stage I.

In general, it has been accepted that the peritectic reaction occurs in Fe–C systems and the transformation from δ to γ phases is closely related to casting defects. However, in situ observation revealed that the massive-like transformation from the δ to the γ phase could dominate the initial stage of solidification. Observation of the transformation mode by X-ray imaging will help to reveal how casting defects form.

Shear deformation of a semisolid was observed in situ on grain scale. The rearrangement of solid grains, induced by shear deformation, produced liquid-filled spaces in the semisolid. In addition, the semisolid acted like a largely cohesionless granular material. These results are useful for revealing the deformation mechanism of semisolids.

Acknowledgments This study was supported by the Global COE Program (Centre of Excellence for Advanced Structural and Functional Materials Design) from MEXT, and a Grant-in-Aid for Scientific Research (A). The synchrotron radiation experiments were performed as a long-term project (2007A0014-2009B0014), and as general projects at BL20B2 and BL20XU beamlines at SPring-8 (JASRI). The in situ observation of solidification in Fe alloys was also supported by "ISIJ Innovative Program for Advanced Technology" from the Institute of Iron and Steel, Japan.

References

1. http://www.spring8.or.jp/
2. Mathiesen RH, Arnberg L, Mo F, Weitkamp T, Snigirev A (1999) Phys Rev Lett 83:5062
3. Mathiesen RH, Arnberg L, Ramsoskar K, Weitkamp T, Rau C, Snigirev A (2002) Metall Mater Trans B 33:613
4. Yasuda H, Ohnaka I, Kawasaki K, Sugiyama A, Ohmichi T, Iwane J, Umetani K (2004) J Cryst Growth 262:645
5. Mangelinck-Noel N, Nguyen-Thi H, Reinhart G, Schenk T, Cristiglio V, Dupouy MD, Gastaldi J, Billia B, Hartwig J (2005) J Phys D 38:A28
6. Mathiesen RH, Arnberg L (2005) Mater Sci Eng A 413:283
7. Mathiesen RH, Arnberg L (2005) Acta Mater 53:947
8. Ohnaka I, Yasuda H, Sugiyama A, Ohmichi T (2005) Trans Indian Inst Met 58:603
9. Schenk T, Thi HN, Gastaldi J, Reinhart G, Cristiglio V, Mangelinck-Noel N, Klein H, Hartwig J, Grushko B, Billia B, Baruchel J (2005) J Cryst Growth 275:201
10. Li B, Brody HD, Black DR, Burdette HE, Rau C (2006) J Phys D 39:4450
11. Li B, Brody HD, Black DR, Burdette HE, Rau C (2006) Meas Sci Technol 17:1883
12. Mathiesen RH, Arnberg L, Bleuet P, Somogyi A (2006) Metall Mater Trans A 37A:2515
13. Yasuda H, Ohnaka I, Sugiyama A, Nagira T, Tsukihara N, Kawasaki K, Umetani K (2006) Proc. Int. Conf. on Modeling of Casting, Welding and Advanced Solidification Processes 375
14. Arnberg L, Mathiesen RH (2007) JOM 59:20
15. Ruvalcaba D, Mathiesen RH, Eskin DG, Arnberg L, Katgerman L (2007) Acta Mater 55:4287
16. Yasuda H, Nagira T, Harada H, Sawai T, Sindoh H, Nishimura K (2007) Proc. 7th Int. Conf. Zinc and Zinc alloy Coated Steel Sheet 545–549
17. Reinhart G, Buffet A, Nguyen-Thi H, Billia B, Jung H, Mangelinck-Noel N, Bergeon N, Schenk T, Hartwig J, Baruchel J (2008) Metall Mater Trans A 39A:865
18. Yasuda H, Yamamoto Y, Nakatsuka N, Nagira T, Yoshiya M, Sugiyama A, Ohnaka I, Umetani K, Uesugi K (2009) Int J Cast Met Res 21:125
19. Wang TM, Xu JJ, Xiao TQ, Xie HL, Li J, Li TJ, Cao ZQ (2010) Phys Rev E 81:042601
20. Boden S, Willers B, Eckert S, Gerbeth G (2009) Int J Cast Met Res 22:30
21. Matsumiya T, Yamada W, Ohashi T, Nittono O (1987) Metall Mater Trans A 18:723–727
22. Yasuda H, Yamamoto Y, Nakatsuka N, Nagira T, Yoshiya M, Sugiyama A, Ohnaka I, Umetani K, Uesugi K (2008) Int J Cast Met Res 22:15
23. Yasuda H, Nagira T, Yoshiya M, Nakatsuka N, Sugiyama A, Uesugi K, Umetani K (2011) ISIJ Int 51:402

24. Yasuda H, Nagira T, Yoshiya M, Uesugi M, Nakatsuka N, Kiire M, Sugiyama A, Uesugi K, Umetani K (2012) IOP Conf. Ser.: Mater Sci Eng 33 (2012) 012053
25. Nagira T, Gourlay CM, Sugiyama A, Uesugi M, Kanazawa Y, Yoshiya M, Uesugi K, Umetani K, Yasuda H (2011) Scr Mater 64:1129
26. NISTIR 5632, National Institute of Standards and Technology, Gaithersburg, MD (1995). (Hubbell JH, Seltzer SM (2004) Available: http://physics.nist.gov/xaamdi 2010/11/15)
27. Goto S, Takeshita K, Suzuki Y, Ohashi H, Asano Y, Kimura H, Matsushita T, Yagi N, Isshiki M, Yamazaki H (2001) Nucl Instrum Methods Phys Res A 467–468:682
28. Cosslett VE, Nixon WC (1953) J Appl Phys 4:616
29. Umetani K, Yagi N, Suzuki Y, Ogasawara Y, Kajiya F, Matsumoto T, Tachibana H, Goto M, Yamashita T, Imai S, Kajihara Y (2000) Proc SPIE 3977:522
30. Yasuda H, Nagira T, Yoshiya M, Sugiyama A, Nakatsuka N, Morita S, Uesugi M, Uesugi K, Umetani K, Kajiwara K (2011) Proc. John Hunt Symposium (2012) 335
31. Kattamis TZ, Coughlin JC, Flemings MC (1967) Trans AIME 239:1504
32. Tseng AA, Horskỳ J, Raudenslỳ M, Kotrbácek P (2001) Mater Des 22:83–92
33. Kikuchi M, Kopp R (2002) Ann CIRP 51:653–676
34. Omar MZ, Palmiere EJ, Howe AA, Atkinson HV, Kapranos P (2005) Mater Sci Eng A 395:53–61
35. Ramadan M, Takita M, Nomura H, EI-Bagoury N (2006) Mater Sci Eng A 430:285–291
36. Püttgen W, Bleck W, Hirt G, Shimahara H (2007) Adv Eng Mater 9:231–245
37. Sugiyama S, Li J, Yanagimoto J (2007) Mater Trans 48:807–812
38. Pierret JC, Rassili A, Vaneetveld G, Lecomte-Beckers J, Cezard P, Bigot R (2008) Int J Mater Form 1:1011
39. Rassili A, Atkinson HV (2010) Trans Nonferrous Met Soc China 20:s1048
40. Young KP, Riek RG, Flemings MC (1979) Met Technol 6:130
41. Flemings MC (1991) Metall Trans 22A:957
42. Tzimas E, Zavaliangos A (1999) Acta Mater 47:517
43. Gourlay CM, Dahle AK (2007) Nature 445:70
44. Gourlay CM, Dahle AK, Nagira T, Nakatsuka N, Nogita K, Uesugi K, Yasuda H (2011) Acta Mater 59:4933
45. Gourlay CM, Meylan B, Dahle AK (2008) Acta Mater 56:3403

Part II
Advanced Materials Research Project for Combined Structural and Functional Applications

Chapter 9
Advanced Materials Design by Microstructure Control Under Magnetic Field

Tomoyuki Kakeshita and Takashi Fukuda

Abstract Solid–solid phase transformations are usually associated with the formation of variants (crystallographic domains). These variants form in equivalent amounts when an external field is not applied. In some alloys and compounds, differences in magnetic energy arise among variants when they are placed under a magnetic field. In such cases, the microstructure comprising such variants can be controlled by the application of a magnetic field. This chapter covers the criterion that is necessary for controlling variants in a magnetic field. Two typical examples of variant control through the use of a magnetic field are shown. The first example is rearrangement of martensite variants by applying a magnetic field to ferromagnetic shape memory alloys. The second example is preferential formation of ordered variants in CoPt and FePd. In both cases, magnetocrystalline anisotropy plays an essential role.

Keywords Magnetic anisotropy • Martensite • Ordering • Transformation

9.1 Introduction

The properties of structural and functional materials are strongly influenced by their microstructure. Therefore, many processes have been developed to obtain a designed microstructure of materials. Among these processes, those that exploit solid–solid phase transformations to control microstructures are widely used. In this chapter, we will show that the microstructure formed by solid–solid transformation can be largely influenced by a magnetic field. Two typical examples are shown. The first is the rearrangement of martensite variants, which is formed by martensitic transformation, under an applied magnetic field. In this case, variants

T. Kakeshita • T. Fukuda (✉)
Division of Materials and Manufacturing Science, Graduate School of Engineering, Osaka University, 2-1 Yamadaoka, Suita, Osaka 565-0871, Japan
e-mail: fukuda@mat.eng.osaka-u.ac.jp

T. Kakeshita (ed.), *Progress in Advanced Structural and Functional Materials Design*, DOI 10.1007/978-4-431-54064-9_9, © Springer Japan 2013

with high magnetic anisotropy energy switch to variants with low magnetic anisotropy energy. In association with this rearrangement, a large magnetic field-induced strain of several percent appears. The second example is the preferential nucleation of an ordered variant in association with a disorder–order transformation under a magnetic field. In this case, the variant with its easy axis orientated to the direction of magnetic field nucleates preferentially. Then in the growth process, a single variant of the ordered phase can be obtained. Before covering these examples, we explain two key concepts necessary for understanding these examples: the formation of variants by cubic-tetragonal transformation and magnetic energy difference between variants.

9.2 Formation of Variants by Cubic-Tetragonal Transformation

Solid–solid phase transformations are usually associated with changes in symmetry. In many cases, the symmetry of the low-temperature phase is lower than that of the high-temperature phase, and the low-temperature phase comprises several variants with different orientations. In this chapter, we consider a cubic (high-temperature phase) to tetragonal (low-temperature phase) transformation only. The crystallographic axes of the cubic phase are orthogonal to each other and are of the same length. In the tetragonal phase, however, one axis (*c*-axis) is longer or shorter than the other two axes (*a*-axes). The *c*-axis can be chosen from three equivalent <001> directions of the cubic phase as shown in the left panel of Fig. 9.1. Consequently, three orientation variants form in association with the cubic-tetragonal phase transformation. We term the three variants X-, Y-, and Z-variants. The number of orientation variants in general can be derived from group theory [1].

The free energies of different variants are equivalent when no external field is applied. Under an external field, however, differences in free energy arise between different variants. This differences influence the microstructure under an applied magnetic field.

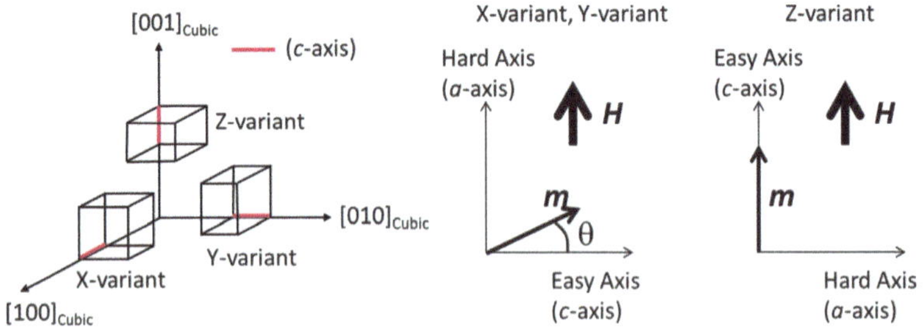

Fig. 9.1 Schematic illustration showing three variants and the orientation of magnetic moment under magnetic field for different variants

9.3 Magnetic Energy Difference Between Variants

The magnetization curve of a crystal usually depends on its crystallographic orientation. In some alloys and compounds with a hexagonal or tetragonal structure, one unique direction, the c-axis, is easy (or hard) to magnetize compared with other directions. Such magnetic anisotropy is termed uniaxial magnetocrystalline anisotropy, and the unique direction is referred to as the easy axis (or the hard axis).

The magnetic anisotropy energy U_A of a ferromagnetic system with uniaxial magnetocrystalline anisotropy is given as [2]

$$U_A = K_u \sin^2\theta + K_u^{'} \sin^4\theta + K_u^{''} \sin^6\theta + \cdots, \tag{9.1}$$

where θ is the angle between the c-axis and the magnetic moment, and K_u, $K_u^{'}$, and $K_u^{''}$ are constants. In many cases, the square term gives a satisfactory approximation of the anisotropic energy, and quadruplicate and higher terms can be neglected. The sign of K_u is positive when the unique axis is the easy axis, while K_u is negative when the unique axis is the hard axis. In the following, we assume for simplicity that the c-axis is the easy axis.

Let us consider a tetragonal phase formed by a cubic-to-tetragonal transformation. The tetragonal phase comprises three variants (X-, Y-, and Z-variants) as described above. We apply a magnetic field in the direction parallel to the c-axis of the Z-variant as shown in Fig. 9.1. The field direction is perpendicular to the c-axis of the X- and Y-variants. We write the magnetic energy per unit volume of the three variants under a magnetic field H as U_X, U_Y and U_Z. They are given by

$$U_Z = -M_s H, \quad \text{and} \quad U_Y = U_X = -M_s H \sin\theta + K_u \sin^2\theta, \tag{9.2}$$

where M_s is the spontaneous magnetization per unit volume. In Eq. (9.2), the quadruplicate and higher terms in Eq. (9.1) are neglected. The angle θ in Eq. (9.2) is obtained by the condition $dU_Y/d\theta = 0$, which yields $\sin\theta = M_s H/2K_u$. The energy difference between the variants is given as

$$\Delta U_{mag} = U_Y - U_Z = -M_s H + \frac{(M_s H)^2}{4K_u} \quad \text{for} \quad H \leq H_c = \frac{2K_u}{M_s}, \quad \text{and}$$
$$\Delta U_{mag} = K_u \quad \text{for} \quad H > H_c. \tag{9.3}$$

Because we assumed that the c-axis is the easy axis ($K_u > 0$), the relation $U_Y > U_Z$ holds under an applied magnetic field. A similar derivation can be made for $K_u < 0$, and in this case, $U_Y < U_z$ holds.

The energy difference ($U_Y > U_Z$) caused by magnetocrystalline anisotropy influences the microstructure through the following two processes. First, the Z-variant grows consuming Y- or X-variants. This is a rearrangement of variants under a magnetic field. Second, the Z-variant forms preferentially from the cubic phase compared with the Y- or X-variants. In the following sections, we will see examples of these two cases.

9.4 Rearrangement of Variants Under Magnetic Field in Ferromagnetic Shape Memory Alloys

In this section we review the rearrangement of variants under an applied magnetic field in three ferromagnetic shape memory alloys: disordered Fe-31.2Pd (at.%), ordered Fe_3Pt (degree of order =0.75), and ordered Ni_2MnGa.

The three above mentioned alloys exhibit a thermoelastic cubic-to-tetragonal martensitic transformation (strictly speaking, the pseudotetragonal phase in Ni_2MnGa) [3–5]. The martensitic transformation temperature T_M is 230 K in an Fe-31.2Pd alloy, 85 K in an Fe_3Pt and 202 K in a Ni_2MnGa. Figure 9.2 shows the temperature dependence of the lattice parameters of the three alloys [6, 7]. The lattice parameters show a clear discontinuity at T_M for Ni_2MnGa. However, for Fe_3Pt and Fe-31.2Pd, the lattice parameters change gradually below T_M. The tetragonality c/a at temperatures sufficiently below T_M is almost the same among the three alloys and is about 0.94 at 77 K (at 13 K for the Fe_3Pt).

Figure 9.3 shows the magnetization curves of a single variant measured under a magnetic field applied in the a- and c-axes. In the case of the Fe-31.2Pd alloy, the a-axis is easy to magnetize compared with the c-axis, implying that $K_u < 0$. However, in the case of the Fe_3Pt and Ni_2MnGa, the c-axis is easy to magnetize compared with the a-axis, implying that $K_u > 0$. The value of $|K_u|$ is obtained from the area enclosed by the two magnetization curves measured for the a-axis and c-axis. The temperature dependence of $|K_u|$ for the three alloys is shown in Fig. 9.4. The value of $|K_u|$ decreases with increasing temperature. Two factors affect this temperature dependence of $|K_u|$. One is the temperature dependence of tetragonal distortion $(1 - c/a)$, and the other is the temperature dependence of spontaneous magnetization. The significant temperature dependence of $|K_u|$ for the Fe-31.2Pd and Fe_3Pt is due to the significant change in c/a of the martensite phase.

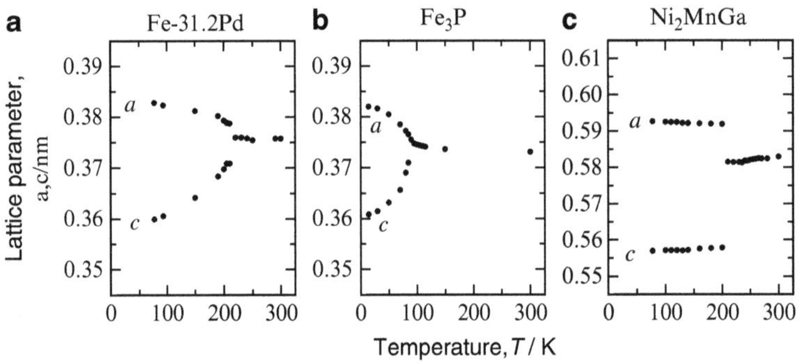

Fig. 9.2 Temperature dependence of lattice parameters for Fe-31.2Pd [6], Fe_3Pt [6], and Ni_2MnGa [7]

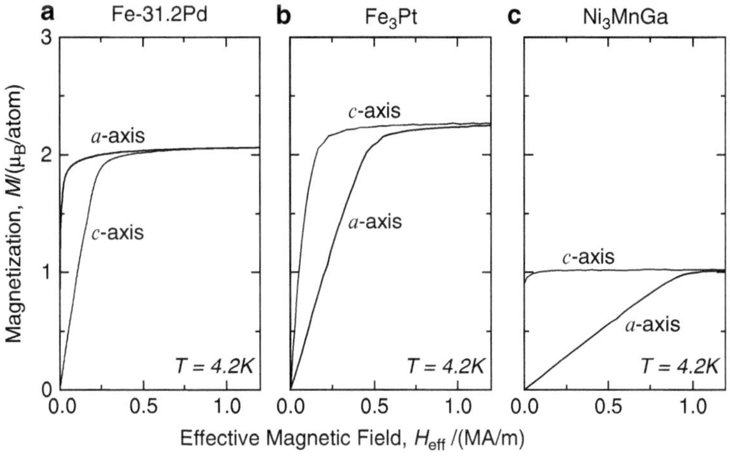

Fig. 9.3 Magnetization curves measured along a- and c-axes of Fe-31.2Pd [8], Fe_3Pt [8] and Ni_2MnGa [9]

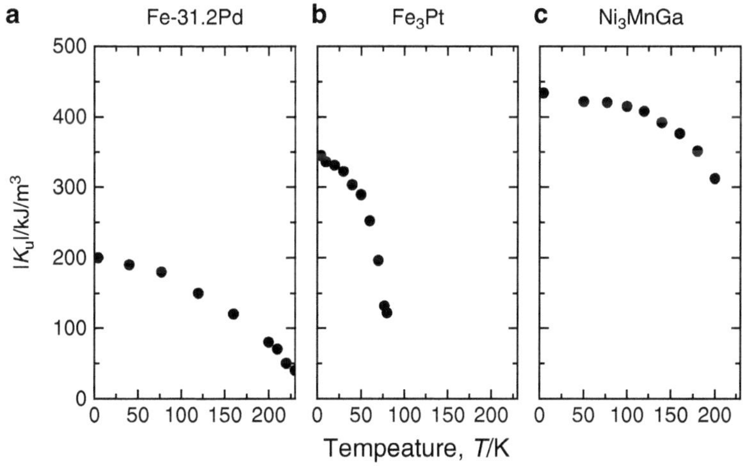

Fig. 9.4 Uniaxial magnetocrystalline anisotropy constant K_u of Fe-31.2Pd [10], Fe_3Pt and Ni_2MnGa [9]

Owing to magnetocrystalline anisotropy, as shown in Figs. 9.3 and 9.4, these alloys exhibit rearrangement of martensite variants under a magnetic field. Figure 9.5 shows an example of the rearrangement of martensite variants in the Fe-31.2Pd alloy. The twinned variants (a) change to a single variant (c) upon the application of magnetic field H. In association with the rearrangement of variants, a large magnetic field-induced strain of several percent appears. Figure 9.6 shows

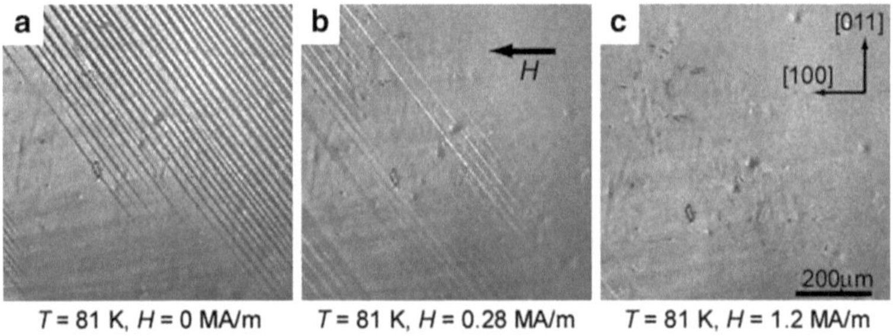

Fig. 9.5 Rearrangement of martensite variants due to applied magnetic field observed in Fe-31.2Pd alloy. The observation was made at 81 K [6]

the magnetic field-induced strain obtained by applying a magnetic field to the easy axis of one variant and hard axis to other variants. In case of Fe-31.2Pd, the specimen expands in the field direction. On the other hand, in the case of Fe_3Pt and Ni_2MnGa, the specimen contracts in the field direction. This means that the X- or Y-variant grows consuming the Z-variant in Fe-31.2Pd, whereas the Z-variant grows consuming X- and Y-variants in Fe_3Pt and Ni_2MnGa. Such a rearrangement of variants can be expected from magnetic anisotropy.

In the following discussion, we consider the effective magnetic field strength at which the rearrangement of variants occurs. The rearrangement of variants occurs by twinning deformation; usually, the rearrangement is made by applying an external stress. Suppose that the rearrangement of variants occurs under a constant shear stress τ_{req}. Then for the complete rearrangement of variants, the external stress does work as given by the product $\tau_{req}s$, where s is the twinning shear. In the cases of tetragonal martensites described above, the twinning plane is {011}, and the twinning shear is given as [13]

$$s = \frac{1 - (c/a)^2}{(c/a)}. \tag{9.4}$$

If the rearrangement of variants occurs through the application of a magnetic field, the same work as $\tau_{req}s$ should be done by the magnetic field. Consequently, ΔU_{mag} given in Eq. (9.3) should equal $\tau_{req}s$. Then, from Eq. (9.3), the effective magnetic field necessary for the rearrangement of the variants is given as

$$H_s = \frac{2K_u}{M_s}\left(1 - \sqrt{1 - \frac{s \cdot \tau_{req}}{K_u}}\right). \tag{9.5}$$

The open squares in Fig. 9.7 show the temperature dependence of H_s evaluated using Eq. (9.5). In the evaluation, the values of M_s and K_u are obtained from Figs. 9.3 and 9.4. The value of s is obtained from the lattice parameter shown in Fig. 9.2 using Eq. (9.4). In addition, the value of τ_{req} is obtained by plotting the

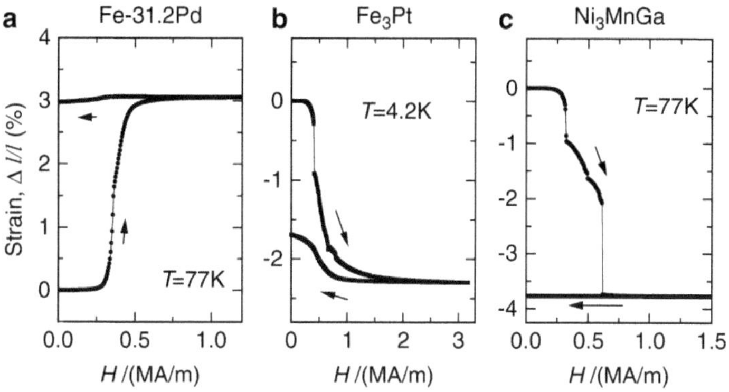

Fig. 9.6 Magnetic field-induced strain in Fe-31.2Pd [11], Fe_3Pt [12], and Ni_2MnGa [7] caused by rearrangement of martensite variants

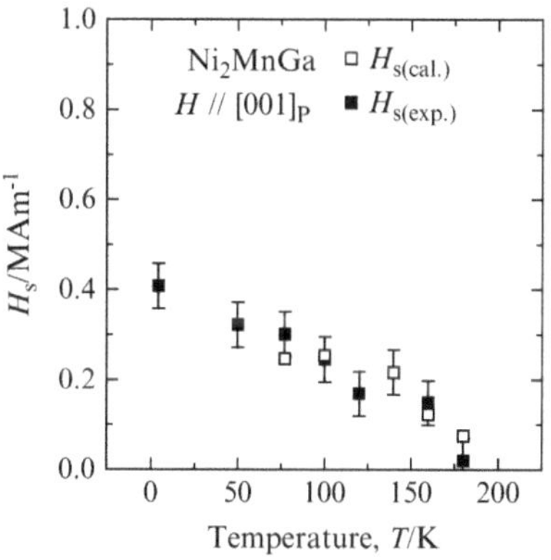

Fig. 9.7 Onset magnetic field for rearrangement of martensite variants in Ni_2MnGa [14]

stress–strain curve. In Fig. 9.6, the experimentally obtained value of H_s is also shown by solid squares. Notice that the calculated value of H_s is in good agreement with the experimentally obtained value.

Equation (9.5) implies that the rearrangement of variants is impossible when $\tau_{req} > K_u/s$. The value K_u/s can be regarded as the maximum shear stress exerted on the twinning plane by the application of the magnetic field, and it is written as $\tau_{mag}{}^{m}$. The value of $\tau_{mag}{}^{m}$ and τ_{req} are plotted as a function of temperature for the three alloys in Fig. 9.8. As known form Fig. 9.7, $\tau_{req} < \tau_{mag}{}^{m}$ is satisfied for all the examined temperature range in the three alloys. Consequently, the rearrangement of variants due to an applied magnetic field is possible at any temperature for the three alloys.

More information of rearrangement of martensite variants by a magnetic field can be found elsewhere [15–18].

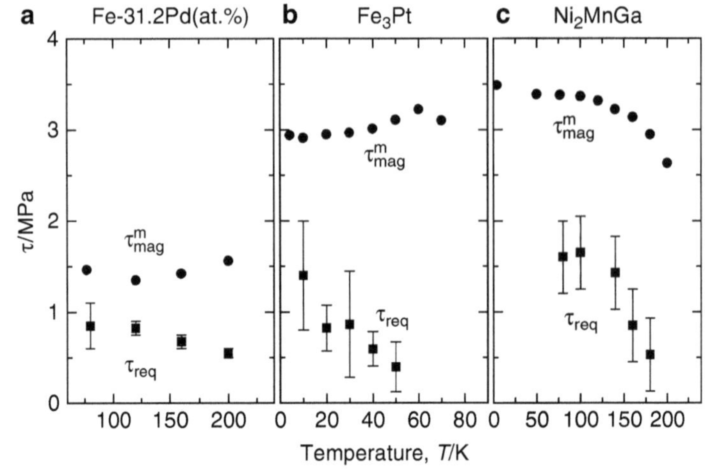

Fig. 9.8 Temperature dependence of maximum magnetic shear stress and stress required for twinning plane movement in Fe-31.2Pd [10], Fe_3Pt and Ni_2MnGa [9]

9.5 Selective Formation of Preferable Variants in CoPt and FePd

The disorder–order transformation in FePd and CoPt is a representative diffusional transformation in which the microstructure formation is influenced by an applied magnetic field because of the large magnetocrystalline anisotropy. The crystal structure changes from an A1-type (cubic) disordered structure to an $L1_0$-type (tetragonal) ordered structure, and the ordered phase has three lattice corresponding variants (X-, Y-, Z-variants as shown in Fig. 9.1). The ordered phase is characterized by high uniaxial magnetocrystalline anisotropy with an "easy" *c*-axis. The disorder–order transformation in FePd and CoPt proceeds via nucleation and growth, and the application of a magnetic field is expected to be especially effective during the nucleation stage of the disorder–order transformation.

In the following, we will see the preferential formation of the Z-variant shown in Fig. 9.1 in an Fe-55Pd (at.%) alloy. As mentioned above, the application of a magnetic field is expected to be especially effective during the nucleation stage. Consequently, we apply a magnetic field only during the early stage of ordering. Figure 9.9 illustrates typical heat-treatment for controlling the microstructure by using a magnetic field [19]. The heat-treatment is composed of two steps. The first step corresponds to the nucleation sage and the second strep to the growth stage. During the first stage, magnetic field is applied in the Z-direction, and ordering heat-treatment is made near the Curie temperature of the ordered phase $T_C^{(o)}$. During the second stage, a magnetic field is not applied, and ordering heat-treatment is carried out at an elevated temperature. Incidentally, the Curie temperature of the disordered

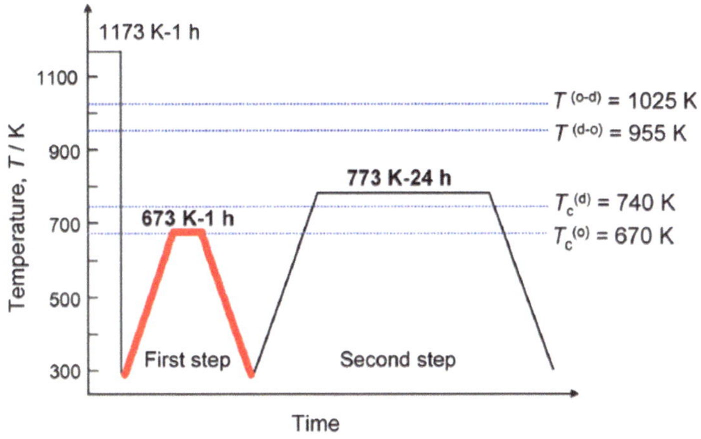

Fig. 9.9 Schematic illustration of two-step heat-treatment to obtain single variant of ordered phase in Fe-55Pd [19]

phase $T_C{}^{(d)}$ is 740 K, and that of the ordered phase $T_C{}^{(o)}$ is 670 K, the disorder–order transformation temperature $T_{(d\text{–}o)}$ is 955 K for Fe-55Pd [19, 20].

Figure 9.10 show the magnetization curves of the Fe-55Pd alloy measured at 300 K in the *X*-, *Y*-, and *Z*-directions after the first step of ordering (a)–(d) and those after the second step (a′)–(d′). It should be noted in Fig. 9.10a, b that when H_1 is 4 T or higher, the magnetization curve of the *Z*-direction is obviously easy to magnetize compared to the *X*- and *Y*-directions after the first step. Once such a difference is achieved, the magnetization curve measured in the *Z*-direction after the second step is that of the easy axis, and the magnetization curve measured in the *X*- and *Y*-directions are that of the hard axis as seen in Fig. 9.10a′–c′. This means that a single variant state is realized when *H*1 is 4 T and higher. On the other hand, when *H*1 is 0 T, no significant difference is observed in the magnetization curve after the first step as seen in Fig. 9.10d. In this case, the magnetization curves after the second step of ordering are as the mixture of easy and hard axes for all the *X*-, *Y*-, and *Z*-directions as seen in Fig. 9.10d'.

Figure 9.11 shows the volume fraction of the Z-variant, f_Z, after the second step heat-treatment plotted as a function of applied magnetic field strength for the first step. In the figure, the results for the Co-50Pt (at.%) alloy is also shown. For both the Fe-55Pd and Co-50Pt alloys, the value of f_Z is about one-third when H_1 is 0 T, and it increases with increasing H_1. Notice that there is a jump in f_Z near $H_1 = 0.3$ T in the case of the Co-50Pt alloy and near $H_1 = 3$ T in the case of the Fe-55Pd alloy. This result suggests that there is a critical condition for the selected formation of variants. Furthermore, notice in Fig. 9.11 that the lowest value of H_1 for obtaining the single variant state of the Fe-55Pd is higher than that of the Co-50Pt alloy. This is due to the difference in the magnetocrystalline anisotropy constant.

We now describe the reason for the influence of the magnetic field on the nucleation stage of the disorder–order transformation. We denote the nucleation

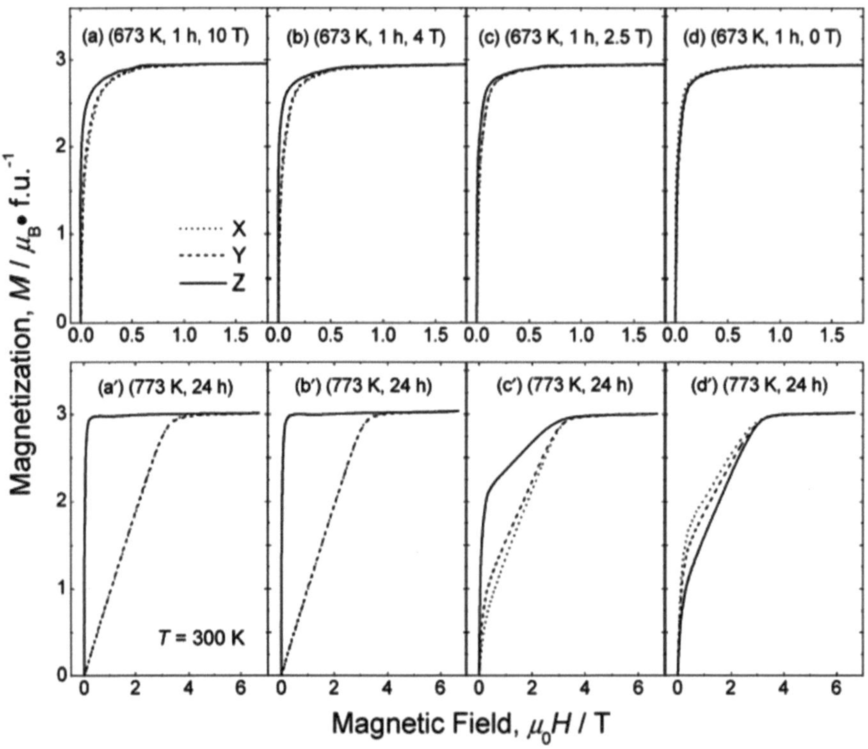

Fig. 9.10 Magnetization curves of Fe-55Pd measured at 300 K along the X-, Y-, Z-directions [19]. Measurements were made after the first step of ordering at 673 K for 1 h under applied magnetic fields of 10 T (**a**), 4 T (**b**), 2.5 T (**c**), 0 T (**d**). Measurements were after the second step of ordering at 773 K for 24 h (**a′**), (**b′**), (**c′**) (**d′**) [19]

probability of the three variants (X-, Y-, Z-variants) of the ordered phase from the disordered phase as P_X, P_Y, and P_Z. If we assume that nucleation proceeds via an ordinary thermal activation process, the nucleation ratio P_Z/P_Y is given as

$$\frac{P_Z}{P_Y} = \exp\left(\frac{-(\Delta_Z - \Delta_Y)}{k_B T}\right). \tag{9.6}$$

Here, Δ_X, Δ_Y, and Δ_Z are potential barriers for the formation of the X-, Y-, and Z-variants, respectively. In the absence of an applied magnetic field, $\Delta_X = \Delta_Y = \Delta_Z$ is satisfied as illustrated in Fig. 9.12a; therefore, $P_X = P_Y = P_Z$. Conversely, when a magnetic field H_1 is applied along the Z-direction, Δ_Z would be lower than Δ_Y ($=\Delta_X$) as illustrated in Fig. 9.12b. We expect this because the magnetic energy of the Z-variant is lower than that of the Y- and X- variants due to magnetocrystalline anisotropy. Then $P_Z > P_Y$ ($=P_X$) under an applied magnetic field. In the case of FePd, for example, electron microscope observations reveal that the size of the nuclei is about 2 nm^3 and P_Z/P_Y is about 2 when ordering occurs under a magnetic

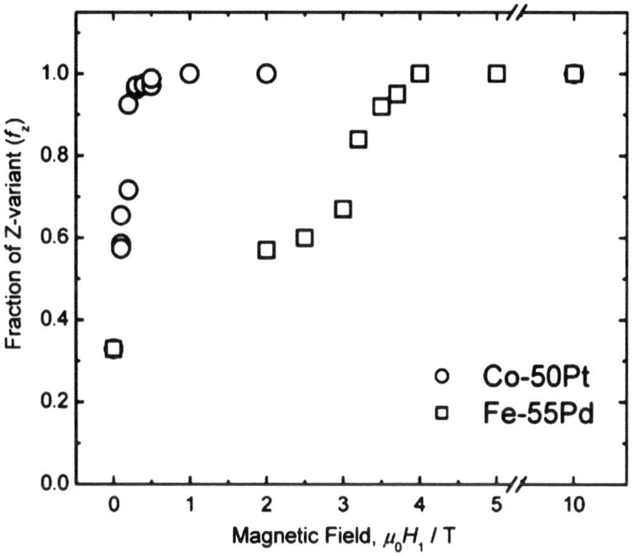

Fig. 9.11 Fraction of Z-variant after second step ordering in Fe-55Pd and Co-50Pt [19]

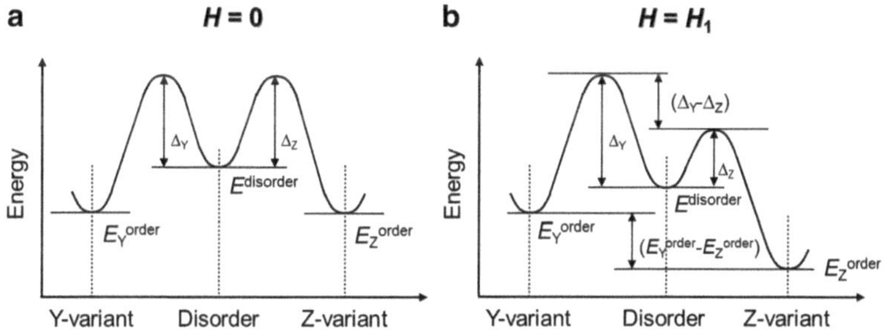

Fig. 9.12 Schematic illustration of potential barriers for nucleation of ordered phase [15]

field of 10 T at 673 K [21]. From this, $(\Delta_Z - \Delta_Y)$ is estimated to be about 800 kJ/m^3 at 637 K. This value is the same order as the estimated magnetocrystalline anisotropy energy of FePd at 673 K under 10 T (~500 kJ/m^3).

When preferential nucleation is achieved under an applied magnetic field, a single variant of the ordered phase can be obtained during the growth process through elastic interaction. More information on the selected growth of preferable variants under an applied magnetic field in $L1_0$-type FePd can be found elsewhere [22–24].

Acknowledgments The authors appreciate the financial support from MEXT, Japan through the Global COE Program "Center of Excellence for Advanced Structural and Functional Materials Design."

References

1. Aizu K (1968) Possible species of "ferroelastic" crystals and of simultaneously ferroelectric and ferroelastic crystals. J Phys Soc Jpn 27:387
2. Morrish AH (2001) The physical principles of magnetism. IEEE Press, New York, Chapter 6
3. Sugiyama M, Oshima R, Fujita FE (1984) Martensitic transformation in the Fe-Pd alloy system. Trans Jpn Inst Met 25:585
4. Muto S, Oshima R, Fujita FE (1988) Nucleation and growth in martensitic transformations of ordered Fe_3Pt alloys. Metall Trans A 19:2931
5. Righi L et al (2006) Incommensurate modulated structure of the ferromagnetic shape-memory Ni_2MnGa martensite. J Solid State Chem 179:3525
6. Fukuda T, Sakamoto T, Kakeshita T, Takeuchi T, Kishio K (2004) Rearrangement of martensite variants in iron-based ferromagnetic shape memory alloys under magnetic field. Mater Trans 45:188
7. Okamoto N, Fukuda T, Kakeshita T, Takeuchi T, Kishio K (2004) Rearrangement of variants in Ni_2MnGa under magnetic field. Sci Technol Adv Mater 5:29
8. Fukuda T, Kakeshita T (2008) Giant magnetic field induced strain in ferromagnetic shape memory alloys and its condition. Mater Sci Technol 24:890
9. Okamoto N, Fukuda T, Kakeshita T, Takeuchi T (2006) Magnetocrystalline anisotropy constant and twinning stress in martensitic phase of Ni_2MnGa. Mater Sci Eng A 438-4440:948
10. Kakeshita T, Fukuda T (2006) Energy evaluation for twinning plane movement under magnetic field in ferromagnetic shape memory alloys. Int J Appl Electromagnet Mech 23:45
11. Koeda J, Nakamura Y, Fukuda T, Kakeshita T, Takeuchi T, Kishio K (2001) Giant magnetostriction in Fe-Pd alloy single crystal exhibiting martensitic transformation. Trans Mater Res Soc Jpn 26(1):215
12. Johmen M, Tabata T, Fukuda T, Kakeshita T, Takeuchi T, Oshima R, Muto S, Kishio K (2001) Trans Mater Res Soc Jpn 26(1):271
13. Christian JW (2002) The theory of transformations in metals and alloys. Pergamon, Oxford
14. Okamoto N (2006) Dr. Thesis, Chapter 7, Osaka University
15. Chernenko VA, Barandiaran JM (eds) (2010) Ferromagnetic shape memory alloys II. Trans Tech Publications, Switzerland
16. O'Handley RC (2000) Modern magnetic shape memory materials: principles and applications. Wiley, New York
17. Chernenko VA (ed) (2008) Advances in shape memory materials: magnetic shape memory alloys. Trans Tech Publications, Switzerland
18. Buschow KHJ (ed) (2011) Handbook of magnetic materials, vol 19. North Holland, Amsterdam, Chapter 4
19. Farjami S, Fukuda T, Kakeshita T (2009) Selective formation of an ordered variant in $Fe_{45}Pd_{55}$ alloy under magnetic field. J Phys Conf Ser 156:012011
20. Farjami S, Fukuda T, Kakeshita T (2009) Ordering process and variant selection under magnetic field in $L1_0$-type Fe-55Pd alloys. ISIJ Int 49:1610
21. Farjami S, Fukuda T, Kakeshita T. Microstructure evolution to reach the single variant in an ordered Fe-55at.%Pd alloy. J Alloys Compd (http://dx.doi.org/10.1016/j.jallcom.2012.02.009)
22. Oshima R, Tokoro H (1998) Effect of magnetic field on early stage of ordering process of FePd alloys. J Jpn Inst Met 62:317–326
23. Tanaka K, Ichitsubo T, Amano M, Koiwa M, Watanabe K (2000) Formation of mono-variant $L1_0$ structure on ordering of FePd under magnetic field. Mater Trans JIM 41:917
24. Tanaka K, Ichitsubo T, Koiwa M (2001) Effect of external field on ordering of FePd. Mater Sci Eng A312:118

Chapter 10
Eco-Friendly Materials Recycling Processing

Toshihiro Tanaka and Masanori Suzuki

Abstract The authors have investigated eco-friendly recycling processes. Large amounts of slag and waste glass are generated every day from such processes as steelmaking. These are very stable multi-component oxide materials. How should we recycle these resources to create value-added materials by eco-friendly processing? We investigated the use of a hydrothermal reaction to make low-temperature-foaming glass. Under hydrothermal conditions of 30–40 MPa and 200–300°C with H_2O, glass powders can be sintered to form solidified glass materials containing about 10 mass% H_2O. When the glass containing H_2O is heated again under normal pressure, the glass expands, releasing H_2O to form a porous microstructure. This glass can be used in filters to remove impurities from polluted air and water, or in insulators to control heat transfer. In this chapter, we describe trials of our eco-friendly recycling process.

Keywords Exergy • Glass • Hydrothermal reaction • Waste

10.1 Introduction

The authors have investigated how to design eco-friendly materials recycling processes. For example, large amounts of slags are discharged by the iron- and steelmaking industries, and are mainly recycled for use as construction materials such as road-bed materials. Suitable recycling processes also need to be developed to promote waste glass recycling. Since slags and glasses consist mainly of SiO_2, CaO, Al_2O_3, MgO, and FeO, which are the general components of ceramic materials, high-temperature sintering processes can be used to produce solidified

T. Tanaka (✉) • M. Suzuki
Division of Materials and Manufacturing Science, Graduate School of Engineering, Osaka University, 2-1 Yamadaoka, Suita, Osaka 565-0871, Japan
e-mail: tanaka@mat.eng.osaka-u.ac.jp

T. Kakeshita (ed.), *Progress in Advanced Structural and Functional Materials Design*, DOI 10.1007/978-4-431-54064-9_10,

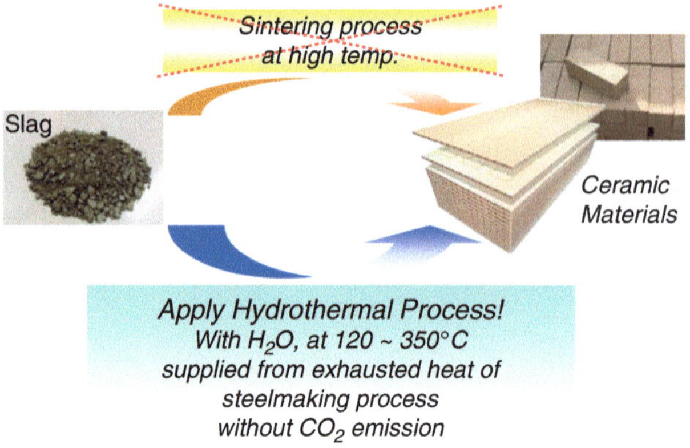

Fig. 10.1 Application of hydrothermal process for recycling of slag

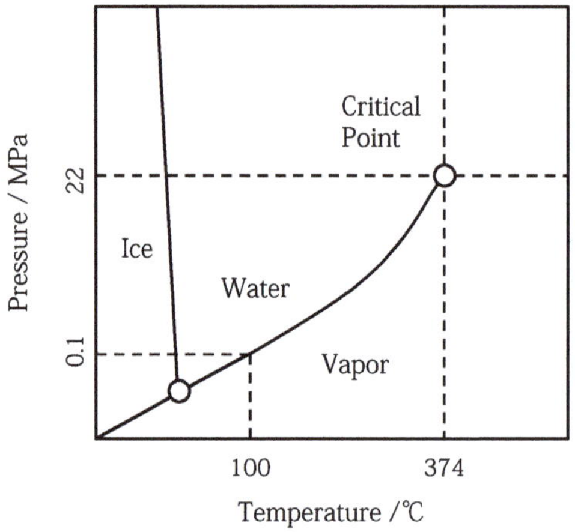

Fig. 10.2 Equilibrium phase diagram of H_2O

materials from slags or glasses. However, we have to keep in mind that heating processes consume energy and sometimes result in CO_2 emissions. We have therefore focused on the use of hydrothermal reactions to solidify slag or glass powders to produce functional ceramic materials such as architectural materials, as shown in Fig. 10.1 [1]. Hydrothermal reactions occur with H_2O under high pressure, that is, with H_2O at 120–350°C, as shown in Fig. 10.2. This temperature could be obtained using exhausted heat from iron- and steelmaking processes, or from waste-melting furnaces. Hydrothermal reactions are ideal eco-friendly processes for dealing with slag-recycling issues, as Jung, Hashida, Ishida, Yamasaki et al. have pointed out [2], and they have already used hydrothermal reactions to solidify slag powders with additives. To obtain functionally useful hydrothermally solidified materials, we have tried to make porous materials from slags or waste glasses using the hydrothermal reactions described below.

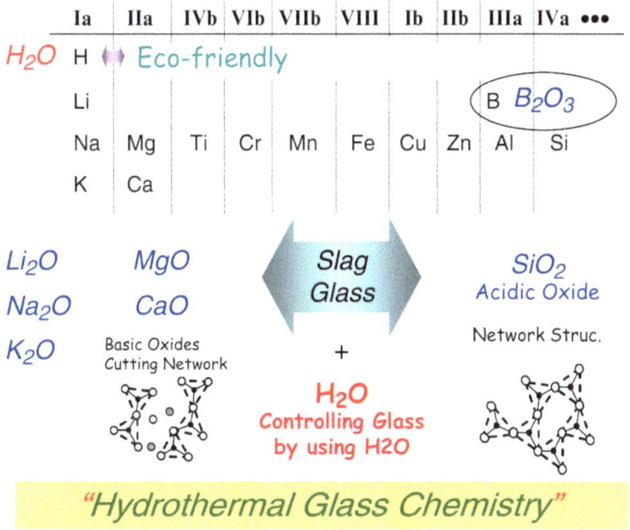

Fig. 10.3 Hydrothermal Slag/Glass Chemistry

Slags and glasses consist mainly of SiO_2-based network structures. The microstructures of molten slags in iron- and steelmaking processes can be controlled by the addition at high temperature of alkali metal or alkaline-earth metal oxides to change the chemical and physical properties, such as basicity and viscosity, of the molten slags, as shown in Fig. 10.3. Under hydrothermal conditions, the microstructures of slags and glasses could be controlled using H_2O; this new approach is called "hydrothermal slag/glass chemistry".

Even when it is possible to solidify the glass or slag powder to make materials, we have to add additional functions to the solidified glass or slag materials because glasses and slags are regarded as having low exergy values. The exergy value indicates how valuable a material is, and is defined by the following equation:

$$Exergy = \Delta H - T_0 \cdot \Delta S \tag{10.1}$$

where ΔH is the enthalpy and ΔS is the entropy of a material and T_0 is room temperature. When a material has a large ΔH and small ΔS, the exergy of the material is large. This means that the material is regarded as valuable and can generate useful work.

Glasses and slags are generally stable multi-component oxide materials. Oxides are more stable than metals, which means that the enthalpies of oxides are lower than those of metals. In addition, glasses and slags are mixtures of many cations and anions, which means that their mixing entropies are very large. Thus, glasses and slags have low exergy values. This suggests that it is very difficult to create value-added materials from low-exergy glasses and slags in recycling processes.

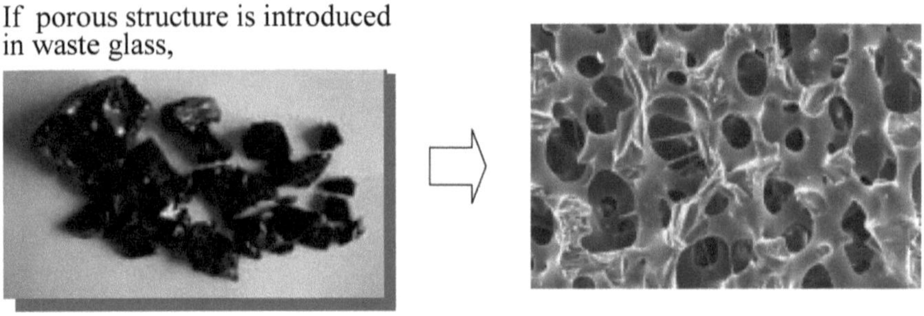

Fig. 10.4 Making porous material from glass or slag with low value of exergy

We assumed in the above discussion that materials are of infinite size and uniform structure. If interfaces can be created in the structure, we can obtain materials with additional valuable functions. A porous structure is one such valuable interfacial structure. For example, porous glass or slag materials (see Fig. 10.4) can be used as insulators for controlling heat transfer, and as filters for removing impurities from polluted air or water. They can also be used as water-retaining materials for walls and sidewalks. These materials adsorb and retain water on rainy days; the water adsorbed in the porous structure is then vaporized on sunny days, thereby decreasing the temperatures of the walls and sidewalks. Such materials are expected to contribute largely to creating an eco-friendly society.

If porous materials can be made from waste glasses or slags by hydrothermal reactions, this gives an eco-friendly process for creating value-added materials. We have been attempting to make various kinds of porous materials based on slags and glasses. In this chapter, we describe an example of the fabrication of a low-temperature-foaming glass using hydrothermal glass chemistry.

10.2 Fabrication of Low Temperature Foaming Glass

Matamoros-Veloza et al. [3] introduced H_2O into waste glass composed mainly of SiO_2, Na_2O, and CaO by hydrothermal synthesis; they obtained a hydrated glass compact. When the prepared glass was heated, it started to expand and foam at around 650°C, with the release of H_2O, and became porous. Glass expansion is an appropriate approach to making porous materials, but foaming at lower temperatures would be beneficial. Since glass containing H_2O can be made at around 200°C by hydrothermal reactions, foaming or expansion at around this temperature is desirable.

In hydrothermal reactions of soda–silicate-based glass, the constituents of the glass had a significant influence on the H_2O content of the glass under a given set of hydrothermal conditions. Moreover, it was found [4–6] that an increase in the H_2O content lowers the glass-transition temperature, as shown in Fig. 10.5. For the fabrication of low-temperature-foaming glass, a 63 mass% SiO_2/27 mass% Na_2O/10 mass% B_2O_3 glass, which has a suitably low glass-transition temperature

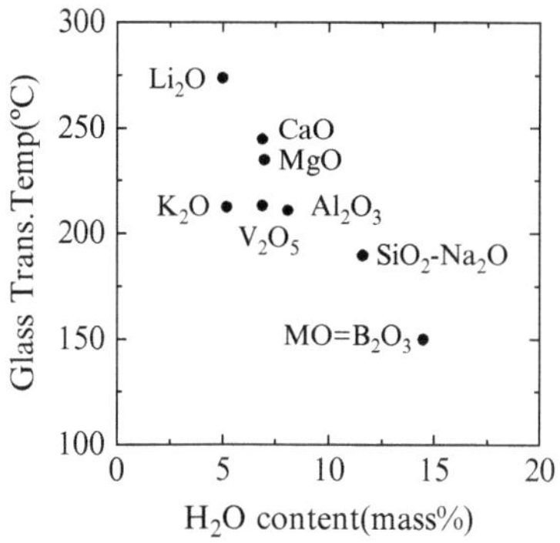

Fig. 10.5 Relationship between glass transition temperature and H_2O content in 63mass%SiO_2-27mass% Na_2O-10mass%MO glass (quoted from ISIJ International)

of around 150°C after hydrothermal treatment, as reported in our previous studies [4–6], was selected as the source material. The glass was subjected to hydrothermal treatment at 250°C and its H_2O-releasing and foaming behaviors after heat-treatment at 150–400°C were investigated [7].

10.2.1 Experimental

The initial glass sample was prepared from reagent grade quartz, Na_2CO_3, and H_3BO_3 powders. The powders were mixed in the ratios 63 mass% SiO_2/27 mass% Na_2O/10 mass% B_2O_3 and melted in a Pt–20 %-Rh crucible at 1,200°C for 3 h in air, and then rapidly cooled on a Cu cooling-block. The glass was subjected to hydrothermal hot-pressing (HHP). The HHP experimental apparatus is shown in Fig. 10.6. The glass powders were well mixed with a small amount of purified H_2O and charged in an autoclave. After the mixture had been pressed at 40 MPa, the autoclave was heated to 250°C within 20 min and then immediately cooled to room temperature within the same length of time.

The HHP-treated $SiO_2/Na_2O/B_2O_3$ glass prepared was cut into cubic blocks of about 6 mm. Each block was placed on a Pt pan and heated in air for 5 min in a horizontal electrical resistance furnace controlled to 150–400°C.

10.2.2 Results and Discussion

To investigate the macroscopic changes in the HHP-treated $SiO_2/Na_2O/B_2O_3$ glass, a block of the glass was heat-treated at 150–350°C in air. The samples after heat-treatment are shown in Fig. 10.7. Macroscopic expansion, namely foaming, of the hydrated glass was observed for the samples heated to above 180°C. The higher the heating temperature was, the larger the glass expansion. Low-temperature foaming was successfully obtained [7] at temperatures lower than that previously reported by Matamoros-Veloza et al. of around 650°C for soda-lime silicate glass [3]. X-ray diffraction analysis confirmed that the foamed glasses possessed a glass structure at all temperatures.

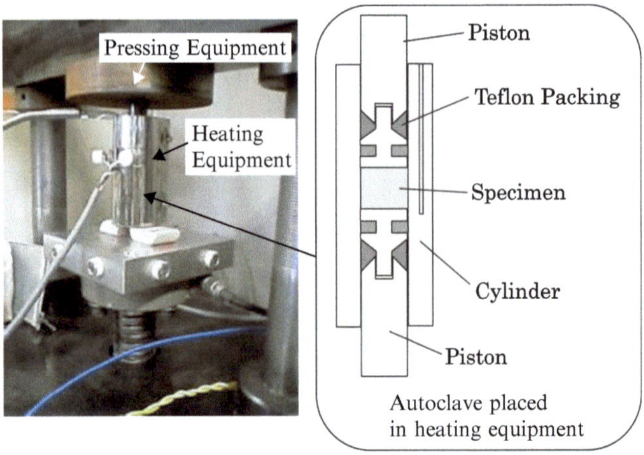

Fig. 10.6 Hydrothermal Hot Pressing (HHP) machine

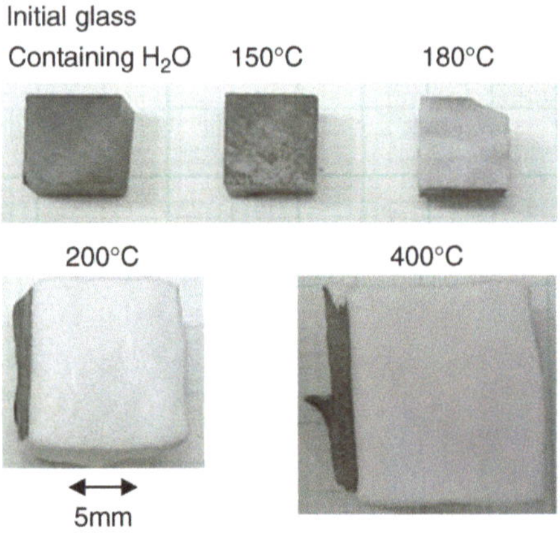

Fig. 10.7 Change in macroscopic shapes of the HHP treated 63mass% SiO_2-27mass% Na_2O-10mass% B_2O_3 glass after firing at 150–400°C (quoted from ISIJ International)

The apparent densities of the foamed glasses were determined from the sample shapes under the assumption of isotropic expansion, and are summarized in Fig. 10.8 [7], with the weight losses during the heat-treatment. The apparent density decreased drastically at 200°C as a result of foaming, and continued to gradually decrease as the heating temperature increased. The lowest apparent density of 0.25 g/cm^3 was obtained when the heat-treatment was conducted at 400°C. The weight losses were larger at higher heating temperatures, and the value of 11 % at 400°C was almost in accordance with the H_2O content of the HHP-treated glass. As shown in Fig. 10.9 [7], when a piece of glass containing H_2O, set in a tube, is heated, the glass expands to fit the inner shape of the tube. This means that the obtained glasses can be used as filters for removing impurities from water or air flowing in a pipe.

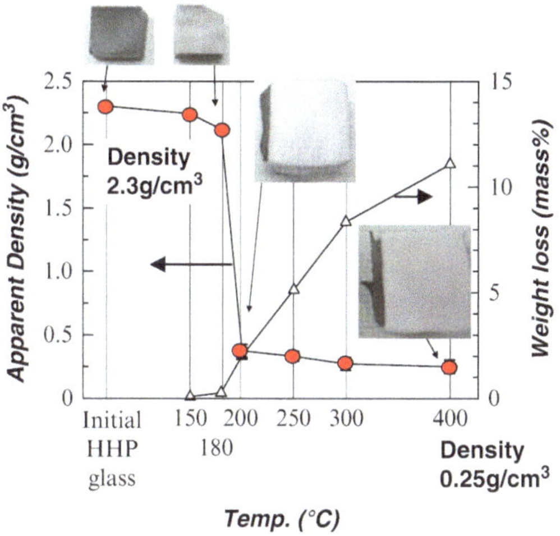

Fig. 10.8 Apparent densities and weight loss after firing of the HHP treated 63mass% SiO_2- 27mass %Na_2O-10mass% B_2O_3 glass

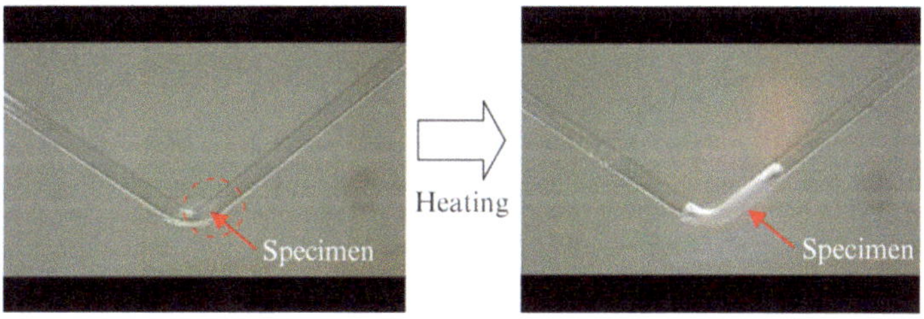

Fig. 10.9 Expansion of a glass containing H_2O in a tube (quoted from ISIJ International)

10.3 Concluding Remarks

The fabrication of low-temperature-foaming glasses using hydrothermal reactions was described as an example of an eco-friendly recycling process. HHP-treated $SiO_2/Na_2O/B_2O_3$ glass was heated at 150–400°C in air to determine the macroscopic changes produced by heating. Foaming behavior was observed even at 200°C; this foaming temperature was much lower than that previously reported for a hydrated glass. The above procedure was carried out at around 200°C, and this temperature could be achieved using exhausted heat in factories, within a short time, e.g., 1 h, using waste glass as the source material and H_2O, which is recognized to be one of the safest materials. The final products can be used in several ways to contribute to an eco-friendly society. The procedure can therefore be considered to be an eco-friendly recycling process.

In addition to the above procedures, we have investigated the following approaches:

- Production of porous ceramics from slags using hydrothermal slag chemistry [8];
- Production of porous glasses by spinodal decomposition [9–12]; and
- Production of surface porous metals by oxidation and reduction [13–15].

Acknowledgements This study was partially supported by Priority Assistance for the Formation of Worldwide Renowned Centers of Research—The Global COE Program (Project: Center of Excellence for Advanced Structural and Functional Materials Design) from the Ministry of Education, Culture, Sports, Science and Technology (MEXT), Japan.

References

1. Tanaka T, Maeda S, Takahira N, Hirai N, Lee J-H (2006) Advanced eco-materials processing from by-products. Mater Sci Forum 512:305–308
2. Jing Z, Ishida EH, Jin F, Hashida T, Yamasaki N (2006) Influence of quartz particle size on hydrothermal solidification of blast furnace slag. Ind Eng Chem Res 45:7470
3. Matamoros-Veloza Z, Yanagisawa K, Rendon-Angeles JC, Yamasaki N (2002) Preparation of porous materials from hydrothermal hot pressed glass compacts. J Mater Sci Lett 21:1855
4. Nakamoto M, Lee J-H, Tanaka T, Ikeda J, Inagaki S (2005) Use of slag containing water as lubricant in high straining rolling for ultrafine-grained steels. ISIJ Int 45:1567–1571
5. Nakamoto M, Lee J-H, Tanaka T (2006) Design of lubricants using waste slag in large strain addition strip processing for ultra-grained steels. Mater Sci Forum 512:319–324
6. Sato S, Yoshikawa T, Nakamoto M, Tanaka T, Ikeda J (2008) Application of hydrothermal treatment on BF slag and waste glass for preparing lubricant materials in high strain rolling for ultrafine-grained steel production. ISIJ Int 48:245–250
7. Yoshikawa T, Sato S, Tanaka T (2008) Fabrication of low temperature forming glass materials using hydrothermal treatment. ISIJ Int 48:130–133
8. Yoshikawa T, Hirano S, Hirai N, Tanaka T (2008) Preparation of porous ceramics by the hydrothermal reaction of blast furnace slag for use in a water-retentive materials. ISIJ Int 48:1322–1324
9. Suzuki M, Tanaka T (2006) Prediction of phase separation in silicate glass for the creation of value-added materials from waste slag. ISIJ Int 46:1391–1395
10. Suzuki M, Tanaka T (2008) Composition dependence of microstructures formed by phase separation in multi-component silicate glass. ISIJ Int 48:405–411
11. Suzuki M, Tanaka T (2008) Materials design for the fabrication of porous glass using phase separation in multi-component borosilicate glass. ISIJ Int 48:1524–1532
12. Suzuki M, Tanaka T (2010) Distribution and coordination sate of titanium oxides in microstructures formed by spinodal decomposition in multicomponent borosilicate glass. ISIJ Int 50:509–514
13. Takahira N, Tanaka T, Hara S, Lee J-H (2005) Unusual wetting of liquid metals on iron substrate with oxidized surface in reduced atmosphere. Mater Trans 46:3008–3014
14. Takahira N, Yoshikawa T, Tanaka T, Holappa L (2007) Wettability of liquid In and Bi on flat and porous solid iron substrate. Mater Trans 48:2708–2711
15. Takahira N, Yoshikawa T, Tanaka T, Holappa L (2007) Unusual wetting of liquid bismuth on a surface-porous copper substrate fabricated by oxidation-reduction process. Mater Trans 48:3126–3131

Chapter 11
Advanced Materials Design by Electrochemical Approach: Self-Organizing Anodization

Hiroaki Tsuchiya

Abstract The fabrication of nano-scale structures and patterns has attracted much attention due to their technological impacts in applications. The present chapter highlights the electrochemical fabrication of nanoporous and nanotubular structures on metal and alloy surfaces based on self-organization. Electrochemical anodization of valve metals and their alloys forms nanoporous or nanotubular oxide layers when anodization is carried out in fluoride-containing electrolytes under optimized conditions. Morphology of porous/tubular oxide layer, that is, diameter and thickness, can be tuned by tailoring electrochemical conditions. Structures obtained strongly depend also on substrate composition—nanoporous oxide layers are formed on Al, Nb, Ta and W whereas nanotubular oxide layers are obtained on Ti, Zr and Hf. Some interesting phenomena—morphological transition from pores to tubes and two-size scale self-organization—are observed when alloys consisting of valve metals are anodized.

Keywords Nanopore • Nanotube • Valve metal oxide • Anodization • Self-organization

11.1 Introduction

Over the decade the formation of self-organized nanostructures and patterns has attracted scientific and technological interests due to their wide range of applications. The significance of these nanostructures originates from the nature of self-organizing processes. These processes essentially represent parallel techniques for surface processing on the nano-scale. In the processes no active

H. Tsuchiya (✉)
Division of Materials and Manufacturing Science, Graduate School of Engineering, Osaka University, 2-1 Yamadaoka, Suita, Osaka 565-0871, Japan
e-mail: tsuchiya@mat.eng.osaka-u.ac.jp

T. Kakeshita (ed.), *Progress in Advanced Structural and Functional Materials Design*,
DOI 10.1007/978-4-431-54064-9_11,

manipulation is essentially required. These are the advantages of self-organizing nano-fabrication process compared to slow and complicated sequential writing techniques. Therefore, a large part of materials science targets self-organizing nano-scale fabrication techniques.

In the field of materials science, one of highly promising approaches to form nanostructures is a very simple electrochemical anodic oxidation, so-called anodization. Well-established examples in this field are highly ordered porous aluminum oxide (porous alumina) [1–3]. Since the remarkable work of Masuda et al. [2], in particular, the fabrication of porous alumina has stimulated considerable research efforts due to many applications of ordered porous alumina structures, for example, photonic crystal or template for the deposition of other materials [4, 5].

It has recently been reported that self-organized porous/tubular oxide layers are obtained for other valve metals such as Ti [6–10], Zr [11], Hf [12], Nb [13], Ta [14] and W [15]. These porous oxide layers have a wide range of functional properties. Ordered porous/tubular structures of valve metal oxides can be formed by anodization of the metals in electrolytes containing fluorides. The present chapter describes pore formation on valve metals by anodization, the key electrochemical factors affecting porous/tubular morphology and the effects of metallurgical aspects that lead to morphological transition.

11.2 Anodization to Form Porous Oxide Layers

In this section the basic of anodization of valve metal is briefly described. In contrast to other metals, on valve metals, compact oxide layers with considerable thickness (some hundred nm) can be grown in most of "fluoride-free" aqueous electrolytes. The formation and growth of oxide layers by anodization of valve metals can be simply described by following reaction (11.1).

$$M + 2H_2O \rightarrow MO_2 + 4H^+ + 4e^- \qquad (11.1)$$

In the system valve metal oxidation (anodic reaction) and reduction of H_2O (corresponding cathodic reaction) take place at the metal / oxide interface and the counter electrode, respectively. When a constant voltage is applied on anode in a fluoride-free electrolyte, therefore, an oxide layer starts to grow which leads to a decrease of the obtained current in current-time curve as shown in Fig. 11.1a because the field strength across the oxide layer continuously decreases. The field maintains inward transport of O^{2-} and outward transport of M ions and thus in principle an infinite growth of the oxide layer would occur. However, the limiting situation is established when the growth rate of the oxide layer drops to the chemical dissolution rate of the oxide layer (very small in most of electrolytes) in the electrolyte. This means that the thickness of the oxide layer is not significantly varied with an extended anodization at a constant voltage. Therefore, the thickness of the oxide layer at the steady state is proportional to the field, that is, to applied voltage.

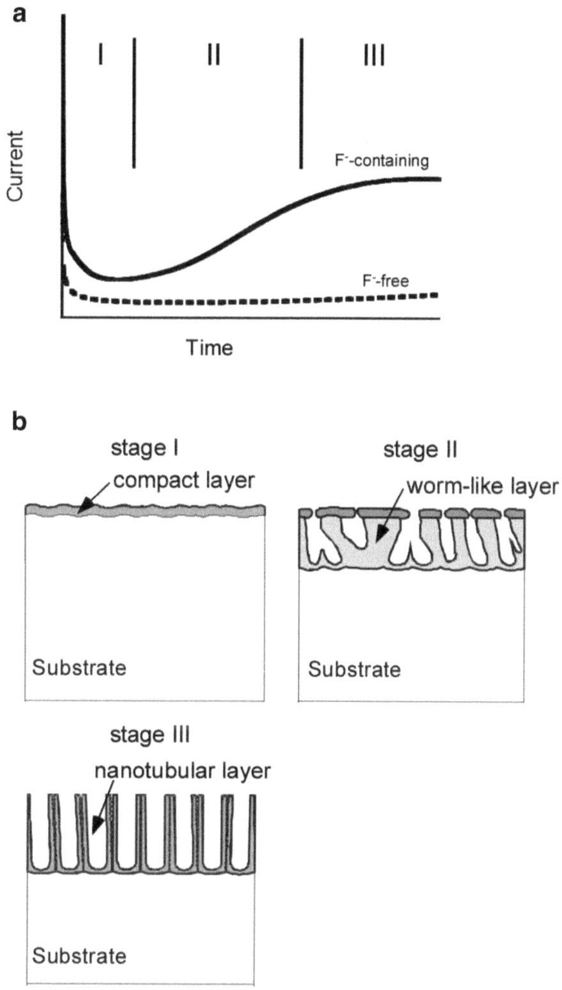

Fig. 11.1 Schematic illustrations of (**a**) typical current-time curves during anodization and (**b**) tubular oxide layer formation process [16]

In fluoride-containing electrolytes, however, deviations from the typical anodization behavior of valve metals can be observed as shown in Fig. 11.1a. This is attributed to the situation induced by fluorides where the electrochemically-formed oxide layer by reaction (11.1) is chemically dissolved by the formation of soluble fluoride complexes according to reaction (11.2).

$$MO_2 + 6HF \rightarrow [MF_6]^{2-} + 2H_2O + 2H^+ \quad (11.2)$$

It is clear that the current-time curve can be divided into three phases when anodized in fluoride-containing electrolytes. After an initial current decay (phase (I)) the current increases (phase (II)) and then reaches the steady state (phase (III)). These current behavior in the phases correspond to different stages of pore formation.

Figure 11.1b schematically illustrates the pore formation process [16, 17]. In the first stage a compact oxide layer is formed and the growth of the oxide layer leads to the current decay in phase (I). In the second stage, pores start to randomly grow underneath the compact oxide layer due to the localized dissolution of the oxide layer by fluoride in the electrolyte. This results in the increased active area and thus the current increases in phase (II). After some period, pores are initiated on the entire surface and a worm-like structure of the oxide layer is formed. Then the individual pores start interfering each other and competing for available current. Under optimized conditions a situation where the pores equally share the available current is established and the current reaches the steady state in phase (III). As a result, self-organized porous structure is obtained.

11.3 Morphology of Anodic Oxide Layers on Valve Metals

This section introduces the morphology of anodic oxide layers on valve metals and describes how electrochemical conditions for anodization affect resulting morphology of anodic oxide layers. Figure 11.2 shows SEM images of anodic oxide layers formed on Ti by anodization in different fluoride-containing electrolytes. It is clear that anodic oxide layers formed on Ti exhibit tubular structure. As shown in Fig. 11.2a, b the tubular oxide layer with the average diameter of 100 nm and the thickness of approximately 500 nm was formed in an acidic electrolyte containing fluorides [7, 16]. It was found from a set of experiments that in acidic electrolytes, tubes grows with time, but with further anodization the thickness of tubular layer levels off to reach a limiting thickness of several hundred nm. During anodization a continuous growth of oxide occurs at the bottom of tubes whereas chemical dissolution of the oxide simultaneously occurs at the surface. Therefore, the limiting thickness of tubular layer means that the tubular layer continuously consumes the substrate without thickening of the layer. The thickness of TiO_2 nanotubular layer can be increased by altering the electrochemical conditions. Effect of anodization voltage was examined using H_3PO_4 containing a small amount of HF. In the electrolyte, tubular layers were formed up to 25 V and the thickness of the tubular layer at 25 V was 1 μm. In this case the tube diameter was also increased to 120 nm. This means that altering the anodization voltage changes diameter and length of tubes at the same time [18]. On the other hand, electrolyte also affects tube morphology. Figure 11.2c, d show SEM images of TiO_2 nanotubular layer formed in a neutral $(NH_4)_2SO_4$ electrolyte containing NH_4F. It is apparent that the diameter of tubes formed in the neutral electrolyte is similar to that in the acidic electrolyte when anodized at a same voltage whereas the thickness of the tubular layer in the neutral electrolyte is approximately 2.5 μm, that is, about five times thicker compared to that in the acidic electrolyte [8, 16]. This clearly indicates that pH of the electrolyte strongly affects the thickness of tubular layer formed. As already described, during anodization in fluoride-containing electrolytes, the field-aided TiO_2 formation at the interface between the Ti substrate and growing TiO_2 layer and the dissolution of formed TiO_2 layer at the interface between TiO_2 and

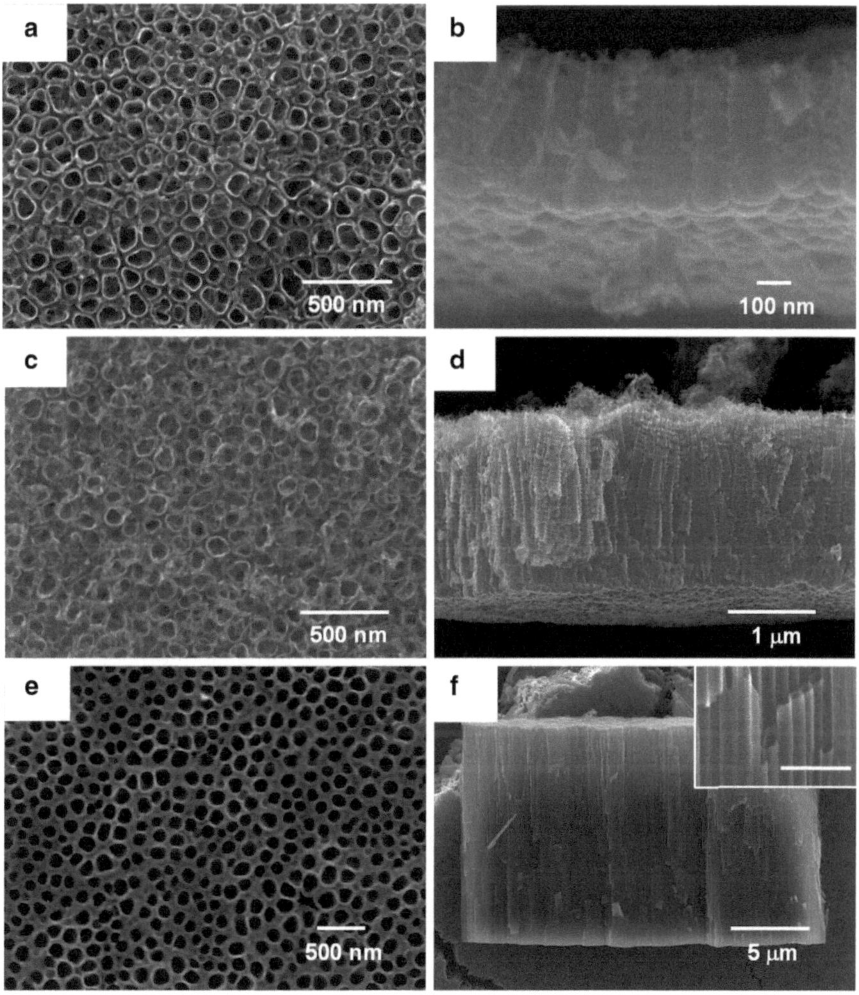

Fig. 11.2 SEM images of nanotubular TiO_2 layers formed by anodization in (**a**, **b**) H_2SO_4/HF, (**c**, **d**) $(NH_4)_2SO_4$/NH_4F and (**e**, **f**) ethylene glycol containing NH_4F and H_2O; (**a**, **c**, **e**) top-view, (**b**, **d**, **f**) cross-section [16]. The *inset* is magnified cross-section of (f). The scale bar corresponds to 500 nm

electrolyte simultaneously occur. The field-aided TiO_2 formation at the tube bottom is accompanied by a generation of acidity according to reaction (11.1). When anodized, this reaction leads to a permanent acidification at the tube bottom. This indicates that there might be a pH gradient established inside and outside the tubes. The dissolution of TiO_2 in fluoride-containing electrolyte is strongly affected by pH of the electrolyte. For higher pH, the dissolution is drastically slower compared to lower pH. The lower pH at the tube bottom maintains the field-aided TiO_2 formation at the tube bottom, that is, tube growth. When the anodization is carried out in a neutral electrolyte, tube growth takes place at the tube bottom while the rest of tubes remains stable due to lower dissolution rate. This results in thicker tubular layer formation in the neutral electrolyte compared to in the acidic electrolyte. The formation of tubes with higher aspect ratio can be achieved when anodized in organic solvents such as ethylene glycol and glycerol [9, 16]. An example is shown in Fig. 11.2e, f. These tubes were grown in ethylene glycol electrolyte containing a small amount of NH_4F and H_2O. It is clear that the tubes have a comparable diameter to tubes formed in aqueous electrolytes (see, Fig. 11.2a, c). However, the tubes formed in the organic solvent grow to a significantly longer length. Another feature observed on the tubes formed in organic solvent is a smooth appearance over their entire length. These findings clearly demonstrate a strong influence of electrolyte viscosity on tube morphology. It could be useful to describe crystallinity of TiO_2 nanotubular layer because applications of TiO_2 require suitable crystal structure. As-formed TiO_2 nanotubular layers are in the amorphous state. However, the tubes can be converted to anatase or a mixture of anatase and rutile by annealing [19]. Recently, we found that amorphous anodic TiO_2 nanotubulars show a tube diameter dependent phase stabilization upon annealing. For tubes with diameter <30 nm the conversion to rutile phase was observed while for tubes with larger diameter anatase was formed [20]. This size effect was induced by the presence of the metallic substrate.

On the other valve metals, self-organized nanostructures can be formed by anodization in fluoride-containing electrolytes, but different morphologies are obtained depending on the metals. Figure 11.3 summarizes the morphology of self-organized nanostructures obtained for other valve metals than Ti [11–16]. On Zr and Hf, long (tens of micrometers) and smooth tubes can be easily formed without optimizing electrochemical condition. In contrast to TiO_2 nanotubular layer, furthermore, nanotubular oxide layers formed on Zr and Hf have crystalline structure directly after anodization. The diameter and length of tubes formed on Zr and Hf also increases with applied voltage, similar to Ti. On Nb, Ta and W, on the other hand, porous oxide layers are formed by anodization. Also in these cases, morphology of oxide layers is strongly affected by electrochemical conditions such as HF concentration and anodization period. Recently it was demonstrated that highly ordered porous oxide layers can be formed also on Al even in "neutral" electrolytes if the electrolytes contain fluorides.

Valve metal oxides possess a variety of functionalities. Therefore, some applications of tubes also have been examined. One can see them in literature [21, 22].

11.4 Metallurgical Aspects on Morphology of Anodic Oxide Layers

In the previous section, one can see that nanotubular or nanoporous oxide layers are formed by anodization in fluoride-containing electrolytes and the morphology is strongly affected by electrochemical condition as well as substrate. The present

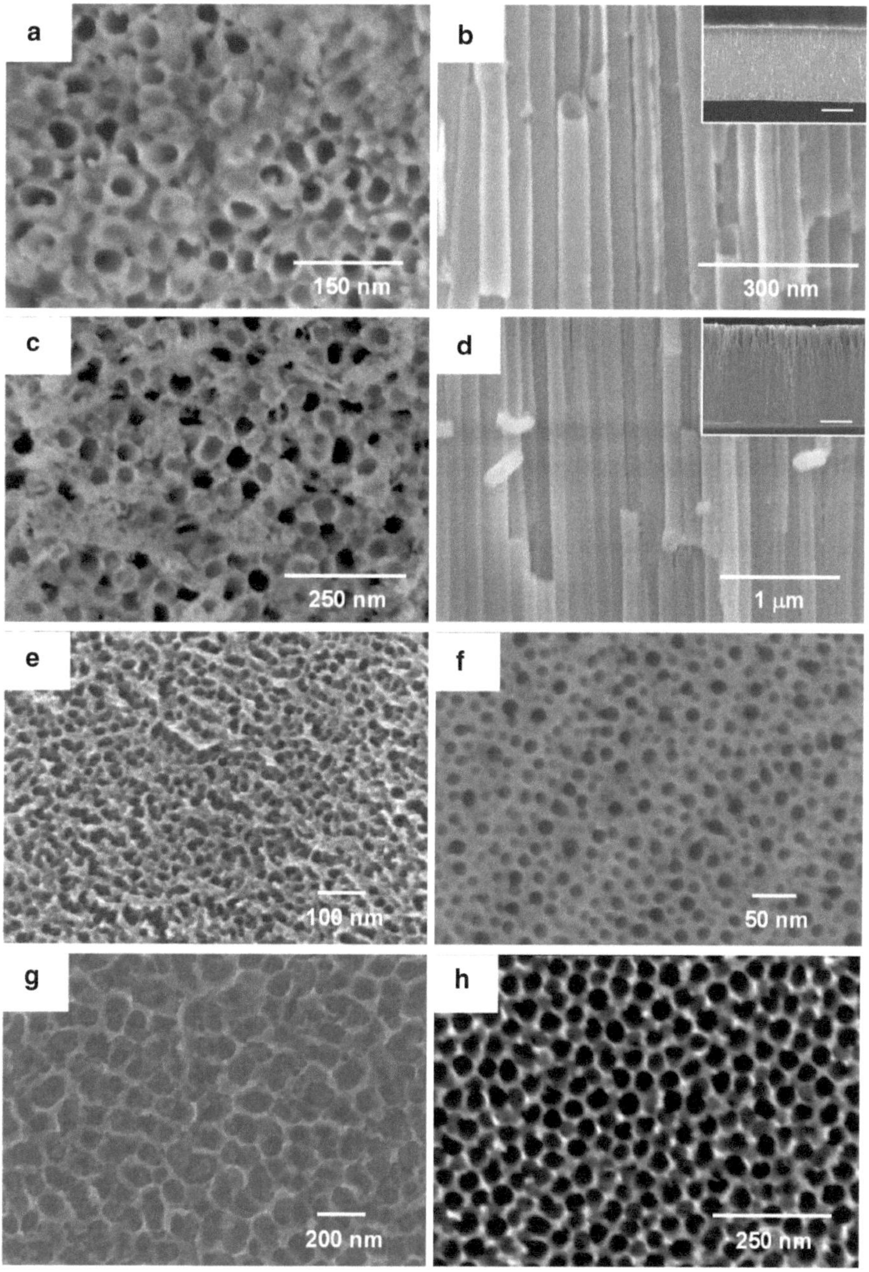

Fig. 11.3 SEM images of oxide layers formed on (**a**, **b**) Zr, (**c**, **d**) Hf, (**e**) Nb, (**f**) Ta, (**g**) W and (**h**) Al by anodization in fluoride-containing electrolytes; (**a**, **c**, **e**–**h**) *top-view*, (**b**, **d**) cross-section [16]. The *insets* are magnified cross-sections of (b) and (d). The scale bars for the *inset* (b) and (d) are 5 μm and 10 μm, respectively

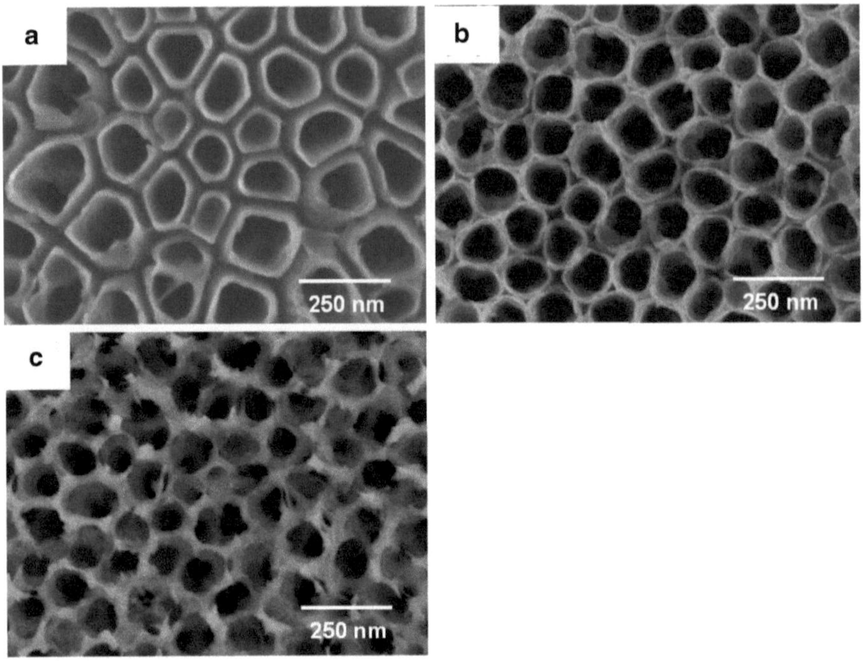

Fig. 11.4 *Top-view* SEM images of oxide layers formed by anodization in a fluoride-containing electrolyte; (**a**) Ti_3Al, (**b**) TiAl and (**c**) $TiAl_3$ [16]

section shows interesting features observed on some alloy systems. However, anodization of two phase alloys such as Ti6Al4V and Ti6Al7Nb suffers from two problems: (1) the selective dissolution of less stable phase and (2) the different reaction rates on different phases [23]. These lead to inhomogeneous surface structure. Therefore, alloys with a single phase microstructure have been extensively studied, for examples, Ti–Zr, Ti–Al and Ti29Nb13Ta4.6Zr [24–26]. Note that these alloys consist of elements on which nanotubular or nanoporous structures have been successfully grown in fluoride-containing electrolytes as shown in the previous section. On the investigated alloys, the formation of self-organized nanostructured oxide layers can be observed over a wide range of anodization voltage (in particular, wider than for pure Ti).

Figure 11.4 shows SEM images of oxide layers formed on various Ti–Al alloys by anodization in a fluoride-containing electrolyte [16, 24]. The anodization was carried out under the same condition (electrolyte, voltage and duration) for all alloys. However, the morphology of formed oxide layers strongly depends on alloy composition. It is clear from the figure that tubular oxide layers are formed on Ti_3Al and TiAl whereas on $TiAl_3$ a porous oxide layer is observed. This means that a morphological transition in the self-organized nanostructures from tubes to pores takes place depending on alloy composition. The threshold composition for the morphological transition is anodization voltage dependent, for examples, at 10 V

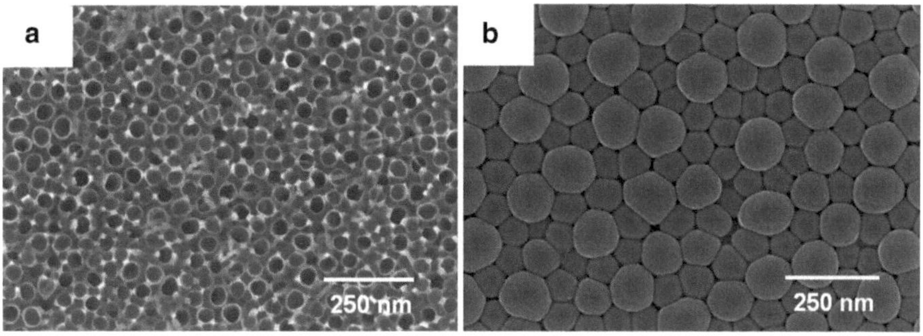

Fig. 11.5 SEM images of an oxide layer formed on Ti29Nb13Ta4.6Zr; (**a**) *top-view*, (**b**) *bottom-view* [16]

the transition occurs between pure Ti and Ti_3Al and furthermore at 20 V the transition occurs between Ti_3Al and TiAl. It is concluded that the occurrence of the tube separation effect is attributed to increased stress within the growing oxides due to increased volume expansion when altering the composition from Al to Ti and supported by sensitization of the cell boundaries by fluoride species. Note that the morphological transition from tubes to pores can be observed on the other alloys such as Ti–Ta and Ti–Nb. However, on Ti–Zr alloy system, only tubular oxide layers are formed independent of alloy composition. Therefore, one can deduce that there is a requirement for morphological transition, that is, alloys are required to consist of tube-forming element such as Ti and pore-forming element such as Al, Nb and Ta. The formation of self-organized nanostructured (nanotubular or nanoporous) oxide layers can be observed on various valve metals and their alloys. However, the self-organized structured oxide layers typically consist of either one discrete size of pores (or tubes) or a continuous size distribution of pores.

Figure 11.5 shows multi-scale self-organized oxide nanotubular layer with two discrete size and geometry obtained on Ti29Nb13Ta4.6Zr alloy by optimized anodization [16, 26]. It is clear that a self-organized doublet nanotubular layer was formed. The layer consists of arrays with two different diameter tubes—50 nm tubes and 30 nm tubes. Apparently a regular assembly is observed where 50 nm tubes are satellite by 30 nm tubes. This unique feature, that is, multi-scale self-organization looks clearer from the bottom-view image as shown in Fig. 11.5b. Here arrangements consisting of 100 nm and 50 nm tubes at the bottom-ends are apparent.

11.5 Summary

The present chapter describes the formation of self-organized nanotubular and nanoporous oxide layers by a simple anodization. Key is to add a small amount of fluorides into anodization electrolyte. The morphology of formed oxide layers strongly depends on electrochemical conditions such as anodization voltage, duration and electrolyte as well as substrate composition. These nanostructured oxide layers can be utilized as functional electrodes.

Acknowledgements The present work is supported by "Priority Assistance of the Formation of Worldwide Renowned Centers of Research—Global COE Program (Center of Excellence of Advanced Structural and Functional Materials Designs)" form the Ministry of Education, Sports, Culture, Science and Technology of Japan and the Grant-in-Aid for Scientific Research (B) (Project No. 22360307) from Japan Society for the Promotion of Science. Some of the results were obtained under the collaboration with Prof. Schmuki's group (University of Erlangen-Nuremberg, Germany).

References

1. Huber A, Huber TE, Sadoqi M, Lubin JA, Manalis S, Prater CB (1994) Science 263:800
2. Masuda H, Fukuda K (1995) Science 268:1466
3. Li AP, Mueller F, Birner A, Nielsch K, Goesele U (1998) J Appl Phys 84:6023
4. Wehrspohn RB, Schilling J (2001) MRS Bull 26:623
5. Steinhart M, Wendorff JH, Greiner A, Wehrspohn RB, Nielsch K, Schilling J, Choi J, Gösele U (2002) Scinece 296:1997
6. Zwilling V, Darque-Ceretti E, Boutry-Forveille A, David D, Perrin MY, Aucouturier M (1999) Surf Interface Anal 27:629
7. Beranek R, Hildebrand H, Schmuki P (2003) Electrochem Solid-State Lett 6:B12
8. Macak JM, Tsuchiya H, Schmuki P (2005) Angew Chem Int Ed 44:2100
9. Macak JM, Tsuchiya H, Taveira L, Aldabergerova S, Schmuki P (2005) Angew Chem Int Ed 44:7463
10. Macak JM, Schmuki P (2006) Electrochim Acta 52:1258
11. Tsuchiya H, Macak JM, Taveira L, Schmuki P (2005) Chem Phys Lett 410:188
12. Tsuchiya H, Schmuki P (2005) Electrochem Commun 7:49
13. Sieber I, Hildebrand H, Friedrich A, Schmuki P (2005) Electrochem Commun 7:97
14. Sieber I, Kannan B, Schmuki P (2005) Electrochem Solid-State Lett 8:J10
15. Tsuchiya H, Macak JM, Sieber I, Taveira L, Ghicov A, Sirotna K, Schmuki P (2005) Electrochem Commun 7:295
16. Tsuchiya H (2011) Recent development in research of macro- and nanoporous metals, pp. 249–258, Nakajima H (ed)
17. Taveira LV, Macak JM, Tsuchiya H, Dick LFP, Schmuki P (2005) J Electrochem Soc 152: B405
18. Bauer S, Kleber S, Schmuki P (2006) Electrochem Commun 8:1321
19. Tsuchiya H, Macak JM, Müller L, Kunze J, Müller F, Greil P, Virtanen S, Schmuki P (2006) J Biomed Mater Res 77A:534
20. Bauer S, Pittrof A, Tsuchiya H, Schmuki P (2011) Electrochem Commun 13:538
21. Macak JM, Tsuchiya H, Ghicov A, Yasuda K, Hahn R, Bauer S, Schmuki P (2007) Curr Opin Solid State Mater Sci 11:3
22. Ghicov A, Schmuki P (2009) Chem Commun 20:2791
23. Macak J, Tsuchiya H, Taveira L, Ghicov A, Schmuki P (2005) J Biomed Mater Res 75A:928
24. Berger S, Tsuchiya H, Schmuki P (2008) Chem Mater 20:3245
25. Tsuchiya H, Akaki T, Nakata J, Terada D, Tsuji N, Koizumi Y, Minamino Y, Schmuki P, Fujimoto S (2009) Electrochim Acta 54:5455
26. Tsuchiya H, Macak JM, Ghicov A, Schmuki P (2006) Small 2:888

Chapter 12
Advanced Materials Design by Irradiation of High Energy Particles

Takeshi Nagase

Abstract The MeV electron irradiation by high-voltage electron microscopy (HVEM) can introduce the simplest type of irradiation defects in materials, and sometimes leads to a phase transition with negligible temperature change and contamination. This technique makes it possible to continuously observe the phase transition process using electron microscopy simultaneously as defects are introduced. Therefore, HVEM can provide a unique opportunity to carry out in-depth studies on the phase transition introduced by the accumulation of defects under a significantly simplified condition. In this paper, the following phase transitions related to non-equilibrium phases under MeV electron irradiation are discussed: (1) solid state amorphization (SSA) in metallic compounds, (2) crystallization of metallic glasses, and (3) crystal-to-amorphous-to-crystal (C–A–C) transition.

Keywords Amorphization • Crystallization • Defect • Free volume • High voltage electron microscopy (HVEM) • Irradiation • Phase transition

12.1 Defects in Crystalline and Amorphous Phases

A perfect crystal, with every atom of the same type and in the correct position, does not exist. All crystals have some defects at finite temperature. Although the term "defect" is commonly used, we should keep in mind that crystalline defects are not always bad. Defects play a crucial role in determining the properties of many materials of scientific and technological interest, and the nature of solid-state

T. Nagase (✉)
Research Center for Ultra-High Voltage Electron Microscopy, Osaka University, 7-1 Mihogaoka, Ibaraki, Osaka 567-0047, Japan

Division of Materials and Manufacturing Science, Graduate School of Engineering, Osaka University, 2-1 Yamadaoka, Suita, Osaka 565-0871, Japan
e-mail: t-nagase@uhvem.osaka-u.ac.jp

T. Kakeshita (ed.), *Progress in Advanced Structural and Functional Materials Design*, DOI 10.1007/978-4-431-54064-9_12,

phase transitions. For example, the followings are easily expected: the relationships between (1) vacancies and diffusion, (2) dislocations and the mechanical properties of crystalline materials, (3) the defect level and band gap, (4) interstitials (interstitial-type dislocation loops) and irradiation embrittlement, etc. Confusion arises about whether it is possible to define the concept of "defect" in an amorphous phase because of the lack of a long-range periodic structure in this phase. The concept of "free volume" is widely used in metallic glasses, while it has been suggested that the free volume theory may not be adopted for metallic glasses [1, 2]. Recent experimental and theoretical research has indicated that the concept of atomic stresses and strains is more suitable for explaining the nature of glass than a theory constructed using a one component defect of the free volume in metallic glasses [3–7]. In the present paper, the defects in materials will be discussed in an amorphous phase as well as in a crystalline phase.

Defects can be introduced by various processes in a crystalline phase: (1) thermal quenching leads to the supersaturation of vacancies, (2) phase transition leads to the formation of defects such as martensite transformation, (3) mechanical deformation leads to the accumulation of dislocations, and (4) high-energy particle irradiation can introduce defects by the mechanical atomic displacement of constituent elements through the elastic collision of high-energy particles and constituent elements, etc. Among the various defect introduction processes, high-voltage electron microscopy (HVEM) has significant advantages over other processes. These advantages include (1) the simplest type of irradiation defect introduction because of single atom displacement, (2) negligible contamination and oxidation, (3) a significant low-temperature increase in the case of metallic materials, (4) an extremely high dose rate, and (5) in site TEM observation of the defect-introduced structural change. These advantages and the research works that have used HVEM were summarized in a review paper on HVEM [8–12].

Under MeV electron irradiation, only single or, at most, double atom displacements of constituent elements can occur by the knock-on mechanism. Figure 12.1 shows a schematic illustration of the atomic defects in crystalline and amorphous phases introduced by the electron knock-on effect. In the crystalline phases [(a) and (b)], not only a vacancy but also an interstitial is introduced under the irradiation, while the existence of an interstitial can be ignored in materials without irradiation. A vacancy type of a free volume like defect and an interstitial type of anti free volume like defect [6, 13–15] are introduced in an amorphous phase under the irradiation [(a) and (c)]. One can notice that the concept of defects based on vacancy and interstitial (free-volume like and anti free volume like defects) may not be always useful in multi-component alloy system such as high entropy materials [16–18] and metallic glasses, and this will be discussed in other papers.

There is a threshold acceleration voltage (U_d) for the single atom displacement by the electron knock-on effect. Under an irradiation with an acceleration voltage lower than U_d, no mechanical atom displacement based on an elastic collision between an electron and constituent atom is introduced. Table 12.1 summarizes the threshold energy (E_d), U_d, and cross section (σ) for the atomic displacement of pure elements (updated on 20 November 2011). Most of the E_d and U_d values were taken from [20, 21]. A list of the systematic experimental data was firstly summarized by

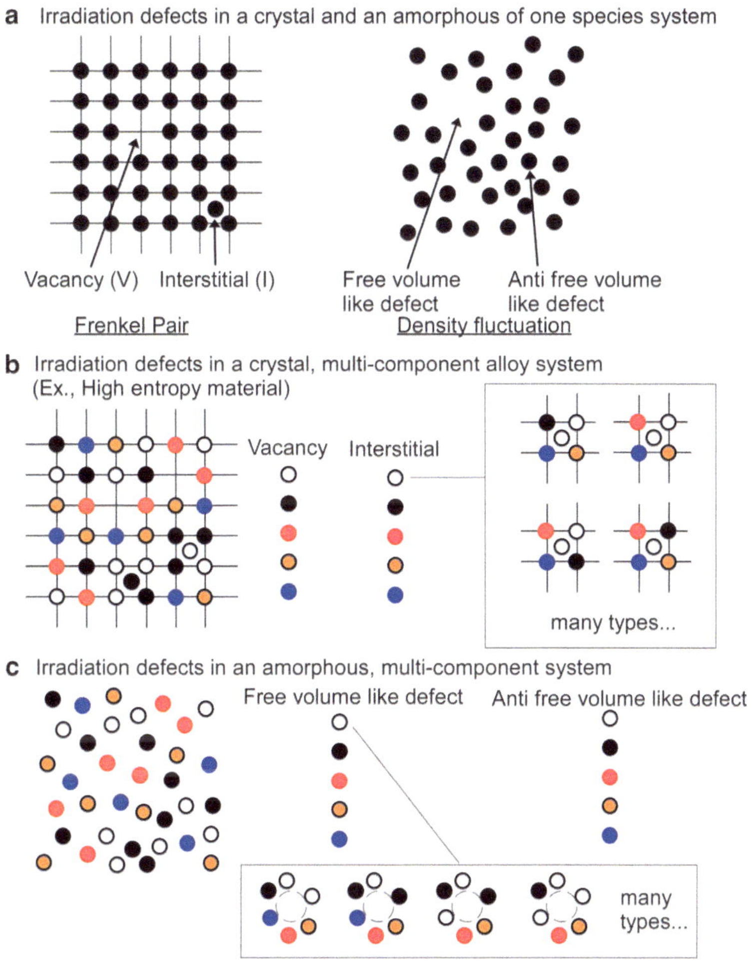

Fig. 12.1 Schematic illustration of MeV-electron irradiation-induced defects formed by single atom displacement. (**a**) Irradiation defects in crystalline and amorphous phases of one species system [6, 13–15]. (**b**) Irradiation defects in a crystal of a multi-component system such as a High-Entropy (HE) material [16–18]. (**c**) Irradiation defects in an amorphous phase of a multi-component system such as a metallic glass

Urban [20, 21] and then slightly modified by Fujita [22]. There are no experimental data about E_d and U_d in many elements, despite their significant importance. In elements with no experimental data, E_d was estimated from the melting temperature (T_m) because E_d has a tendency to increase with an increase in T_m [19]. The σ values were calculated using the McKinley–Feshbach formula, which is frequently used in irradiation damage analysis [23–25]. It should be emphasized that mechanical atom displacement cannot be achieved by 1 MeV electron irradiation in many atom species. However, 2.0 MeV can achieve this displacement for almost every element.

Table 12.1 Threshold energy (E_d), threshold acceleration voltage (U_d), and cross section (σ) for atomic displacement of pure element [19]

				Threshold energy		Threshold voltage		Cross section	
			Melting temp.	Exp.[a]	Calc.[b]	Exp.[a]	Calc.[b]	At 1 MV	At 2 MV
Element	Atomic number	Atom weight	T_m (K)	E_d (eV)	E_d (eV)	U_d (kV)	U_d (kV)	σ (barns)	σ (barns)
Be	4	9.012	1,560		22		90	11	11
B	5	10.81	2,365		28		150	8	9
C	6	12.01	3,825	33		200		11	12
Mg	12	24.31	922	14		100		53	57
Al	13	26.98	934	14		150		55	60
Si	14	28.09	1,687	13		140		67	73
P	15	30.97	317		12		160	74	81
Ti	22	47.88	1,946	19		320		49	66
V	23	50.94	2,202	26		430		28	45
Cr	24	52.00	1,857		24		440	29	48
Mn	25	54.94	1,245		19		360	50	72
Fe	26	55.85	1,811	20		370		49	73
Co	27	58.93	1,770	22		420		41	66
Ni	28	58.69	1,728	24		440		38	64
Cu	29	63.55	1,358	19		400		55	84
Zn	30	65.39	693	17.5		380		65	97
Ga	31	69.72	30		10		260	151	186
Ge	32	72.59	1,211	15		370		81	118
As	33	74.92	817		16		400	72	111
Y	39	88.91	1,801		24		600	31	76
Zr	40	91.22	2,128		26		660	22	67
Nb	41	92.91	2,750	33.5		800		8	46
Mo	42	95.94	2,895	30		750		12	55
Pd	46	106.4	1,827	34		890		4	45
Ag	47	107.9	1,235	24		700		24	84
Cd	48	112.4	594	19		610		46	118
Sn	50	118.7	505	12		450		113	226
Sb	51	121.8	630		15		540	86	176
La	57	138.9	920		17		660	52	153
Nd	60	144.2	1,290		19		730	33	134
Er	68	167.3	1,802		24		940	3	95
Hf	72	178.5	2,504		29		1,130	–	60
Ta	73	180.9	3,293	32		1,210		–	46
W	74	183.8	3,695	35		1,300		–	35
Re	75	186.2	3,455		36		1,340	–	32
Pt	78	195.1	2,045	33		1,290		–	40
Au	79	197.0	1,338	33		1,300		–	40

(continued)

Table 12.1 (continued)

				Threshold energy		Threshold voltage		Cross section	
			Melting temp.	Exp.[a]	Calc.[b]	Exp.[a]	Calc.[b]	At 1 MV	At 2 MV
Element	Atomic number	Atom weight	T_m (K)	E_d (eV)	E_d (eV)	U_d (kV)	U_d (kV)	σ (barns)	σ (barns)
Pb	82	207.2	601	11.5		1,490		114	348
U	92	238.0	1,406	34		1,500		–	26

Most of the values for E_d and U_d were taken from [20, 21]. A list of the systematic experimental data was firstly summarized by Urban [20, 21] and slightly modified by Fujita [22] (updated on 20 November 2011)

[a]Experimental data reported to date

[b]Estimated data by calculation

12.2 Solid-State Amorphization (Crystal-to-Amorphous Transition) by MeV Electron Irradiation

It is well known that the accumulation of the simplest types of crystal lattice defects under MeV electron irradiation using HVEM can lead to the formation of non-equilibrium phases through a variety of equilibrium to non-equilibrium solid-phase transitions: (1) the transition from an ordered intermetallic compound to a random solid solution [26, 27], (2) the transition from a fully ordered compound to a compound with a reduced value for long-range order parameter S [28], (3) the transition from one intermetallic compound to another intermetallic compound with a different crystal structure [28], (4) the solid-state amorphization (SSA) of intermetallic compounds [29–31], and (5) the transition from a single-phase intermetallic compound to a mixture of an amorphous phase and a different intermetallic compound [32]. This section focuses on the MeV electron irradiation induced SSA (crystal-to-amorphous transition, C–A transition).

Figure 12.2 shows a typical example of MeV-electron irradiation-induced SSA behavior: SSA in a B2 intermetallic compound in $Ti_{50}Ni_{46}Fe_6$ alloy [33]. The crystalline contrast in the BF image and the diffraction spot in the SAD pattern before irradiation (a) disappeared because of the irradiation, resulting in the appearance of a featureless contrast in the BF image and halo rings in the SAD pattern after the irradiation at $7.5 \times 10^{24}\ m^{-2}$ (c). The B2 phase cannot maintain its original structure under irradiation, resulting in the occurrence of SSA. No formation of black dot contrast owing to the formation of dislocation loops can be observed during SSA (b), whereas black dot contrast formation is a typical feature of crystalline materials (pure metals, alloys, and intermetallic compounds) without SSA [34].

Table 12.2 summarizes the occurrences of SSA in intermetallic compounds by MeV electron irradiation reported to date (updated on 20 November 2011). This list was firstly developed by Mori [37], and most of the data were taken from that list.

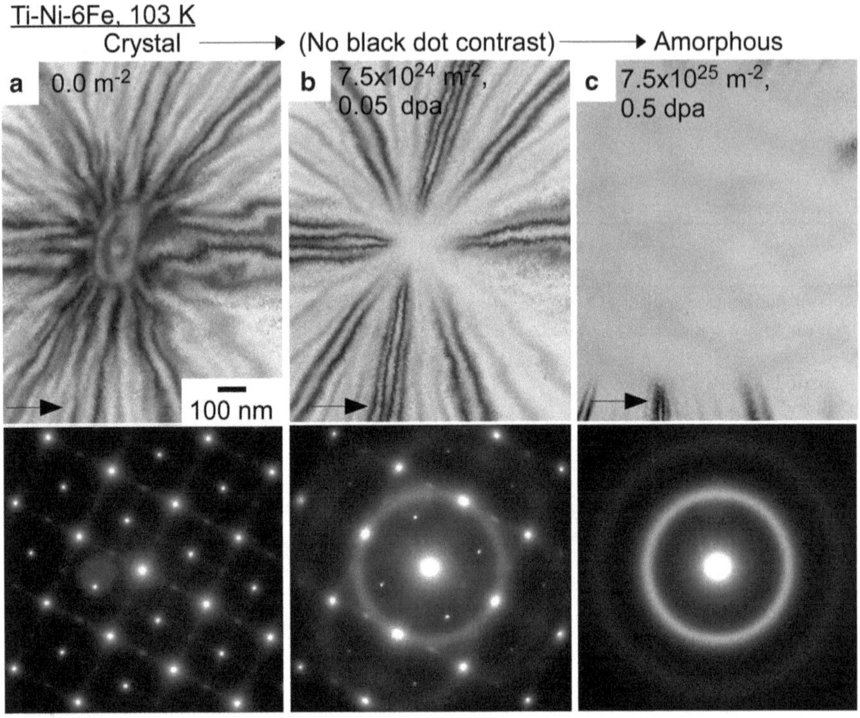

Fig. 12.2 Typical example of solid-state amorphization (crystal-to-amorphous transition) of intermetallic compound introduced by MeV electron irradiation. Change in TEM microstructure and corresponding SAD pattern in [0 0 1] direction of B2 phase in $Ti_{50}Ni_{46}Fe_6$ (Ti–Ni–6Fe) alloy at 103 K at a dose rate of 1.7×10^{24} m^{-2} s^{-1}. The *arrows* in the BF images mark the same position: (**a**) before irradiation, (**b**) 5 s after irradiation (7.5×10^{24} m^{-2}, 0.05 dpa), (**c**) 60 s after irradiation (7.5×10^{25} m^{-2}, 0.5 dpa) [33]

The occurrence of SSA by mechanical milling was taken from [35], and an amorphous phase formation by liquid quenching was taken from [36]. Many intermetallic compounds exhibit SSA, indicating that this phenomenon commonly occurs in metallic materials.

The tendency of metallic materials to undergo SSA under electron irradiation is related to the position of these compounds in the temperature–composition (T–C) phase diagram [37–39]. Intermetallic compounds that lie close to the liquidus valley in the T–C diagram show a strong tendency to undergo SSA, while those that are far from the liquidus valley do not. This criterion can be adopted, not only for metallic compounds, but also for non-metallic compounds [38, 40]. It should be noticed that this tendency is consistent with that predicted by the generalized Lindemann melting (GLM) criterion [41]. Although the criterion of the position in the T–C phase diagram is the most reliable criterion for SSA, it is difficult to predict the occurrence of SSA using only the T–C diagram criterion. To find a more quantitative parameter for predicting SSA, the occurrence of SSA was plotted using

Table 12.2 Crystal stability under MeV electron irradiation in intermetallic compounds

	Experimental data				Experimental data		
Compounds	E-IR	LQ	MA	Compounds	E-IR	LQ	MA
Al_9Co_2	•	×		Al_2Au	×	×	
Al_7Cr	•	•		Al_5Co_2	×	×	
Al_5Cr	•	•		Al_9Cr_4	×	×	
Al_4Cr	•	×		Al_8Cr_5	×	×	
Al_3Fe	•	×	•	Al_2Cu	×	×	
Al_6Mn	•	•		$AlCu(\eta_2)$	×	×	
Al_4Mn	•	•		Al_5Fe_2	×	×	•
$Al_{10}V$	•	×		Al_2Fe	×	×	•
$Al_{45}V_7$	•	•		AlFe	×	×	•
$Al_{23}V_4$	•	•		Al_3Mn	×	×	
Al_2Zr	•	×	×	$Al_{11}Mn_4$	×	×	
Al_3Zr_2	•	×	×	AlMn (γ_2)	×	×	
AlZr	•	×	×	$Al_{12}Mo$	×	×	
Al_4Zr_5	•	×	×	Al_8Mo_3	×	×	
Al_3Zr_4	•	×	×	Al_3Ni	×	×	
Al_2Zr_3	•	×	•	Al_3Ni_2	×	×	
$AlZr_2$	•	×	•	AlNi	×	×	×
BCo_2	•	×	•	$AlNi_3$	×	×	×
BCo_3	•	•	×	Al_3Ti	×	×	×
BFe_3	•	•	×	Al_3V	×	×	
B_3Ni_4 (o)	•	•		Al_8V_5	×	×	
BNi_2	•	•		$Al_{12}W$	×	×	
Co_2Ti	•	×	×	Al_3Zr	×	×	×
Cr_2Zr	•	×		$AlZr_3$	×	×	•
Cr_2Ti	•	×		BCo	×	×	•
Cu_3Ti_2	•	•	•	BFe_2	×	×	×
Cu_4Ti_3	•	•	•	BNi	×	×	
CuTi	•	•	•	B_3Ni_4 (m)	×	×	
$CuTi_2$	•	•	•	BNi_3	×	×	
$Cu_{10}Zr_7$	•	•	•	CoTi	×	×	×
CuZr	•	•	•	Cu_4Ti	×	×	•
$CuZr_2$	•	•	×	FeTi	×	×	
$Fe_{17}Nd_2$	•	•		$NbNi_3$	×	×	
Fe2Ti	•	×		Ni_3Ti	×	×	×
$FeZr_2$	•	•	•	$Fe_4Nd_{1.1}B_4$	×	×	
$FeZr_3$	•	•	•				
Mn_2Ti	•	×					
MoNi	•	×	•				
Nb_7Ni_6	•	•	•				
NiTi	•	•	•				
$NiTi_2$	•	•	•				
Ni_3Zr	•	•	•				
NiZr	•	•	•				
$NiZr_2$	•	•	•				
$PdZr_2$	•	•	•				
Pt_3Zr_5	•	×					

(continued)

Table 12.2 (continued)

	Experimental data				Experimental data		
Compounds	E-IR	LQ	MA	Compounds	E-IR	LQ	MA
$Fe_{23}Nd_2B_3$	•	×					
$Fe_{14}Nd_2B$	•	×					
$Fe_{81}Zr_9B_{10}$	•	•					

Process	
E-IR	Electron irradiation
MA	Mechanical alloying
LQ	Liquid quenching
Amorphous phase formation	
•	Yes, formed
×	No, not formed
(Open cell)	No reports

The latest data on the occurrence of solid-state amorphization (crystal-to-amorphous transition) by MeV electron irradiation. This list was firstly developed by Mori [28], and most of the data are taken from that list. The occurrence of solid-state amorphization by mechanical milling is taken from [35], and an amorphous phase formation by liquid quenching is taken from [36] (updated on 20 November 2011)

a map for the chemical mixing enthalpy (ΔH_{chem}) and mismatch entropy normalized using the Boltzmann constant (S_σ/k_B), which was suggested by Takeuchi and Inoue [42, 43]. This map is used for the evaluation of the glass forming ability (GFA) by liquid quenching; ΔH_{chem} corresponds to the heat of mixing, while S_σ/k_B corresponds to the difference in the atomic radii of the constituent elements. The results are shown in Fig. 12.3 [44]. The occurrence of SSA by irradiation cannot be explained completely by the ΔH_{chem}-S_σ/k_B map. However, the following tendencies can be found: the intermetallic compounds that undergo SSA show a tendency to have a large negative ΔH_{chem} and large positive S_σ/k_B. All the intermetallic compounds with $\Delta H_{chem} < 35$ kJ/mol exhibit irradiation-induced SSA. The occurrence of SSA may be estimated using a combination of the T–C phase diagram and the quantitative parameters of the ΔH_{chem} and S_σ/k_B.

12.3 Crystallization (Amorphous-to-Crystal Transition) by MeV Electron Irradiation

MeV electron irradiation can introduce irradiation defects in an amorphous phase, as shown in Fig. 12.1, resulting in the devitrification (crystallization) of an amorphous phase (amorphous-to-crystal transition) in some metallic glasses, while it can bring about the collapse of the crystalline structure (SSA), as mentioned in Sect. 12.2.

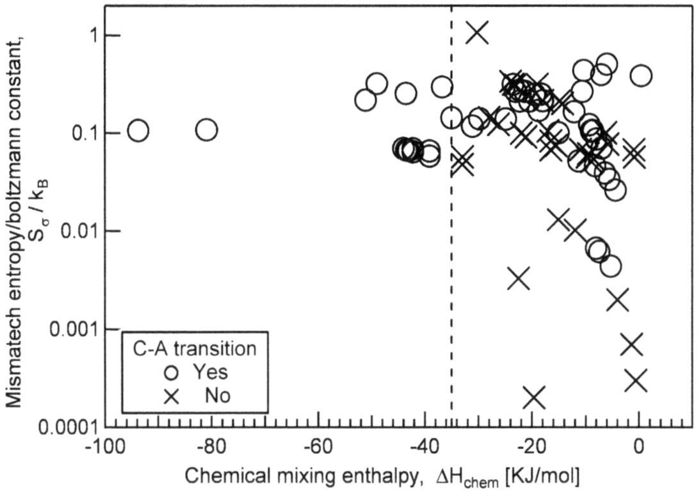

Fig. 12.3 Map of mismatch entropy (S_σ) and mixing enthalpy (ΔH_{chem}) parameters in occurrence of MeV-electron irradiation-induced solid-state amorphization (crystal-to-amorphous transition) [34]. The S_σ and ΔH_{chem} parameters were calculated with reference to Takeuchi's study [42, 43]

Figure 12.4 shows a typical example of the MeV electron irradiation induced crystallization of an amorphous phase: irradiation-induced crystallization in $Fe_{88}Zr_9B_3$ (Fe–9Zr–3B) alloy [46]. Before irradiation (a), BF images show a featureless image, and the SAD pattern shows the halo rings. These features are typical for an amorphous single phase. After 300 s of irradiation, nano-granular contrast in the BF image and discontinuous Debye rings in the SAD pattern began to appear. An amorphous phase cannot maintain its original structure under irradiation; instead, irradiation-induced crystallization was stimulated. Upon further irradiation, the area of the nano-granular contrast spread, but no change can be seen in the size of the nano-crystalline grains. In the SAD pattern, the intensity of the Debye rings increased and that of the halo rings decreased. No coarsening of the crystalline grains can be seen. In Fe–9Zr–3B alloy, the Bcc-solid-solution (α-Fe) phase and unknown intermetallic compounds (maybe Fe_2Zr) were formed by irradiation-induced crystallization.

Table 12.3 summarizes the occurrences of the MeV-electron irradiation-induced crystallizations reported to date, together with data on the onset total dose for crystallization, cross section (σ) for atomic displacement in an amorphous phase estimated by method 1 (M-1) and method 2 (M-2), and the onset dpa (updates on 20 November 2011) [19]; M-1 represents the calculation method for σ by the linear combination of pure elements, and M-2 represents the modified calculation method for σ by using the melting temperature. These methods were explained in [19]. As can be seen, electron-irradiation-induced crystallization can be observed in many metallic glasses, indicating that this phase transition is common in metallic glasses, just as SSA is in compounds.

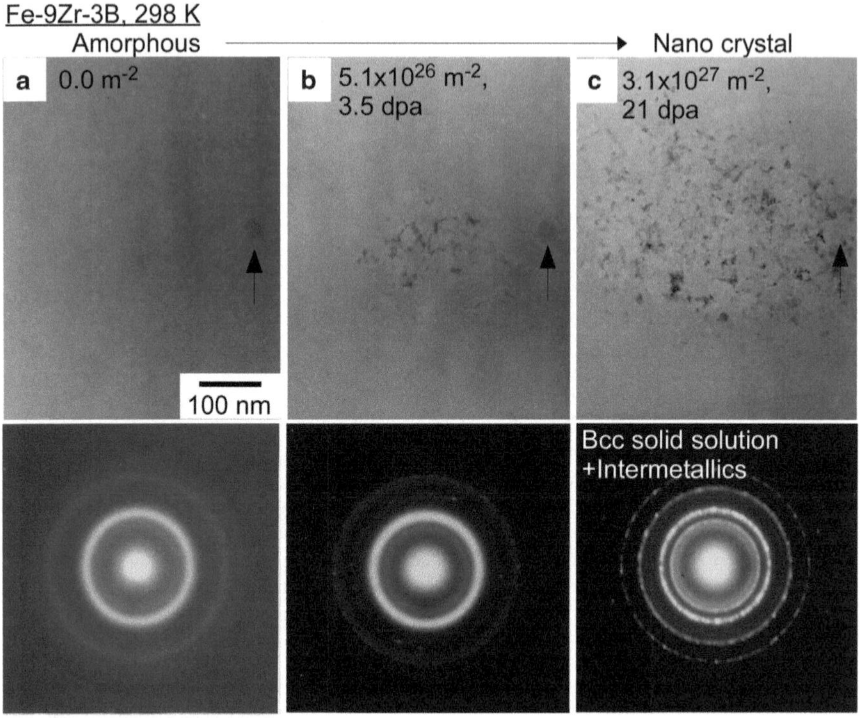

Fig. 12.4 Typical example of MeV-electron irradiation-induced-crystallization (crystal-to-amorphous transition) of amorphous phase. Change in the TEM microstructure and corresponding SAD pattern of an amorphous phase in $Fe_{88}Zr_9B_3$ (Fe–9Zr–3B) alloy at 298 K at a dose rate of 1.7×10^{24} m^{-2} s^{-1}. The *arrows* in the BF images mark the same position: (**a**) before irradiation, (**b**) at 300 s (5.1×10^{26} m^{-2}, 3.5 dpa), and (**c**) at 1.8×10^3 s (3.1×10^{27} m^{-2}, 21 dpa) [45]

To find a quantitative parameter for predicting the occurrence of irradiation-induced crystallization in metallic glasses, we tried to investigate it using a map of the mismatch entropy (S_σ) and mixing enthalpy (ΔH_{chem}) parameters. The results are shown in Fig. 12.5. Because of the lack of systematic data for the irradiation-induced crystallization, in particular, the lack of data for metallic glasses with a small negative ΔH_{chem} value and small positive S_σ/k_B value, a prediction of the occurrence of irradiation-induced crystallization cannot be performed using just this map. As shown in Table 12.3, the Ni–Nb-based metallic glasses with the occurrence of irradiation-induced crystallization show extremely high values for the onset total dose and onset dpa, and some Ni–Nb-based metallic glasses do not exhibit irradiation-induced crystallization. This implies that Ni–Nb-based metallic glasses have high phase stability against irradiation. This tendency can be explained by the high thermal crystallization temperature (T_x) [19].

Table 12.3 Stability of amorphous phase under MeV electron irradiation in metallic glasses
(a) Experimental data at 298 K at 2.0 MeV by use of UHVEM in Osaka University

	Experimental data	Onset TD	σ (barns)		Onset dpa (dpa)	
Alloy composition (at.%)	E-IR	ϕ ($\times 10^{26}$ m^{-2})	M-1[a]	M-2[b]	M-1[a]	M-2[b]
$Co_{80}B_{20}$	•					
$Co_{75}Si_{10}B_{15}$	•	96	58	64	56	62
$Fe_{85}B_{15}$	•					
$Fe_{88}Zr_9B_3$	•	2.0	71	69	1.4	1.4
$Fe_{86}Zr_9B_5$	•	3.9	69	69	2.7	2.6
$Fe_{81}Zr_9B_{10}$	•	7.2	66	65	4.8	4.7
$Fe_{76}Zr_9B_{15}$	•	10	63	62	6.3	6.2
$Fe_{71}Zr_9B_{20}$	•	12	60	65	7.2	7.8
$Fe_{82.2}Nd_{7.1}B_{10.7}$	•	1.1	71	70	0.8	0.8
$Fe_{77}Nd_{4.5}B_{18.5}$	•	6.0	64	64	3.8	3.8
$Fe_{71}Nd_9B_{20}$	•	8.5	66	65	5.6	5.6
$Fe_{44}Nd_{11}B_{44}$	×		51	47		
$Ni_{60}Nb_{20}Ti_{20}$	•	118	61	82	72	97
$Ni_{60}Nb_{20}Zr_{20}$	•	93	61	98	57	91
$Ni_{75}Si_{10}B_{15}$	•	13	57	70	7.4	9.1
$Ni_{60}Nb_{40}$	×		57	85		
$Ni_{60}Nb_{20}V_{20}$	×		57	95		
$Ni_{60}Nb_{20}Ta_{20}$	×		57	87		
$Ni_{60}Nb_{20}Y_{20}$	•	13	63	90	8.2	12
$Zr_{66.7}Cu_{33.3}$	•	2.2	73	95	1.6	2.1
$Zr_{66.7}Ni_{33.3}$	•	2.7	66	95	1.8	2.6
$Zr_{65}Al_{7.5}Cu_{27.5}$	•	4.6	71	98	3.3	4.5
$Zr_{60}Al_{15}Ni_{25}$	•	26	65	94	17	24
$Zr_{65}Al_{7.5}Ni_{10}Cu_{17.5}$	•	4.3	69	102	3.0	4.4
$Zr_{66.7}Pd_{33.3}$	•	4.9	60	101	2.9	4.9
$Zr_{80}Pt_{20}$	•	1.1	62	104	0.7	1.1
$Pd_{80}Si_{20}$	×		51	110		
$Pd_{40.5}Ni_{10.3}Cu_{30.6}P_{18.6}$	×		62	156		

Crystallization of an amorphous phase

•	Yes, observed
×	No, not observed

(b) Experimental reports about the electron irradiation in metallic glasses out of Osaka University

Alloy composition (at.%)	Experimental data E-IR	Acceleration voltage (MV)	Temperature (K)	Dose rate (m^{-2} s^{-1})
$Fe_{61}Cr_{17}Ni_8W_{14}$	•	1.2 or 1.5	750	(5–8) × 10^{23}
$Fe_{80}P_{13}C_7$	×	1.0	Heating to 723	About 1 × 10^{23}
$Ni_{75}Si_8B_{17}$	Acceleration[c]	1.0	Heating to 663	(2.6–2.7) × 10^{23}
$Ni_{75}Si_8B_{15}C_2$	Acceleration[c]	1.0	Heating to 633	(2.6–2.7) × 10^{23}

(continued)

Table 12.3 (continued)

(b) Experimental reports about the electron irradiation in metallic glasses out of Osaka University

Alloy composition (at.%)	Experimental data E-IR	Acceleration voltage (MV)	Temperature (K)	Dose rate ($m^{-2} s^{-1}$)
$Ni_{80}P_{10}B_{10}$	Acceleration[c]	1.0	Heating to 668	(2.6–2.7) × 10^{23}
$Ni_{80}P_{20}$	Acceleration[c]	1.0	Heating to 645	(2.6–2.7) × 10^{23}

The occurrences of MeV-electron irradiation-induced crystallization (amorphous-to-crystal transition) reported to date [23], together with data on the onset total dose for the crystallization, cross section (σ) for atomic displacement in an amorphous phase estimated by method 1 (M-1) and method 2 (M-2), and the onset dpa. M-1 represents the calculation method for σ by a linear combination of pure elements. M-2 represents the modified calculation method for σ by using the melting temperature. (a) Experimental data at 298 K obtained using an HU-2000 or H-3000 UHVEM at Osaka University. The irradiation was performed at 298 K with a dose rate of the order of 10^{24} m^{-2} s^{-1}. (b) Experimental reports out of Osaka University on electron irradiation by use of HVEM in metallic glasses (updated on 20 November 2011)

[a]Cross section for atom displacement was calculated by the linear combination of pure elements

[b]Cross section of atom displacement was modified by the melting temperature

[c]Acceleration, Acceleration of crystallization during heating under the irradiation

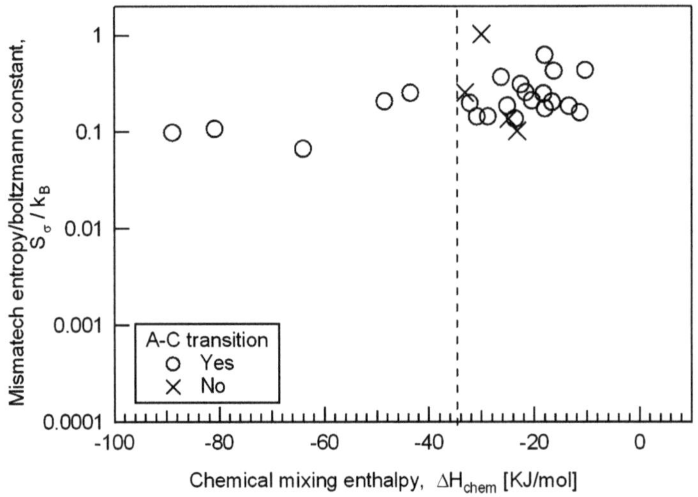

Fig. 12.5 Map of mismatch entropy (S_σ) and mixing enthalpy (ΔH_{chem}) parameters in occurrence of MeV-electron irradiation-induced crystallization (amorphous-to-crystal transition) [46]. The S_σ and ΔH_{chem} parameters were calculated with reference to Takeuchi's study [43, 44]

12.4 Crystal-to-Amorphous-to-Crystal Transition (C–A–C) by MeV Electron Irradiation

Recently, a unique disordering-ordering phase transition, i.e., a crystalline-to-amorphous-to-crystalline (C–A–C) transition, was found in some intermetallic compounds under MeV electron irradiation using HVEM: a new crystalline phase with a crystal

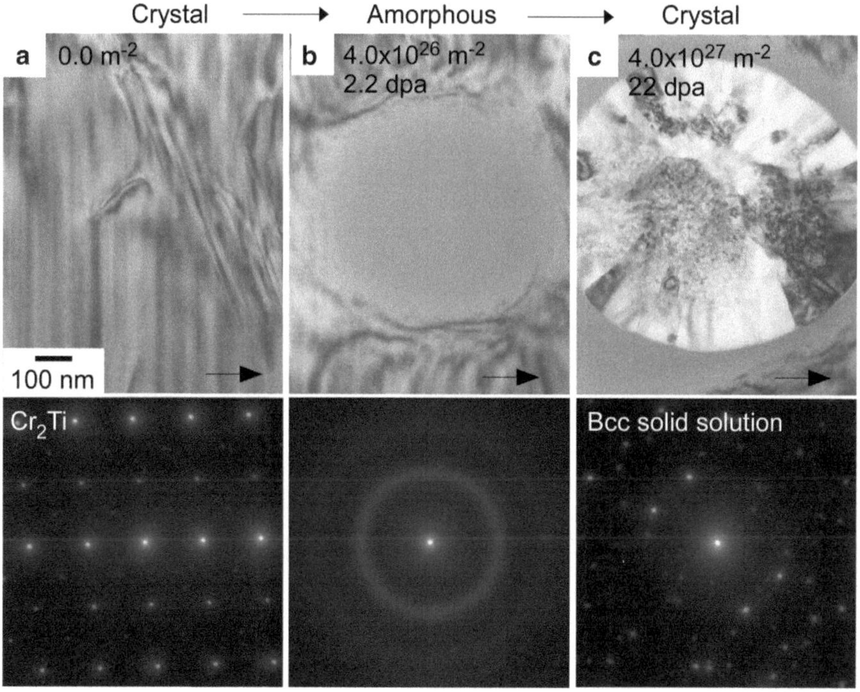

Fig. 12.6 Typical example of MeV-electron irradiation-induced crystal-to-amorphous-to-crystal (C–A–C) transition in intermetallic compounds. Change in TEM microstructure and corresponding SAD pattern of Cr_2Ti in $Cr_{65}Ti_{35}$ alloy at 103 K at a dose rate of 6.7×10^{24} m^{-2} s^{-1}. This C–A–C transition was found by Anada et al. The *arrows* in the BF images mark the same position: (**a**) before irradiation, (**b**) at 60 s (4.0×10^{26} m^{-2}, 2.2 dpa), and (**c**) at 600 s (4.0×10^{27} m^{-2}, 22 dpa) [48]

structure different from the original intermetallic compound appears from an amorphous phase, which is formed by SSA of the compound [45, 47]. The C–A–C transition is of significance: (1) From the viewpoint of fundamental material science, it provides evidence that even in the same material, the topological disordering in a crystalline phase and the topological ordering in an amorphous phase can occur under the same irradiation conditions. In the other words, both the crystalline phase formation and the collapse of the crystalline phase beyond the limit of the stability of the crystal can occur under the same irradiation conditions. (2) From the viewpoint of engineering, C–A–C transition may suggest a route to develop advanced materials that show a strong resistance to heavy electron irradiation.

Figure 12.6 shows a typical example of MeV electron irradiation-induced crystal-to-amorphous-to-crystal (C–A–C) transition in an intermetallic compound: the C–A–C transition of the Cr_2Ti intermetallic compound in the $Cr_{65}Ti_{35}$ alloy, which was found by Anada et al. [48]. The Cr_2Ti intermetallic compound cannot maintain its original crystalline structure, an irradiation-induced SSA occurred and an amorphous single phase was formed [(a) and (b)]. With continued irradiation,

Table 12.4 Occurrences of crystal-to-amorphous-to-crystal (C1–A–C2) transitions and quasi-crystal-to-amorphous-to-crystal (Q1–A–C2) transitions reported to date

(a) Crystal-to-amorphous-to-crystal (C1–A–C2) transition

		Crystalline structure		
		C1	C2-main phase	C2-minor phase
Compounds	Temperature (K)	(Before)	(After C–A–C)	
Zr_2Cu	298	t16(C11b)	cF4(A1) – F.c.c.S.S	Residual-Am.
	103			Residual-Am.
Zr_2Pd	298	t16(C11b)	cF4 (A1) – F.c.c.S.S	Residual-Am.
	103			Residual-Am.
Zr_5Pt_3	298	hP16	cF4(A1) – F.c.c.S.S	Residual-Am.
$Fe_{17}Nd_2$	298	hR19	c12 (A2) – Bcc S.S.	Residual-Am. + I.M.
	103			Residual-Am.
Cr_2Ti	103	cF12(C15)	c12 (A2) – Bcc S.S.	
$Nd_2Fe_{14}B$	298	tP68	c12 (A2) – Bcc S.S.	Residual-Am. + I.M.
	103			Residual-Am.
$Nd_2Fe_{23}B_3$	298	c1224	c12 (A2) – Bcc S.S.	Residual-Am. + I.M.
	103			Residual-Am.
α-Mn type	298	α-Mn type[a]	c12 (A2) – Bcc S.S.	Residual-Am. + I.M.
$Fe_{81}Zr_9B_{10}$	103			Residual-Am.

(b) Quasicrystal-to-amorphous-to-crystal (Q1–A–C2) transition

		Crystalline (quasi-crystalline) structure		
		Q1	C2-main phase	C2 minor phase
Compounds	Temperature (K)	(Before)	(After C–A–C)	
$Zr_{66.7}Pd_{33.3}$	298	Nano quasicrystal	cF4(A1) – Fcc. S.S.	Residual-Am.
	103			Residual-Am.

Electron irradiation was performed at 2.0 MeV at a dose rate on the order of 10^{24} m^{-2} s^{-1} (updated on 20 November 2011)

S.S. solid solution, *Residual-Am.* residual amorphous phase after C–A–C transition, *I.M.* intermetallic compounds whose crystalline structure is not clarified

[a]α-Mn type structure shows a complex structure with body-centered symmetry [49]

further changes in the BF images and SAD patterns were noticed (c). Crystalline grains appeared within the amorphous phase in the BF image, and in the SAD pattern, discontinuous Debye rings and/or crystalline diffraction spots appeared together with the disappearance of halo rings. A crystal-to-amorphous (C–A) transition initially occurred and was followed by an amorphous-to-crystal (A–C) transition, i.e., a crystal-to-amorphous-to-crystal (C–A–C) transition was observed in the Cr_2Ti intermetallic compound.

Table 12.4 summarizes the C–A–C transitions reported to date, together with similar quasi-crystal-to-amorphous-to-crystal (Q–A–C) transitions (updated on 20 November 2011). Occurrences of C–A–C transitions have been found in seven intermetallic compounds to date, indicating that this type of transition is common in metallic materials, similar to irradiation-induced SSA and crystallization. As can be seen, intermetallic compounds with various crystalline structures exhibit C–A–C transitions, indicating that the occurrence of C–A–C transition cannot be explained simply by the initial crystalline structure. The indicators for predicting the occurrence of C–A–C transition have not yet been clarified. Further experimental and theoretical works must be performed to understand the origin and dominant factors of C–A–C transition.

12.5 Summary

The experimental data on the occurrences of solid-state amorphization (SSA) of crystal-to-amorphous (C–A) transitions, crystallization in amorphous-to-crystal (A–C) transitions, and crystal-to-amorphous-to-crystal (C–A–C) transitions obtained to date were summarized in Tables 12.2, 12.3, and 12.4, respectively. The tendencies for these transitions to occur were discussed, especially in relation to quantitative parameters for the prediction of their occurrence. The origin of C–A–C transition has not yet been elucidated. However, systematic research and the accumulation of experimental results will clarify the nature of C–A–C transition.

Acknowledgments This study was supported by Priority Assistance for the Formation of Worldwide Renowned Centers of Research—The Global COE Program (Project: Center of Excellence for Advanced Structural and Functional Materials Design) of the Ministry of Education, Culture, Sports, Science and Technology, Japan. The author greatly thanks Prof. H. Mori and Prof. Y. Umakoshi in Osaka University for the fruitful discussions, valuable suggestions, and comments. Many experimental results about irradiation-induced amorphization and crystallization were obtained by Dr. A. Nino in Akita University, Dr. W. Qin in University of Saskatchewan, T. Hosokawa, A. Sasaki and T. Sanda. The recent experimental results about the irradiation-induced C–A–C transition were obtained by S. Anada in Osaka University.

Appendix: Technical Terms

(1) Anti-free volume-like defect [6, 13–15]

In an amorphous phase, not only vacancy-type defects but also interstitial-type defects can be considered, as shown in Fig. 12.1a. Anti-free volume-like defects correspond to interstitial-type defects. Petrusenko et al. reported MeV electron irradiation damage and suggested the existence of vacancy-type defects and interstitial-type defects in metallic glasses based on the experimental results. The recovery of introduced defects in metallic glasses has two threshold temperatures because of the changes in the relaxation mechanism under 298 K: the first was related to with complexes containing interstitial-type defects in metallic glass, while the second was a result of the relaxation of vacancy-containing complexes [14].

(2) High-entropy materials (HE materials) [16–18]
This class of alloys consists of multi-component materials with an approximately equiatomic ratio of components. Thus, these alloys have a high entropy of mixing, which distinguishes them from conventional alloys. Solid solutions with multi-principal elements have generally been found to be more stable than intermetallic compounds at elevated temperatures because of their large entropies of mixing. Some researchers have defined a high-entropy material as one that has at least five principal elements, each of which has an atomic concentration between 5 % and 35 %; for example, the $Fe_{20}Ni_{20}Cu_{20}Co_{20}Cr_{20}$ alloy.

References

1. Cohen MH, Turnbull D (1959) J Chem Phys 31:1164–1169
2. Cohen MH, Grest GS (1979) Phys Rev B 20:1077–1098
3. Egami T, Maeda K, Vitek V (1980) Philos Mag A 41:88–901
4. Egami T, Srolovitz D (1982) J Phys F Met Phys 12:2141–2164
5. Srolovitz D, Egami T, Vitek V (1982) Phys Rev B 24:6936–6944
6. Egami T, Maed K, Srolovitz D, Vitek V (1980) J Phys 41(C8):272–275
7. Egami T, Poon SJ, Zhang Z, Keppens V (2007) Phys Rev B 76:024203_1-024203_6
8. Fujita H (1989) J Electron Microsc Tech 3:243–304
9. Fujita H (1989) J Electron Microsc Tech 12:201–218
10. Seeger A (1999) J Electron Microsc 48:301–305
11. Mori H (2001) J Electron Microsc 60:S189–S197
12. Yasuda H (2011) Kenbikyo 46:160–164 (in Japanese)
13. Petrusenko Y, Bakai A, Borysenko V, Astakhov A, Barankov D (2009) Intermetallics 17:246–248
14. Nagase T, Hosokawa T, Umakoshi Y (2010) Intermetallics 18:767–772
15. Nagase T, Umakoshi Y (2010) Intermetallics 18:1803–1808
16. Ranganathan S (2003) Curr Sci 85:1404–1406
17. Cantor B, Chang ITH, Night PK, Vincent AJ (2004) Mater Sci Eng A 375:213–218
18. Yeh JW, Chen SK, Lin SJ, Gan JY, Chin TS, Shun TT, Tsau CH, Chang SY (2004) Adv Eng Mater 6:299–303
19. Nagase T, Sanda T, Nino A, Qin W, Yasuda H, Mori H, Umakoshi Y, Szpunar JA (2012) J Non-Cryst Solids 358:502–518
20. Urban K (1979) Phys Status Solidi A 56:157–168
21. Urban K (1980) Electron Microsc 4:188–195
22. Fujita H (1989) Hiheikou-zairyo no Riron to Gijyutsu-Seminar Text of Japan Inst Metals. JIM, Sendai 73–82 (in Japanese)
23. Seitz F, Koehler JS (1956) In: Seitz F, Tumbull D (eds) Solid state physics, vol 2. Academic, New York
24. Corbett JW (1966) Electron radiation damage in semiconductors and metals. Academic, New York
25. Oen OS (1988) Nucl Instrum Methods Phys Res B 33:744–747
26. Carpenter GJC, Schulson EM (1981) Scr Metall 15:549–554
27. Carpenter GJC, Schulson EM (1978) J Nucl Mater 73:180–189
28. Yasuda H, Mori H (1999) J Electron Microsc 48:581–584
29. Mori H, Fujita H (1982) Jpn J Appl Phys 21:L494–L496
30. Thomas G, Mori H, Fujita H, Sinclair R (1982) Scr Metall 16:589–592

31. Mogro-Campero A, Hall EL, Walter JL, Ratkowski AJ (1982) In: Picraux ST, Choyke WJ (eds) Metastable materials formation by ion-implantation. North-Holland, New York, pp 203–208
32. Mori H, Fujita H (1991) Ultramicroscopy 39:355–360
33. Nagase T, Sasaki A, Yasuda HY, Mori H, Terai T, Kakeshita T (2011) Intermetallics 19:1313–1318
34. Nagase T, Takizawa K, Wakeda M, Shibutani Y, Umakoshi Y (2010) Intermetallics 18:441–450
35. Suryanarayana C (2001) Prog Mater Sci 46:1–84
36. Mizutani U, Hoshino Y, Yamada H (1986) Amorphous-Gokin Sakusei no Tebiki. Agne, Tokyo (in Japanese)
37. Mori H (1993) In: Sakurai Y, Hamakawa Y, Masumoto T, Shirae K, Suzuki K (eds) Current topics in amorphous materials, physics and technology. Elsevier Science, Amsterdam, pp 120–126
38. Sakata T, Mori H, Fujita H (1989) J Chem Soc Jpn Int 97:1382–1388
39. Mori H, Fujita H (1992) In: Yavari AR (ed) Electron irradiation induced crystal-to-amorphous transition in metallic and non-metallic compounds in ordering and disordering in alloys. Applied Science, London, pp 277–286
40. Inui H, Mori H, Fujita H (1989) Acta Mater 37:1337–1342
41. Okamoto PR, Lam NQ, Rehn LE (1999) Physics of crystal-to-glass transformations. In: Ehrenreich H, Spaepen F (eds) Solid state physics, vol 52. Academic, San Diego
42. Takeuchi A, Inoue A (2000) Mater Trans 41:1372–1378
43. Takeuchi A, Inoue A (2005) Mater Trans 46:2817–2829
44. Nagase T, Hosokawa T, Takizawa K, Umakoshi Y (2009) Intermetallics 17:657–668
45. Nagase T, Umakoshi Y (2003) Scr Mater 48:1237–1242
46. Nagase T, Umakoshi Y, Sumida N (2002) Mater Sci Eng A 323:218–225
47. Nagase T, Nino A, Hosokawa T, Umakoshi Y (2007) Mater Trans 48:1651–1658
48. Anada S, Nagase T, Yasuda H, Mori H (to be submitted)
49. Imafuku M, Sato S, Koshiba H, Matsubara E, Inoue A (2000) Mater Trans JIM 41:1526–1529

Chapter 13
Advanced Analysis and Control of Bone Microstructure Based on a Materials Scientific Study Including Microbeam X-ray Diffraction

Takayoshi Nakano, Takuya Ishimoto, Naoko Ikeo, and Aira Matsugaki

Abstract Bone tissue is predominantly composed of biological apatite (BAp) crystals and collagen (Col) fibers, which shows hierarchical structure at various scale levels. Therefore, to design and develop implants suitable for bone replacement, both bone mineral density (BMD) and bone anisotropic microstructure should be investigated. From the viewpoint of materials scientific study, the bone microstructure based on the orientation degree of BAp *c*-axis which is dependent upon the bone portion, turnover, cell arrangement, etc., was clarified in intact, pathological and regenerated bones. For the analysis of BAp orientation, the microbeam X-ray diffraction method is quite effective on the basis of crystallography of anisotropic hexagonal BAp crystal. Moreover, this method is applicable even to a small region of several 10 μm or more on a side. Therefore, advanced design of implants for bone replacement should take into account anisotropic bone microstructure containing preferential alignment of BAp/Col.

Keywords Anisotropic microstructure • Apatite orientation • Biomaterial • Bone tissue • Microbeam X-ray diffraction • Osteocyte (OCY) • Stress

13.1 Introduction

The bone mechanical function depends on both bone quantity and quality, which correspond predominantly to bone mineral density [BMD: density of biological apatite (BAp)] and the internal microstructure, respectively [1]. BMD is correlated with bone strength, but it does not completely explain the variance in ultimate strength of bone [2]. Thus, novel parameters for representing the bone quality have been explored [3].

T. Nakano (✉) • T. Ishimoto • N. Ikeo • A. Matsugaki
Division of Materials and Manufacturing Science, Graduate School of Engineering, Osaka University, 2-1 Yamadaoka, Suita, Osaka 565-0871, Japan
e-mail: nakano@mat.eng.osaka-u.ac.jp

T. Kakeshita (ed.), *Progress in Advanced Structural and Functional Materials Design*, DOI 10.1007/978-4-431-54064-9_13,

Bone has a well organized and hierarchical structure at various scale levels, and it is dominantly composed of inorganic BAp crystal and organic collagen (Col) fiber, exerting reinforcement and pliability, respectively [4]. Since BAp crystallizes in an anisotropic hexagonal lattice, mechanical properties of BAp crystallite depends upon the crystal orientation [5, 6]. It was indeed reported that stiffness along the *c*-axis is higher than that along the *a*-axis under the nano-indentation measurement [6]. Moreover, it is believed that the BAp *c*-axis roughly associated with the extended direction of collagen fibers [7]. Preferential alignment of the BAp *c*-axis along the extended collagen fibers in the bone must be closely related to the mechanical function of bone; it is also utilized as a possible index for evaluating bone quality in various bones such as intact, regenerated and pathological bones including bones in gene-defected animals [8–10]. The microbeam X-ray diffraction (μXRD) method is a powerful tool for the analysis of the atomic arrangement in the BAp crystallites [10]. Moreover, there are a lot of materials scientific techniques that can be applied to clarify the bone functions apart from traditional methods [11]. This review article will be focused on our group's results showing strong correlations among in vivo external stress distribution, anisotropy of the BAp and Col alignment, and the mechanical function in various bones. In addition, the development and design of bone implants based on the structural anisotropy of bones, which is optimally designed depending on the suitable BAp orientation closely related to the bone mechanical function and stress distribution in vivo.

13.2 Crystallography for Understanding the Atomic Arrangement in Apatite

Natural creatures living in a gravitational environment have anisotropic and multiscale structures for exerting efficient and anisotropic functions in the required direction. In other words, living beings can sense in a specialized direction to demonstrate the absolutely imperative ability to the fullest in the direction. Bone and tree, for example, are typical anisotropic products. Materials composed of various crystals often have crystallographic texture and preferential arrangement of crystallite in some directions in order to exert the best functions. For example, BAp crystallizes in an anisotropic hexagonal crystal system as an ionic crystal with a space group of $P6_3/m$. The dominant constituents and composition are based on hydroxyapatite expressed as a chemical formula, $Ca_{10}(PO_4)_6(OH)_2$, but the ionic sites are replaced by a great amount of CO_3^{2-} ion and small amounts of other ionic elements [12]. BAp is, for example, described to be (Ca, Na, Mg, K, etc.)$_{10}$(PO_4, CO_3, HPO_4)$_6$(OH, Cl, F)$_2$. The arrangement of ions is quite different along the *a*- and *c*-axes in the BAp crystallite, and the *c*-axis of BAp crystallite is roughly distributed along the extending collagen fibril in bone as shown in Fig. 13.1 [7].

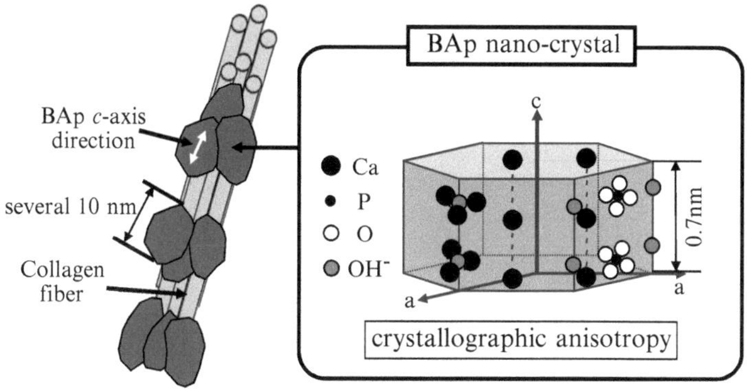

Fig. 13.1 Schematic illustrations of bone anisotropic microstructure composed of biological apatite (BAp) and collagen fiber, and ionic atom arrangement of apatite crystal structure

Crystals are solids with long-range periodicity whose constituent atoms, ions, or molecules are arranged in an orderly repeating pattern extending in all three spatial dimensions [13]. Crystals are clearly distinguished from amorphous materials, and their crystal structure consisting of a three-dimensional (3D) periodic arrangement is deeply related to the mechanical, chemical, and biological functions of the materials. The crystal structure does not necessarily depend on the arrangement of individual atoms; it is expressed by the distribution of imaginary points reflecting the periodicity in crystals, which are called the lattice points. As shown in Fig. 13.2, the arrangement of all of the lattice points is classified into seven crystal systems defined by three vectors, $\vec{a}$, $\vec{b}$ and $\vec{c}$ and the angles between them, α, β and γ, and furthermore are finally divided into 14 types of Bravais lattice on the basis of the distribution of the lattice points. The lattice points certainly have the same atomic environment.

BAp belongs to a hexagonal-based crystal system, and the molecule consisting of some ionic atoms exists at a lattice point, resulting in relatively high molecular weight approximately 1,000, while a single metallic atom in metallic materials occupies the lattice points of a simple lattice.

These atomic, ionic and molecular arrangements are deeply related to the mechanical functions in crystals. For example, fluorapatite, which is isomorphic with BAp, exhibits anisotropic plastic deformation behavior due to the dislocation motion depending on the operative slip system in a single crystalline form at high temperatures [5].

13.3 Typical Optical System of Microbeam X-ray Diffraction

Distribution of BAp *c*-axis orientation largely parallels the direction of extended collagen and can be evaluated by various microbeam XRD systems with collimeters from 20 to 500 μm ϕ and the optics of reflection (Fig. 13.3)

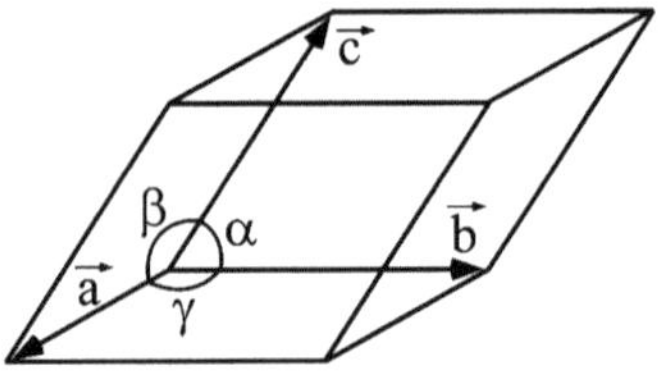

Crystal system	Axial lengths and angles	Bravais lattice
cubic	$a = b = c,\ \alpha = \beta = \gamma = 90^\circ$	simple body-centered face-centered
tetragonal	$a = b \neq c,\ \alpha = \beta = \gamma = 90^\circ$	simple body-centered
orthorhombic	$a \neq b \neq c,\ \alpha = \beta = \gamma = 90^\circ$	simple body-centered base-centered face-centered
rhombohedral	$a = b = c,\ \alpha = \beta = \gamma \neq 90^\circ\ (< 120^\circ)$	simple
hexagonal	$a = b \neq c,\ \alpha = \beta = 90^\circ,\ \gamma = 120^\circ$	simple
monoclinic	$a \neq b \neq c,\ \alpha = \gamma = 90^\circ \neq \beta$	simple base-centered
triclinic	$a \neq b \neq c,\ \alpha \neq \beta \neq \gamma \neq 90^\circ$	simple

Fig. 13.2 Unit cell and crystal system for classification of crystal structures

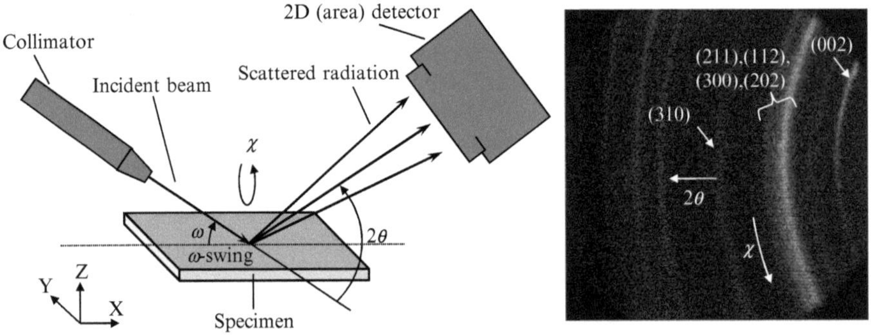

Fig. 13.3 Reflection optics of microbeam X-ray diffraction equipped with two-dimensional (2D) detector. Detected diffraction is from the trabecular bone [14]

and transmission (Fig. 13.4). Since the diffracted beam from the small volume of bone specimen is very weak, one-dimensional (1D) or two-dimensional (2D) detectors are generally utilized, while the detected diffracted X-ray beam does not come from the symmetrical condition against the specimen surface.

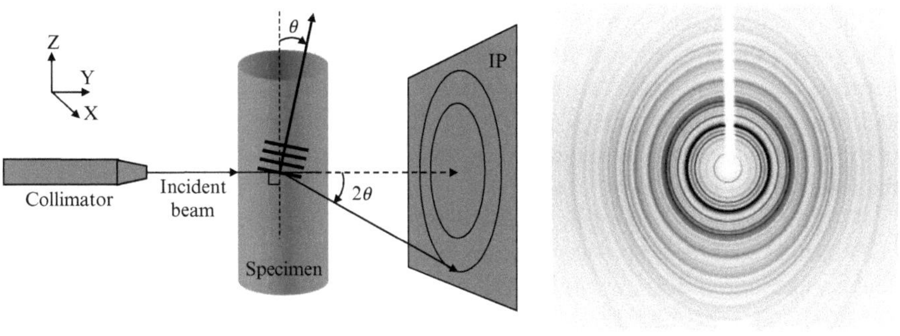

Fig. 13.4 Transmission optics of microbeam X-ray diffraction in Rigaku R-AXIS BQ (Bone Quality) diffractometer equipped with an imaging-plate detector [15]

In the case of the system with reflection optics as shown in Fig. 13.3, the X–Y–Z specimen table is mounted on a chi (χ) axis, and the χ axis is further mounted on an omega (ω) axis. The χ axis is always perpendicular to the ω axis [14]. Incident beam of characteristic X-ray (e.g. Cu-Kα) was generated by rotating anode or filament tube X-ray generator, and the incident beam was focused onto a small beam spot by collimators. In this case, diffracted beams were simultaneously detected by a 2D position sensitive proportional counter (2D PSPC) in which the intensity of the diffracted beam could be detected along the χ and 2θ axes. Distances between the specimen and the collimator and between the specimen and the detector are very important to the detectable angular resolution of diffracted beams in the detector.

Figure 13.4 shows a schematic illustration showing transmission optics in Rigaku R-AXIS BQ (Bone Quality) system developed by Rigaku Co., Ltd. and our group for analyzing the degree of BAp orientation as bone quality. The purpose of this development was to apply the transmission X-ray diffraction method with higher energy characteristic X-ray Mo-Kα radiation on mouse or rat femur without sectioning. The high energy radiation reduced the effect of absorption, resulting in improvements of the signal-to-noise ratio [15].

R-AXIS BQ system in Fig. 13.4 employs an imaging plate (IP) as the 2D X-ray detector (storage phosphors) developed by Fuji Film Co., Ltd. The distance between the detector and the X-ray focus of the specimen is fixed at 127.4 mm in a horizontal direction. The detected area on the imaging plate is 256 mm $\times$ 460 mm with a curvature on the horizontal plane. This provides a 2θ range from $-60°$ to $+144°$ in the horizontal direction and a 2θ range of $\pm 45°$ in the vertical direction. The pixel area of the imaging plate is 100 μm $\times$ 100 μm. A Rigaku ultra X rotating anode X-ray generator with either a copper ($\lambda = 0.15418$ nm) or a molybdenum ($\lambda = 0.07107$ nm) target is prepared accompanied with a graphite monochromator. The monochromator provides substantial monochromatic radiation of the wavelength.

The specimens were oriented on a three-circle Eulerian goniometer with an X–Y–Z stage. The Eulerian angles were ϕ, χ, and ω. The ϕ-axis was closest to the specimen and provided complete specimen rotation around that axis. The χ-axis, the next closest to the specimen, was used to tilt the specimen. In general, the other ω-axis is used as a scanning axis. The specimens were moved to their desired positions by the X–Y–Z stage. The distribution of the X-ray absorption of the bone specimens was measured by an X-ray scintillation counter operating in the integrating mode.

Two diffraction peaks of hexagonal-based BAp, (0 0 2) and (3 1 0), are basically used to analyze BAp c-axis orientation [9]. The (0 0 2) and (3 1 0) diffraction peaks appear around Bragg angles (2θ) of 25.9° and 39.8°, respectively, by Cu-Kα radiation and 11.9° and 18.1°, respectively, by Mo-Kα radiation. The degree of orientation of the BAp c-axis as an integrated intensity ratio of the (0 0 2) diffraction to the (3 1 0) diffraction was defined in this article. The value of the orientation degree in randomly orientated apatite (calcium hydroxyapatite) powders (NIST #2910) is determined in each μXRD system.

13.4 BAp Orientation Analysis in Bones

13.4.1 Unique Alignment in Cortical Intact Bones

The degree of BAp orientation strongly depends on the cortical bone position, which exhibits various geometries as shown in Fig. 13.5. For example, 1D alignment appears in long bones such as the ulna, femur, and tibia along the longitudinal axis, the mandible along the mesiodistal axis, and the vertebra in the cephalocaudal direction [9]. In contrast, the mature calvarial bone, a flat bone, exhibits preferential alignment in two dimensions along its bone surface. Mastication also makes the BAp orientation change from uni- to multi-axial, especially along the biting direction near the tooth root or tooth crown [9]. These unique alignments in intact bones are deeply related to their in vivo stress distribution, especially principal stress of greatest absolute values, because the direction of BAp c-axis alignment roughly corresponds to the direction of the greatest principal stress in vivo.

The calvarial bone grows through a membranous ossification process and basically has 2D BAp c-axis orientation along the flat bone surface [16]. However, our recent study exhibited a complicated change in the BAp orientation depending on the position and growth direction rather than in vivo stress distribution during the bone growth process [16].

Figure 13.6 contains a 2D radar diagram showing that a BAp orientation depends on the position of the calvarial bone of a 5-week-old rat as fitted in the following equation.

$$r = \left(\frac{\cos^2(\theta-\alpha)}{a^2} + \frac{\sin^2(\theta-\alpha)}{b^2}\right)^{-\frac{1}{2}} - c$$

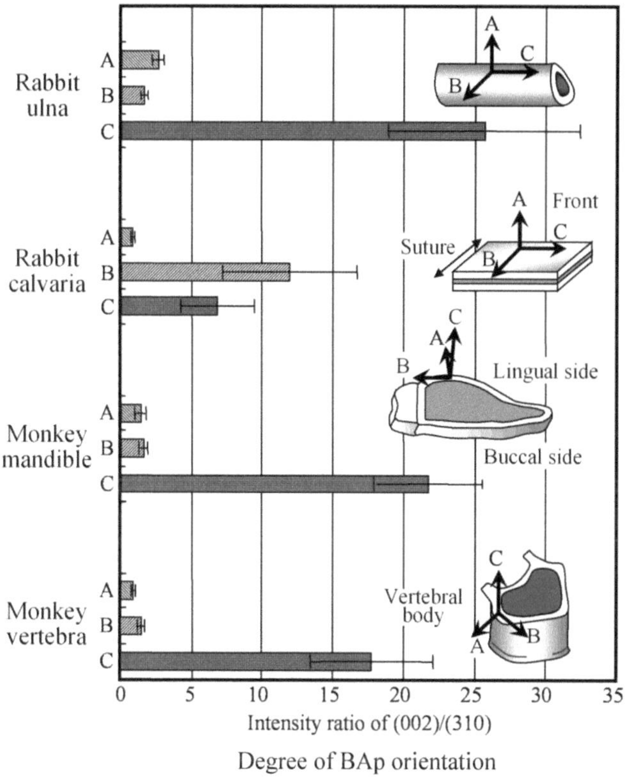

Fig. 13.5 Variations in the relative diffraction intensity ratio of the (0 0 2) diffraction peak to the (3 1 0) peak with different directions, A, B, and C for the ulna, skull bone, dentulous mandible, and lumber vertebra [9]. The BAp orientation strongly depends on the bone portion

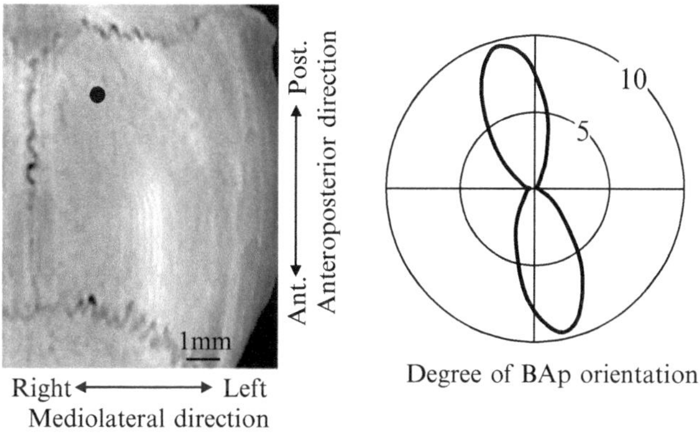

Fig. 13.6 Calvarial bone of a 5-week-old rat and the anisotropic distribution of the degree of BAp *c*-axis orientation in radar diagram along the flat bone [16]. Near the suture of young carvarial bone, the preferential orientation of BAp accords with the bone growth direction

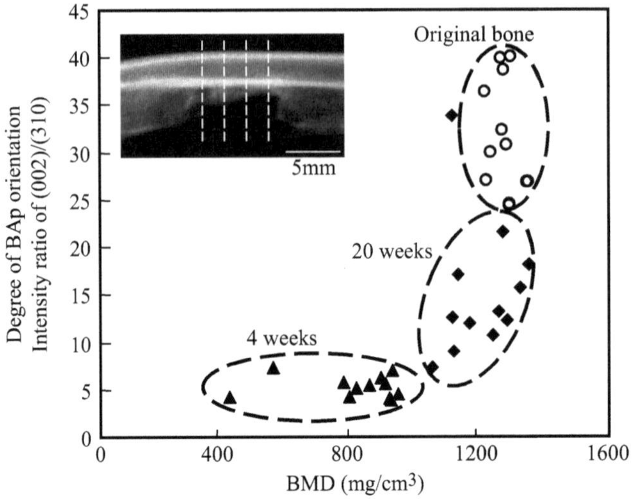

Fig. 13.7 Variations in BAp *c*-axis orientation along bone axis and bone mineral density (BMD) as a function of healing period in the 10 mm-defected ulnar bone of rabbit [19]. BMD recovers prior to the BAp orientation during the healing process

where *r* is the intensity of diffraction, and *a*, *b*, and *c* are constants for fitting the elliptic-like function.

The measured position clearly exhibits 1D alignment on the flat bone surface along the anteroposterior axis parallel to the bone growth direction as shown in Fig. 13.6 [16]. This means that the mature calvarial bone exhibits preferential alignment in two dimensions within its surface.

13.4.2 Variation and Detection During the Healing Process of Defected Bones

Distribution of BAp orientation is an essential microstructural feature that influences mechanical, chemical, and biological functions. Thus, techniques for controlling BAp orientation should be developed, especially with regard to tissue engineering techniques for lost bone tissues [17, 18].

In order to clarify the natural regeneration process of defected long bone on the basis of BAp orientation, a rabbit ulnar osteotomy model was prepared. A 10 mm-long segmental defect was introduced in the ulnar middiaphysis in mature male Japanese White Rabbits (~3 kg) [19]. Both BMD and BAp alignment were analyzed in the same local region. Figure 13.7 shows the correlation between the degree of BAp orientation and BMD in the healed and original ulna. Randomly oriented apatite (hydroxyapatite) powders show relative intensity ratio of approximately two. When the BAp *c*-axis shows the preferential alignment along the longitudinal bone axis, the intensity ratio is maintained above two. Four weeks after the operation, the intensity ratio of (0 0 2)/(3 1 0) in the regenerated bone tissue is much lower than in the original tissue. Although the BMD was almost restored to its original levels after 20 weeks, the recovery of the BAp orientation was insufficient to reach its original level. The recovery of the BAp orientation strongly depends on the regenerated portion. This indicates that BMD recovers prior to the improvement of BAp orientation and the related mechanical property in the regenerated bone tissue.

Thus, reloading on the regenerated portion caused by BMD restoration and subsequent filling of the defects are suggested to promote the generation of appropriate BAp orientation distribution. Moreover, the degree of BAp orientation rather than BMD during the bone healing process corresponds to the recovery of Young's modulus [20].

13.4.3 BAp Orientation of Pathological Bones

Bone disease, including gene-defected models, often changes the degree of BAp orientation. One of the typical cases is the op/op mouse that has defects in the expression of macrophage colony-stimulating factor (M-CSF), resulting in osteopetrosis. This is caused by the lack of osteoclasts, which are a bone cell absorbing bone tissue.

The lack of osteoclasts induces abnormal calcification of the medullary cavity, which are typical features of osteopetrosis [21]. Preferential alignment of the BAp *c*-axis in the osteopetrotic (op/op) mouse always exhibits a lower degree than that in the control mouse, independent of the distance from the periosteum [22]. Moreover, the degree of the BAp *c*-axis orientation on the femoral cross-section shows a quite different tendency between the op/op and control mice. The BAp preferential alignment gradually increases towards the periosteal surface in the op/op mouse due to intramembranous ossification, but that in the control mouse is the lowest near the cortical envelope. This suggests that a decrease in the number of osteoclasts suppresses the normal modeling or remodeling, resulting in degradation of preferential alignment of the BAp *c*-axis as a bone quality parameter in the op/op mouse. Similar change in the degree of BAp orientation was found in the ovariectomized rat model of osteoporosis with estrogen-deficiency [23] and the rat in which mineral apposition rate (MAR) changes due to the turnover rate [24].

13.4.4 Relationship Among In Vivo Stress (Strain) Distribution, BAp Orientation and Young's Modulus Through Osteocyte

Osteocytes (OCYs) (Fig. 13.8) that are arranged in the bone matrix is believed to sense the stress (strain) distribution in vivo and to control bone cells, thus regulating the formation of bone matrix. As described in the previous sections, the externally

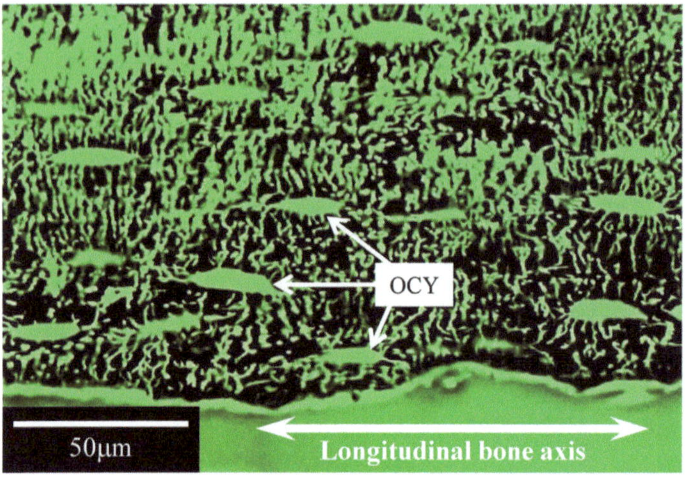

Fig. 13.8 Osteocyte arrangement along longitudinal bone axis in mouse tibia

applied stress distribution produces the degree of preferential alignment of BAp/Col, resulting in the change in Young's modulus. The degree of anisotropy in strain inside of bone caused by anisotropic external load diminishes due to the enhancement of the preferential alignment of BAp/Col and the subsequent increase in Young's modulus as schematically drawn in Fig. 13.9. This suggests that osteocytes can sense a 3D in vivo strain field; OCY prefers isotropic strain fields to anisotropic strain fields.

13.5 Control of BAp Orientation by Using Biomaterials and Other Methodology

The orientation of BAp/Col inside biological bones strongly depends on the in vivo stress distribution and other parameters. Herein, we describe the detailed mechanism for the formation of unique and appropriate BAp orientation in cellular and molecular levels. Moreover, the degree of BAp orientation in bone should be controlled by biomaterials and other methodology.

The principal stress direction and the *c*-axis priority orientation of the BAp, for example, match well; therefore, optimal design of metallic implants to maintain the healthiness of this bone microstructure should be given. Generally, the homeostasis of bone microstructure is maintained and bone remodeling progresses due to osteoblasts that form the bone, osteoclasts that resorb the bone, and OCYs that sense the stress distribution within the bones. Making the direction of the grooves and pores match the principal stress direction gives an optimal environment to the bone cells [25–27]; this, in particular, enables the sensing of the stress by the OCYs to get closer to a more normal state. Broadly classified, there are three necessary

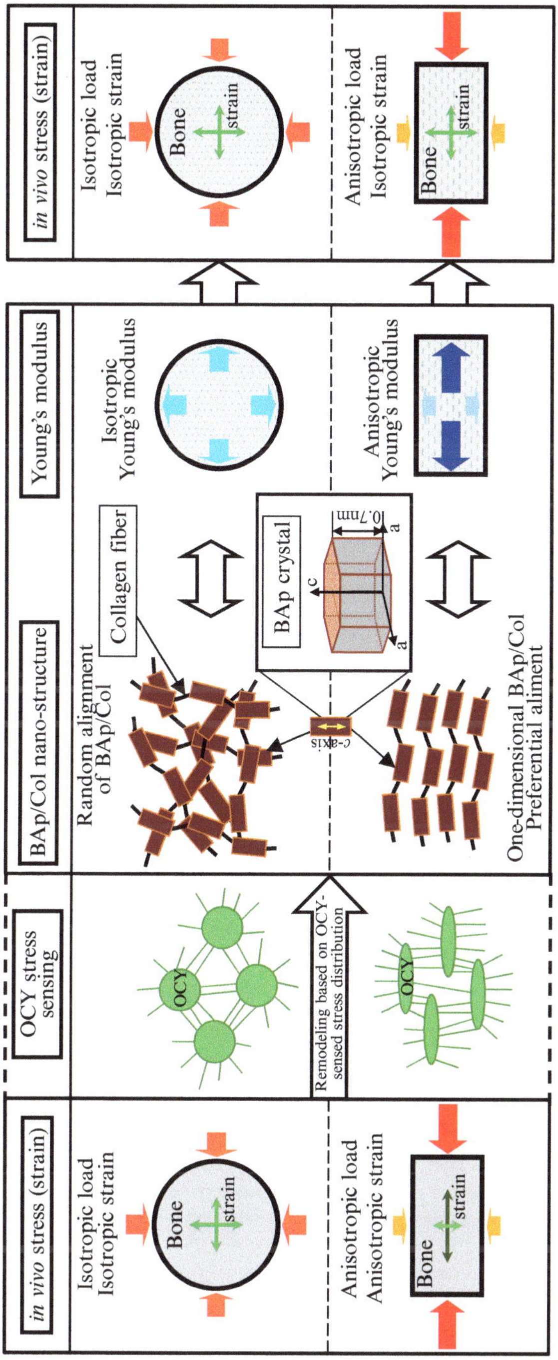

Fig. 13.9 Response among in vivo stress (strain) distribution and preferential orientation of BAp *c*-axis and collagen fiber and Young's modulus through osteocyte

points required for future types of biomaterials: (1) surface design [28], (2) improvement of the properties of the materials themselves for reducing the stress shielding, and (3) switching to tailor-made macro shapes [29].

13.6 Conclusion

This chapter introduced new materials scientific approach to bone microstructure and biomaterials design for bone replacement. Microbeam X-ray diffraction technique is one of the powerful methods for analyzing the preferential degree of BAp crystal and the related collagen fiber orientation in various bones under intact, regenerated, and pathological conditions. Further study from the viewpoint of materials scientific aspect, new strategy for controlling bone microstructure, and the mechanism for appropriate bone formation are evolved, resulting in the development of novel implants, pharmacy, and diagnosis methods for diseased bones in the near future.

Acknowledgments This work was supported by the Funding Program for Next Generation World-Leading Researchers from the Japan Society for the Promotion of Science (JSPS) and the Priority Assistance for the Formation of Worldwide Renowned Centers of Research—The Global COE Program (Project: Center of Excellence for Advanced Structural and Functional Materials Design) from the MEXT, Japan.

References

1. Dougherty G (1996) Quantitative CT in the measurement of bone quantity and bone quality for assessing osteoporosis. Med Eng Phys 18:557–568
2. Snyder BD, Piazza S, Edwards WT, Hayes WC (1993) Role of trabecular morphology in the etiology of age-related vertebral fractures. Calcif Tissue Int 53:S14–S22
3. NIH Consensus Development Panel on Osteoporosis Prevention, Diagnosis, and Therapy (2001) Osteoporosis prevention, diagnosis, and therapy. JAMA 285:785–795
4. Bonfield W, Grynpas MD (1977) Anisotropy of the Young's modulus of bone. Nature 270:453–454
5. Nakano T, Awazu T, Umakoshi Y (2001) Plastic deformation and operative slip system in mineral fluorapatite single crystals. Scr Mater 44:811–815
6. Viswanath B, Raghavan R, Ramamurty U, Ravishankar N (2007) Mechanical properties and anisotropy in hydroxyapatite single crystals. Scr Mater 57:361–364
7. Landis WJ (1995) The strength of a calcified tissue depends in part on the molecular structure and organization of its constituent mineral crystals in their organic matrix. Bone 16:533–544
8. Sasaki N, Matsushima N, Ikawa T, Yamanura H, Fukuda A (1989) Orientation of bone mineral and its role in the anisotropic mechanical properties of bone-transverse anisotropy. J Biomech 22:157–159
9. Nakano T, Kaibara K, Tabata Y, Nagata N, Enomoto S, Marukawa E, Umakoshi Y (2002) Unique alignment and texture of biological apatite crystallites in typical calcified tissues analyzed by microbeam x-ray diffractometer system. Bone 31:479–487

10. Nakano T, Tabata Y, Umakoshi Y (2005) Texture and bone reinforcement. In: Encyclopedia of materials science and technology updates. Elsevier, Oxford, pp 1–8 (Ms: 2061)
11. Fratzl P, Gupta HS, Paschalis EP, Roschger P (2004) Structure and mechanical quality of the collagen–mineral nano-composite in bone. J Mater Chem 14:2115–2123
12. Elliot JC (1994) Structure and chemistry of the apatites and other calcium phosphates. Elsevier, Amsterdam
13. Niinomi M (ed) (2010) Metals for biomedical devices. Woodhead Publishing Limited, Oxford
14. Miyabe S, Nakano T, Ishimoto T, Takano N, Adachi T, Iwaki H, Kobayashi A, Takaoka K, Umakoshi Y (2007) Two-dimensional quantitative analysis of preferential alignment of BAp c-axis for isolated human trabecular bone using microbeam X-ray diffractometer with a transmission optical system. Mater Trans 48:343–347
15. Sasaki K, Nakano T, Ferrara JD, Lee JW, Sasaki T (2008) New technique for evaluation of preferential alignment of biological apatite (BAp) crystallites in bone using transmission X-ray diffractometry. Mater Trans 49:2129–2135
16. Ishimoto T, Sakamoto T, Nakano T (2010) Orientation of biological apatite in rat calvaria analyzed by microbeam X-ray diffractometer. Mater Sci Forum 638–642:576–581
17. Nakano T, Kaibara K, Tabata Y, Nagata N, Enomoto S, Marukawa E, Umakoshi Y (2002) Analysis of hydroxyapatite (HAp) texture in regenerated hard tissues using micro-beam X-ray diffractometer technique. In: Ikada Y, Umakoshi Y, Hotta T (eds) Tissue engineering for therpeutic use, vol 6. Elsevier, Amsterdam, pp 95–104
18. Nakano T, Kaibara K, Ishimoto T, Tabata Y, Umakoshi Y (2012) Biological apatite (BAp) crystallographic orientation and texture as a new index for assessing the microstructure and function of bone regenerated by tissue engineering. Bone 51:741–747
19. Ishimoto T, Nakano T, Umakoshi Y, Yamamoto M, Tabata Y (2006) Role of stress distribution on healing process of preferential alignment of biological apatite in long bones. Mater Sci Forum 512:261–264
20. Ishimoto T, Nakano T, Yamamoto M, Tabata Y (2011) Biomechanical evaluation of regenerated long bone by nanoindentation. J Mater Sci Mater Med 22:969–976
21. Abboud SL, Woodruff K, Liu C, Shen V, Ghosh-Choudhury N (2002) Rescue of the osteopetrotic defect in op/op mice by osteoblast-specific targeting of soluble colony-stimulating factor-1. Endocrinology 143:1942–1949
22. Lee JW, Nakano T, Toyosawa S, Tabata Y, Umakoshi Y (2007) Areal distribution of preferential alignment of biological apatite (BAp) crystallite on cross-section of center of femoral diaphysis in osteopetrotic (op/op) mouse. Mater Trans 48:337–342
23. Shiraishi A, Miyabe S, Nakano T, Umakoshi Y, Ito M, Mihara M (2009) The combination therapy with alfacalcidol and risedronate improves the mechanical property in lumbar spine by affecting the material properties in an ovariectomized rat model of osteoporosis. BMC Musculoskelet Disord 10:paper #66
24. Kashii M, Hashimoto J, Nakano T, Umakoshi Y, Yoshikawa H (2008) Alendronate treatment promotes bone formation with a less anistropic microstructure during intramembranous ossification in rats. J Bone Miner Metab 26:24–33
25. Nakano T, Kan T, Ishimoto T, Ohashi Y, Fujitani W, Umakoshi Y, Hattori T, Higuchi Y, Tane M, Nakajima H (2006) Evaluation of bone quality near metallic implants with and without lotus-type pores for optimal biomaterial design. Mater Trans 47:2233–2239
26. Alvarez K, Hyun SK, Nakano T, Umakoshi Y, Nakajima H (2009) In vivo osteocompatibility of lotus-type porous nickel-free stainless steel in rats. Mater Sci Eng C 29:1182–1190
27. Noyama Y, Nagayama N, Ishimoto T, Kuramoto K, Sakai T, Yoshikawa H, Nakano T (2010) Stress simulation and related bone ingrowth in grooves on implant. Mater Sci Forum 638–642:664–669
28. Matsugaki A, Aramoto G, Nakano T (2012) The alignment of MC3T3–E1 osteoblasts on steps of slip traces introduced by dislocation motion. Biomaterials 33:7327–7335
29. Nakano T, Ishimoto T (2012) Design of biomaterials for bone replacement based on parameters determining bone quality. In: Sasaki K (ed) Interface oral health science 2011. Springer, New York, pp 55–65

Chapter 14
Advanced Materials Design by Controlling Transformation Temperature Using Magnetic Field

Takashi Fukuda and Tomoyuki Kakeshita

Abstract A phase diagram is an essential guide for developing new materials, and a phase boundary can be greatly influenced by a magnetic field. This chapter is devoted to introducing how a magnetic field influences the solid–solid phase transformations. The influence of a magnetic field on γ(fcc)–α(bcc) transformation in pure iron and iron based alloys is shown as prototype examples. The transformation temperature is shown to increase linearly or parabolically depending on the magnetism of the α phase. In addition, the influence of magnetocrystalline anisotropy on the transformation temperature is described by using the results of Ni_2MnGa.

Keywords Curie temperature • Ferromagnetic shape memory alloys • Magnetic anisotropy • Phase equilibrium

14.1 Introduction

In designing new materials, we frequently consult phase diagrams. Binary and ternary phase diagrams of alloys and ceramics at ambient pressure have been widely investigated, and are used for material design. In addition, much effort has been made to construct phase diagrams under pressure because it is a fundamental variable of thermodynamics; many new phases have been found under pressure. The magnetic field is also an intensive variable in thermodynamics and is expected to be widely utilized in the design of materials in the near future. However, phase diagrams under a magnetic field have not been widely studied compared with those under hydrostatic pressure.

T. Fukuda (✉) • T. Kakeshita
Division of Materials and Manufacturing Science, Graduate School of Engineering, Osaka University, 2-1 Yamadaoka, Suita, Osaka 565-0871, Japan
e-mail: fukuda@mat.eng.osaka-u.ac.jp

T. Kakeshita (ed.), *Progress in Advanced Structural and Functional Materials Design*,
DOI 10.1007/978-4-431-54064-9_14, © Springer Japan 2013

In this chapter, we will explore how the magnetic field influences the first order transformation in structural and functional materials. We first review the thermodynamic analysis of transformations under a magnetic field, and then explore the experimental results for some alloys.

14.2 Thermodynamics for Magnetic Field Dependence of Transformation Temperature

The effect of an intensive variable on the equilibrium temperature, T, for a first order transformation is principally given by the Clausius–Clapeyron equation. The equation under hydrostatic pressure, P, can be found in most books on thermodynamics [1]; it is given as

$$\frac{\mathrm{d}T}{\mathrm{d}P} = \frac{\Delta v}{\Delta s}, \tag{14.1}$$

where Δv is the volume change per mole, and Δs is the entropy change per mole associated with the phase transformation. A similar relation can be derived for the equilibrium temperature under a magnetic field as follows.

We consider a system under a magnetic field H. In order to increase the magnetization of the system by dM, the magnetic field has to do work $H{\cdot}dM$ on the system. Then, from the first law of thermodynamics, the infinitesimal change in internal energy dU should be given by

$$\mathrm{d}U = T\mathrm{d}S - p\mathrm{d}V + H\mathrm{d}M. \tag{14.2}$$

The Legendre transformation of the extensive variables to intensive variables (S to T, V to P, and M to H) in Eq. (14.2) gives us the expression for free energy G as

$$\mathrm{d}G = -S\mathrm{d}T + V\mathrm{d}P - M\mathrm{d}H \tag{14.3}$$

We write G, S, V, and M per mole as g, s, v, and m, respectively. Here, g is equal to chemical potential μ. If we consider a fixed pressure condition ($dP = 0$), then Eq. (14.3) becomes

$$(\mathrm{d}g =)\mathrm{d}\mu = -s\mathrm{d}T - m\mathrm{d}H. \tag{14.4}$$

Let us consider two phases, A and B, and four states, A1, A2, B1, and B2, on the H–T phase diagram shown in Fig. 14.1. The two states A1 and B1 are in equilibrium at (H_1, T_1); A2 and B2 are also in equilibrium at (H_2, T_2). The difference between the magnetic fields $H_2 - H_1$ is assumed to be infinitesimal ($=dH$), and similarly for the temperature difference ($T_2 - T_1 = dT$). Phase equilibrium requires that the chemical potential is equal ($\mu_{A1} = \mu_{B1}$, and $\mu_{A2} = \mu_{B2}$). Thus, $\mu_{A2} - \mu_{A1} = \mu_{B2} - \mu_{B1}$. On the other hand, from Eq. (14.4),

$$\mu_{A2} - \mu_{A1} = (\mathrm{d}\mu_A) = -s_A\mathrm{d}T - m_A\mathrm{d}H \quad \text{and} \quad \mu_{B2} - \mu_{B1} (= \mathrm{d}\mu_B) = -s_B\mathrm{d}T - m_B\mathrm{d}H.$$

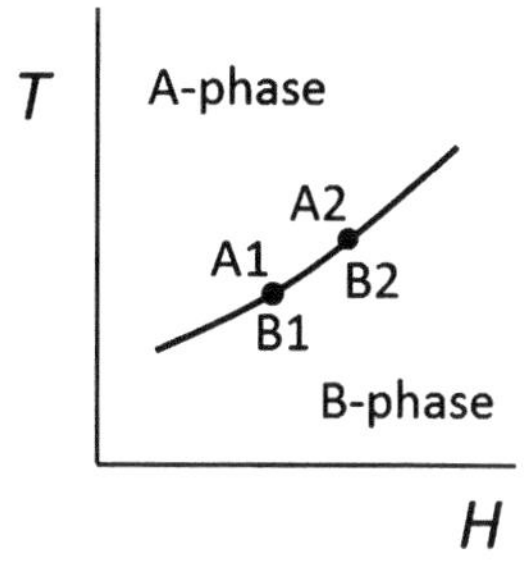

Fig. 14.1 Schematic *H–T* phase diagram composed of two phases A and B

Then, the Clausius–Clapeyron equation under a magnetic field is given by

$$\frac{\mathrm{d}T}{\mathrm{d}H} = -\frac{m_B - m_A}{s_B - s_A} = -\frac{\Delta m}{\Delta s}. \tag{14.5}$$

Equation (14.5) tells us that the gradient of the boundary between the A- and B-phases in the *T–H* phase diagram can be obtained provided that Δm and Δs are given as a function of H and T. If we assume that Δs takes a constant value, and is given by the value at $T = T_0$ under zero magnetic field, the change in the equilibrium temperature ΔT by the application of magnetic field H_1 is obtained by integrating Eq. (14.5) as

$$\Delta T = T(H = H_1) - T(H = 0) = -\frac{1}{\Delta s(T = T_0)} \int_0^{H_1} \Delta m \, \mathrm{d}H. \tag{14.6}$$

In many cases, Eq. (14.6) provides a satisfactory explanation of the magnetic field dependence of equilibrium temperature.

The first order transformation is usually associated with supercooling and superheating. That is, the transformation in the cooling process starts below the equilibrium temperature T_0, and vice versa in the heating process. When the super cooling and super heating are within several Kelvins, Eq. (14.6) gives a satisfactory explanation for the magnetic field dependence of the transformation temperature. However, if the supercooling and superheating exceeds several tens of Kelvins, we have to modify Eq. (14.6).

We derive the modified equation by introducing some assumptions. Consider that the transformation in the cooling process occurs at T_s, which is below T_0 as shown in Fig. 14.2. At this temperature, the difference in the free energy is given by $\Delta g(T_s)$. This energy difference is usually referred to as the driving force necessary for the transformation. The application of a magnetic field influences the free energy difference between the two phases. We write the difference in the free energy under the magnetic field of H_1 as Δg_{H1}. Then, by considering the work done by the magnetic field, Δg_{H1} is given by

$$\Delta g_{H_1}(T) - \Delta g(T) = -\int_0^{H_1} \Delta m \mathrm{d}H. \tag{14.7}$$

Here, we neglect the influence of the volume change by the application of the magnetic field (forced volume magnetostriction).

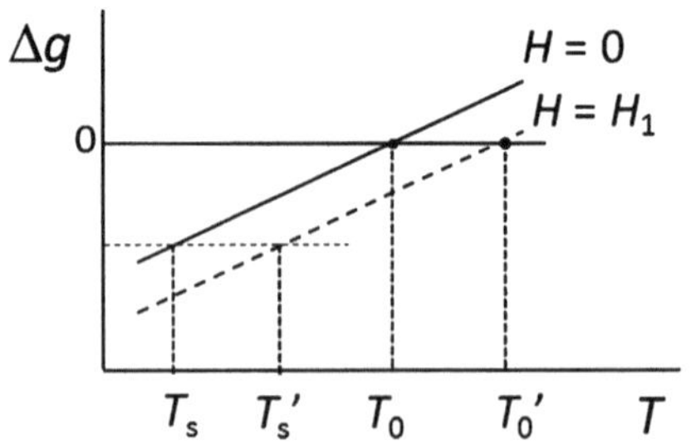

Fig. 14.2 Schematic illustration showing transformation start temperature under magnetic field

Let the transformation start temperature under the magnetic field of H_1 be T_s' and assume that the driving force at T_s' under the magnetic field is equal to $\Delta g(T_s)$. That is, we assume that the driving force is not changed by the application of the magnetic field. This assumption was originally made by Patel and Cohen to explain the stress dependence of the martensitic transformation temperature [2]. Under this assumption, we can derive the following equation to estimate the field-dependence of the transformation temperature using Eq. (14.7).

$$\Delta g(T_s) - \Delta g(T_s') = -\int_0^{H_1} \Delta m \mathrm{d}H \qquad (14.8)$$

If the change in the transformation temperature by the application of the magnetic field is small, the left hand side of the equation can be approximated as $\Delta s(T = T_s)$ multiplied by $(T_s' - T_s)$. Then, the field-dependence of the transformation temperature is given by

$$\Delta T = T_s' - T_s = -\frac{1}{\Delta s(T = T_s)} \int_0^{H_1} \Delta m \mathrm{d}H. \qquad (14.9)$$

We can calculate the field-dependence of the transformation temperature if we know the entropy change at T_s and the magnetic field dependence of Δm.

In the above consideration, we neglected the volume change caused by the application of the magnetic field. This effect becomes especially significant in Invar alloys such as Fe–Ni and Fe–Pt alloys. The details of the effect of the volume change caused by a magnetic field are discussed elsewhere [3].

14.3 Influence of Magnetic Field on γ–α Transformation in Pure Iron

Iron-based alloys, including steels, are the most valuable materials humans have ever encountered. Many of the excellent properties of iron-based alloys are the result of the γ–α transformation. In this section, we will see how the α-γ equilibrium temperature of pure iron is shifted by the application of a magnetic field, and that this behavior can be well explained by Eq. (14.6).

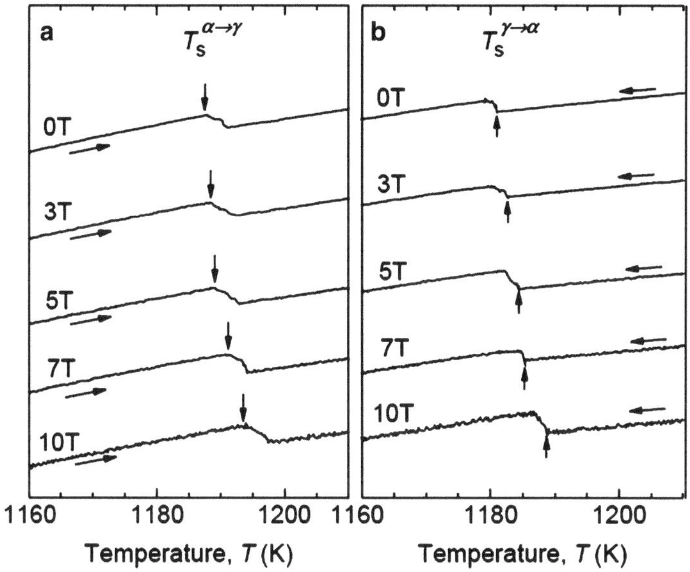

Fig. 14.3 Temperature dependence of electrical resistivity of Fe in heating (**a**) and cooling (**b**) processes under magnetic fields of 0, 3, 5, 7 and 10 T. Arrows indicate transformation-start temperatures [4]

The ground state of pure iron has a so-called BCC structure, which is referred to as the α-phase or ferrite. Pure iron exhibits an allotropic transformation at 1,183 K to the so-called FCC structure, which is referred to as the γ-phase or austenite. Both the α- and γ-phases are paramagnetic at the γ–α equilibrium temperature. However, as the α-phase is ferromagnetic below 1,044 K, we may expect the magnetic field to have a significant influence on the γ–α equilibrium temperature.

Electrical resistivity measurement is a highly effective method to detect the γ–α transformation. Figure 14.3 shows the temperature dependence of the electrical resistivity of pure iron measured in the heating (a) and cooling (b) processes under various magnetic fields [4]. The $\alpha \to \gamma$ transformation start temperature ($T_s^{\alpha\to\gamma}$) and $\gamma \to \alpha$ transformation start temperature ($T_s^{\gamma\to\alpha}$) are detected as bends in the resistivity curves as indicated by an arrow on each curve. These temperatures are summarized in Fig. 14.4. We notice in Fig. 14.4 that both $T_s^{\alpha\to\gamma}$ and $T_s^{\gamma\to\alpha}$ increase with increasing magnetic field. If we assume that the supercooling needed for the $\gamma \to \alpha$ transformation is the same as the superheating for the $\alpha \to \gamma$ transformation, the equilibrium temperature, T_0, will be given by $T_0 = (T_s^{\alpha\to\gamma} + T_s^{\gamma\to\alpha})/2$. The magnetic field dependence of T_0 thus obtained is shown in Fig. 14.5.

In the following, we will show that the field dependence of T_0 shown in Fig. 14.5 is in satisfactory agreement with that calculated by Eq. (14.6). The value of Δs under a magnetic field is approximated to the value under zero field, which is evaluated from a reported latent heat of −0.92 kJ/mol [5]. In evaluating Δm, we neglect the

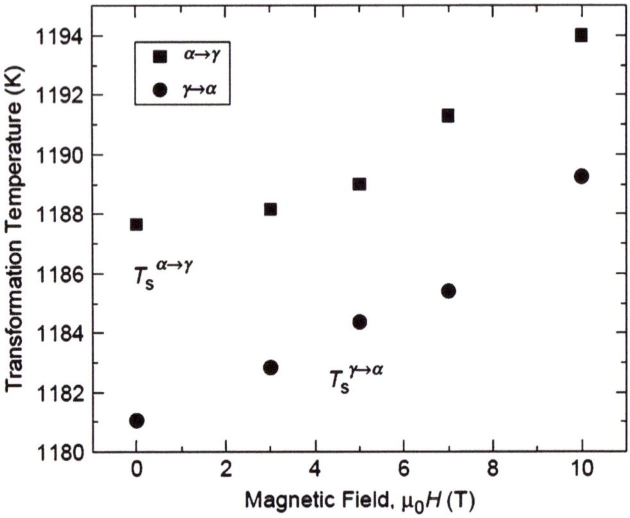

Fig. 14.4 Transformation-start temperatures of Fe plotted as a function of magnetic field [4]

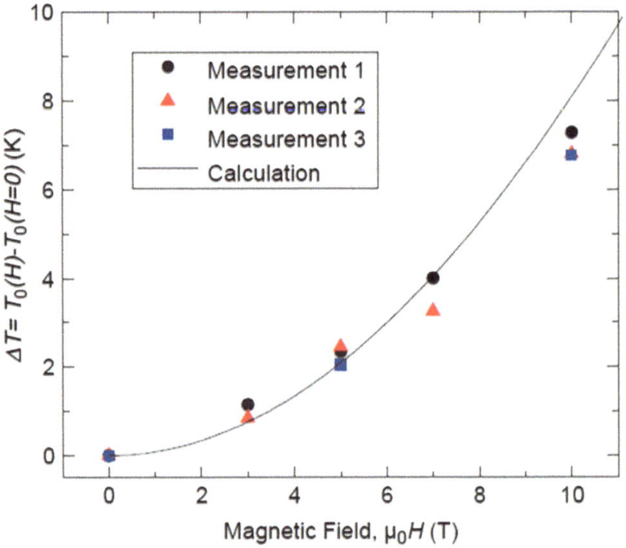

Fig. 14.5 Change in equilibrium temperature plotted as a function of magnetic field of Fe. Lines are calculated by using the Clausius–Clapeyron equation with magnetization of the α-phase derived from the mean field theory [4]

magnetization of the γ-phase m_γ, because m_γ is extremely small compared with the magnetization of the α-phase m_α. The value of m_α is calculated by using the Weiss mean-field theory, where we use the value of 2.219 μ_B/atom for the spontaneous magnetization of the α-phase at 0 K by referring to a data book [6] and assume the total angular momentum number to be 1/2, although this is a rough approximation. The calculated equilibrium temperature under a magnetic field is shown by the solid line in Fig. 14.5. As known from the figure, the calculated result is in satisfactory agreement with the experimental results. In this way, the magnetic field dependence of the γ–α equilibrium temperature in iron is well explained by Eq. (14.6).

14.4 Influence of Magnetic Field on γ–α Transformation in Fe–Rh Alloy

Among various Fe-based alloys, the Fe–Rh system is especially of interest because the Curie temperature, T_c, of the α-phase becomes higher than the $\gamma \leftrightarrow \alpha$ transformation temperatures when the Rh content exceeds a certain value while the relation reverses when the content is below it. For this reason, the field-dependence of the $\gamma \leftrightarrow \alpha$ transformation temperatures in the former case differs from that in the latter case.

Figures 14.6a and 14.7a, b show the temperature dependences of the electrical resistivity of the Fe–2Rh, Fe–5Rh, and Fe–10Rh (at.%) alloys, respectively, measured under magnetic fields of 0 T and 10 T [7]. The resistivity curve under magnetic field of 10 T is shifted upward by a constant value of $\beta = 0.3$ μΩm to separate the curves. Using Figs. 14.6 and 14.7, we determine the Curie temperature, $\gamma \rightarrow \alpha$ transformation temperature ($T_s^{\gamma \rightarrow \alpha}$), and $\alpha \rightarrow \gamma$ transformation temperature ($T_s^{\alpha \rightarrow \gamma}$).

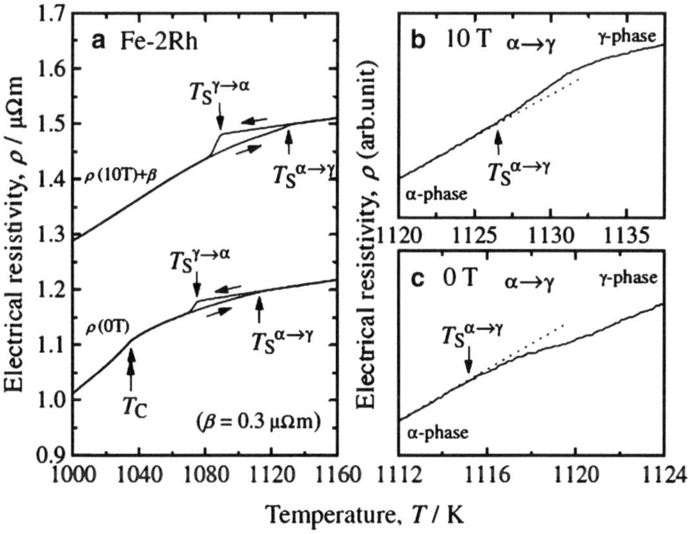

Fig. 14.6 Temperature dependence of electrical resistivity of Fe–2Rh alloy measured under magnetic fields of 0 and 10 T [7]

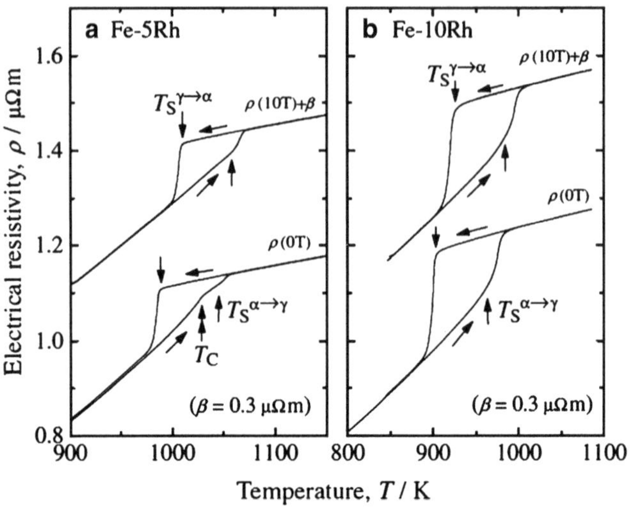

Fig. 14.7 Temperature dependences of electrical resistivity of Fe–5Rh alloy (**a**) and Fe–10Rh alloy (**b**) measured under magnetic fields of 0 and 10 T [7]

First, we determine the Curie temperature of the α-phase. The heating and cooling curves of the Fe–2Rh alloy and Fe–5Rh alloy measured under zero magnetic field exhibit bends at about 1,036 and 1,029 K, respectively, as indicated by the double arrows in Figs. 14.6a and 14.7a. These bends correspond to the Curie temperature, T_c, of the α-phase. In case of the Fe–10Rh alloy, no T_c is detected for the α-phase, but is estimated to be 1,015 K by extrapolating the T_c's of pure Fe (1,044 K), and the Fe–2Rh and Fe–5Rh alloys. Concerning the γ-phase of the present alloys, the Curie temperature is expected to be far below the $\gamma \to \alpha$ transformation temperature. Next, we determine $T_s^{\gamma\to\alpha}$. The $\gamma \to \alpha$ transformation is detected as a sharp decrease in resistivity for all of the alloys, and we show $T_s^{\gamma\to\alpha}$ with an arrow on each cooling curve. Finally, we determine $T_s^{\alpha\to\gamma}$. The resistivity heating curves of the Fe–5Rh and Fe–10Rh alloys show sharp increases in association with the $\alpha \to \gamma$ transformation. Thus, $T_s^{\alpha\to\gamma}$ is easily determined as indicated by the arrows in Fig. 14.7a, b. In case of the Fe–2Rh alloy, $T_s^{\alpha\to\gamma}$ is determined as the temperature at which the heating curve starts to deviate from a linear relation (dotted line), which is shown in Fig. 14.6b, c.

The transformation start temperatures ($T_s^{\alpha\to\gamma}$ and $T_s^{\gamma\to\alpha}$) are plotted using square marks as a function of the magnetic field in Fig. 14.8. In this figure, ΔT is the difference between the transformation start temperature under various magnetic field strengths, $T_s(H)$, and that measured under zero magnetic field $T_s(H = 0)$. As seen in the figure, $T_s^{\alpha\to\gamma}$ and $T_s^{\gamma\to\alpha}$, both increase with increasing magnetic field. Among the six panels in Fig. 14.8, it should be noted that $T_s^{\alpha\to\gamma}$ (a) and $T_s^{\gamma\to\alpha}$ (b) of the Fe–2Rh alloy and $T_s^{\alpha\to\gamma}$ (c) of the Fe–5Rh alloy are above the T_c of the respective alloy. Thus, the α-phase is paramagnetic at these transformation temperatures. In this condition, the transformation temperatures increase

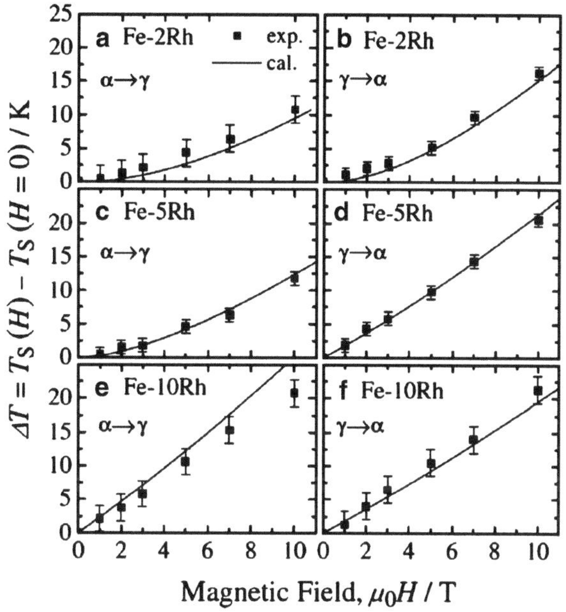

Fig. 14.8 Magnetic field dependence of transformation temperatures in Fe–2Rh, Fe–5Rh and Fe–10Rh alloys [7]

parabolically with increasing magnetic field. On the other hand, it should be noted that $T_s^{\gamma\to\alpha}$ (d) of the Fe–5Rh alloy, and $T_s^{\alpha\to\gamma}$ (e) and $T_s^{\gamma\to\alpha}$ (f) of the Fe–10Rh alloy are below the T_c of the respective alloy. Thus, the α-phase is ferromagnetic at these transformation temperatures. In this case, the transformation temperatures increase linearly with increasing magnetic field. In this way, the field-dependence of the transformation temperature for the former case (α-phase is paramagnetic) is obviously different from that of the latter case (α-phase is ferromagnetic).

Next, we discuss the magnetic field dependence of $T_s^{\alpha\to\gamma}$ and $T_s^{\gamma\to\alpha}$ using thermodynamics. As seen in Figs. 14.5 and 14.6, $T_s^{\alpha\to\gamma}$ is higher than $T_s^{\gamma\to\alpha}$ by about 50 K. This implies that $T_s^{\alpha\to\gamma}$ and $T_s^{\gamma\to\alpha}$ are both largely different from the equilibrium temperature, T_0. Thus, Eq. (14.9) should be used instead of Eq. (14.6) to explain the magnetic field dependence of the transformation temperature. The entropy change in Eq. (14.9) can be evaluated using latent heat L divided by the transformation temperature. $L(\alpha \to \gamma)$ is 1.13, 1.63, and 2.93 kJ/mol for the Fe–2Rh, Fe–5Rh and Fe–10Rh alloys, respectively. $L(\gamma \to \alpha)$ is −1.69, −3.36, and −4.43 kJ/mol for the Fe–2Rh, Fe–5Rh and Fe–10Rh alloys, respectively [7]. For all of the alloys $|L(\gamma \to \alpha)|$ is larger than $|L(\alpha \to \gamma)|$, and the difference is especially large for the Fe–5Rh alloy in which the α-phase is ferromagnetic at $T_s^{\gamma\to\alpha}$, although it is paramagnetic at $T_s^{\alpha\to\gamma}$. The value of Δm in Eq. (14.8) can be obtained by magnetization measurements and extrapolation. The solid lines in Fig. 14.7 are results that were calculated using Eq. (14.8). Obviously, the calculated results agree with the experimental results. Consequently, we may regard Eq. (14.8) as an appropriate expression for the magnetic field dependence of the transformation temperature.

Further experimental data and information on the influence of C, Ni, and Co on γ–α transformation under a magnetic field can be found in the literature [8–11].

14.5 Influence of Magnetocrystalline Anisotropy on Transformation Under Magnetic Field

In the above examples of pure iron and Fe–Rh alloys, the magnetization difference, Δm, did not change its sign under different magnetic fields. However, when the magnetocrystalline anisotropy is large, Δm could change its sign. Such a change comes to interesting behavior in the transformation temperature under magnetic field.

Let us consider that two phases A and B are in equilibrium at T_0. The spontaneous magnetization of the B-phase is higher than that of the A-phase at T_0, but the B-phase is hard to magnetize compared with the A-phase as shown in Fig. 14.9. In such a case, Δm $(= m_B - m_A)$ is negative below H_2, and positive above H_2. Let us also assume that $\Delta s(= s_B - s_A)$ is negative. Under this situation, Eq. (14.5) tells us that dT/dH has the same sign as Δm. Consequently, the transformation temperature initially decreases with increasing H, showing a minimum at $H = H_2$; then, it increases with increasing H.

The phenomenon described above is clearly seen in the M–I transformation in Ni_2MnGa. This alloy is a representative ferromagnetic shape memory alloy that exhibits a large magnetic field-induced strain [12, 13]. In this alloy, the martensite phase (M-phase, low temperature phase) has a large magnetocrystalline anisotropy. The dotted curves in Fig. 14.10 are the magnetization curves of the M-phase measured in different directions [14]. The angle, θ, indicated in the figure is the angle between the easy axis and field direction. Obviously, the M-phase is hard to magnetize as θ increases. On the other hand, the solid curves in Fig. 14.10 are the magnetization curves of the I-phase (high temperature phase). We notice that there is an intersection of magnetization curves between the M-phase and I-phase when $\theta = 45°$, $55°$, and $90°$, while Δm is always positive when $\theta = 0$.

Figure 14.11 shows the change in the M $\rightarrow$ I transformation temperature (ΔT) plotted as a function of magnetic field H. ΔT increases monotonically in (a), where Δm is always positive. On the other hand, ΔT shows a minimum when Δm changes

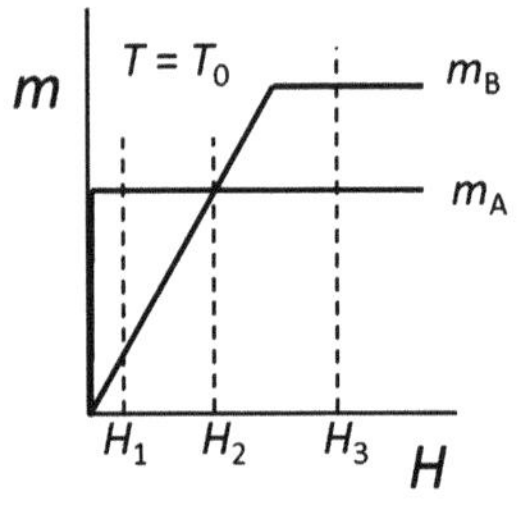

Fig. 14.9 Schematic illustration of magnetization curves of two phases (A, B) at equilibrium temperature T_0. Δm $(= m_B - m_A)$ is negative below H_2, and positive above H_2

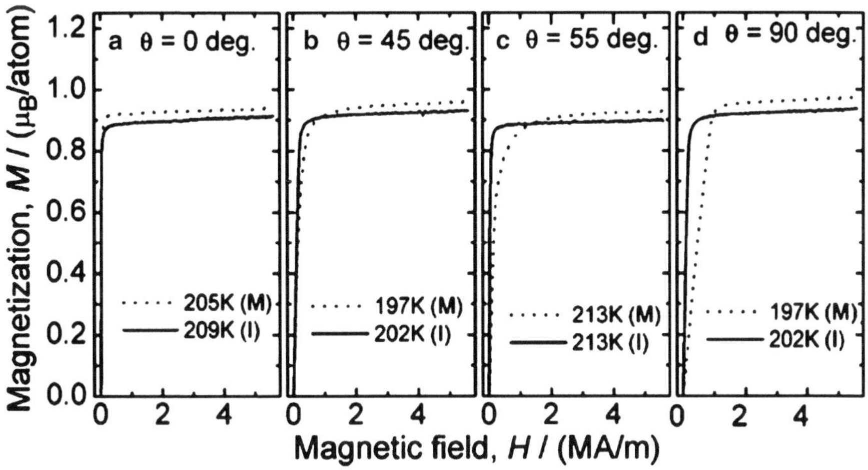

Fig. 14.10 Magnetization curves of Ni_2MnGa measured near equilibrium temperature between I-phase and M-phase [14]

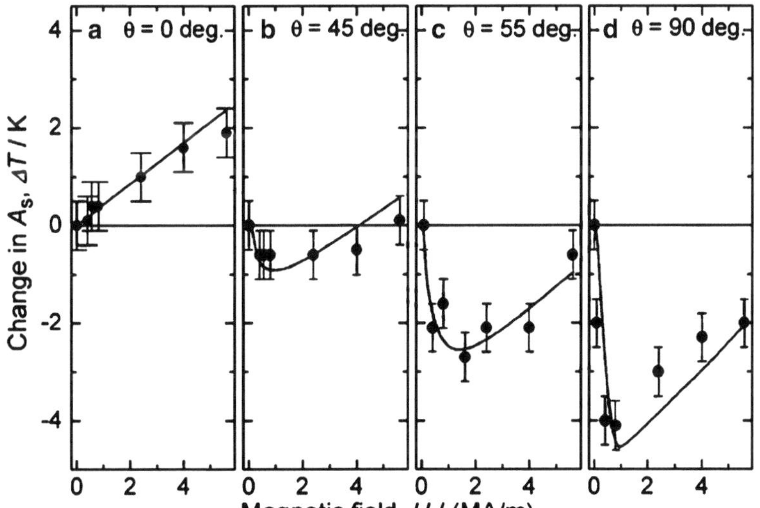

Fig. 14.11 Magnetic field dependence of M → I transformation temperature in Ni_2MnGa [14]. The *solid lines* were calculated using Eq. (14.6)

its sign. The field strength at which $\Delta m = 0$ agrees with the temperature at which ΔT shows a minimum. The solid line in Fig. 14.11 was calculated using Eq. (14.6). The calculated results are in satisfactory agreement with experimental results.

In summary, the magnetic field dependence of the first order transformation temperature is explained by the Clausius–Clapeyron equation (Eq. (14.5)) and its modified form (Eq. (14.8)).

Acknowledgments The authors appreciate the financial support from MEXT, Japan through the Global COE Program "Center of Excellence for Advanced Structural and Functional Materials Design."

References

1. Callen HB (1985) Thermodynamics and an introduction to thermostatistics. Wiley, New Jersey
2. Patel JR, Cohen M (1953) Criterion for the action of applied stress in the martensitic transformation. Acta Metall 1:532
3. Kakeshita T, Saburi T, Kindo K, Endo S (1999) Martensitic transformations in some ferrous and non-ferrous alloys under magnetic field and hydrostatic pressure. Phase Transitions 70:65
4. Kakeshita T, Fukuda T (2006) Magnetic field-control of microstructure and function of materials exhibiting solid-solid phase transformation. Sci Technol Adv Mater 7:350
5. Normanton AS, Bloomfield PE, Sale FR, Argent BB (1975) Calorimetric study of iron-cobalt alloys. Met Sci 9:510
6. Poerschke R (ed) (1991) Data in science and technology, magnetic properties of metals, d-elements, alloys and compounds. Springer, Berlin
7. Farjami S, Yuge M, Fukuda T, Terai T, Kakeshita T (2007) Effect of magnetic field on γ–α transformations in Fe–Rh alloys. Mater Trans 48:2821
8. Garacin T, Rivoirard S, Beaugnon E (2011) Thermodynamic analysis using experimental magnetization date of the austenite/ferrite phase transformation in Fe–xNi alloys ($x = 0$, 2, 4 wt%) in a strong magnetic field. J Phys D Appl Phys 44:015001
9. Hao X, Ohtsuka H (2006) Effect of high magnetic field on transformation temperatures in Fe based alloys. ISIJ Int 46:1271
10. Guo H, Enomoto M (2000) Influence of magnetic field on α/γ equilibrium in Fe–C(−X) alloys. Mater Trans 41:911
11. Fukuda T, Yuge M, Lee J-H, Terai T, Kakeshita T (2006) Effect of magnetic field on γ–α transformation temperature in Fe–Co alloys. ISIJ Int 46(1267)
12. Planes A, Manosa L, Saxena A (eds) (2006) Magnetism and structure in functional materials, Springer series in materials science, vol 79
13. Chernenko VA, Barandiaran JM (eds) (2010) Ferromagnetic shape memory alloys II. Trans Tech Publications, Zurich
14. Fukuda T, Maeda H, Yasui M, Kakeshita T (2009) Influence of magnetocrystalline anisotropy on martensitic transformation under magnetic field on single-crystalline Ni_2MnGa. Scr Mater 60:261

Chapter 15
Advanced Materials Design for Fe-Based Shape Memory Alloys Through Structural Control

Hiroyuki Y. Yasuda

Abstract Materials properties of crystalline materials are closely related to their microstructure and therefore, microstructural control is necessitated to get desirable properties. This chapter deals with a new approach to microstructural control in crystalline materials. In particular, an advanced microstructural control to realize pseudoelasticity of Fe-based intermetallic compounds is described.

Keywords Dislocation • Intermetallic compound • Microstructural control • Ordered domain • Shape memory alloys

15.1 Introduction

Microstructural control is one of the effective ways used to improve material properties such as mechanical, electrical, magnetic and chemical properties. For example, in steels, large variety of microstructure such as ferrite, austenite, martensite and bainite leads to the variation in mechanical properties and therefore, the steels can be tailored for specific applications [1]. It is also well known that a grain refinement generally leads to an increase in yield stress in crystalline materials through the Hall–Petch law [2, 3]. In addition, the magnetic properties of electrical steels and Nd–Fe–B permanent magnets are closely related to the crystallographic texture [4, 5]. Recently, microstructural control on nano- and meso-scales has been extensively examined for further improvement of materials properties [6]. Moreover, even lattice defects such as point defects and dislocations have been studied from the viewpoint of microstructural control [7, 8]. In this chapter, one of the examples of advanced microstructural control to realize pseudoelastic Fe-based intermetallic compounds is described [9–11].

H.Y. Yasuda (✉)
Division of Materials and Manufacturing Science, Graduate School of Engineering,
Osaka University, 2-1 Yamadaoka, Suita, Osaka 565-0871, Japan
e-mail: hyyasuda@mat.eng.osaka-u.ac.jp

T. Kakeshita (ed.), *Progress in Advanced Structural and Functional Materials Design*, 181
DOI 10.1007/978-4-431-54064-9_15, © Springer Japan 2013

15.2 Pseudoelasticity in Fe-Based Intermetallic Compounds

Shape memory alloys exhibit two fascinating phenomena: shape memory effect and pseudoelasticity (Fig. 15.1) [12]. In the case of shape memory effect, strain can be recovered by heating followed by unloading. In contrast, pseudoelasticity is a phenomenon by which large strain is recovered during unloading without the need for a change in temperature. In general, the shape memory effect and pseudoelasticity are based on thermoelastic martensitic transformation as shown in Fig. 15.1b [12]. If a parent phase is cooled to a temperature below the martensite-finish temperature, the martensite phase containing self-accommodated variants is formed. The self accommodation of variants occurs to minimize the shape change of the specimen. The martensite phase deforms by the movement of the variant interface to accommodate the applied stress. On the other hand, if the deformed martensite is heated to a temperature above austenite-finish temperature, the shape of the specimen is recovered by the reverse transformation resulting in the shape memory effect. In the case of pseudoelasticity, stress-induced martensitic transformation takes place during loading. On the other hand, the reverse transformation occurs during unloading, which leads to pseudoelasticity. This phenomenon is called "transformation pseudoelasticity". Many non-ferrous alloys exhibit the shape memory effect and pseudoelasticity, such as Ti–Ni and Cu–Al–Ni alloys [12]. In Fe-based alloys, however, pseudoelasticity rarely takes place since the martensites are non-thermoelastic with large lattice dilatation during the transformation. But recently, Fe_3Al intermetallic compounds with the $D0_3$ structure was found to exhibit large pseudoelasticity [9, 10, 13]. In Fe_3Al, however, martensitic transformation never occurs in the crystals. The peculiar motion of a dislocation

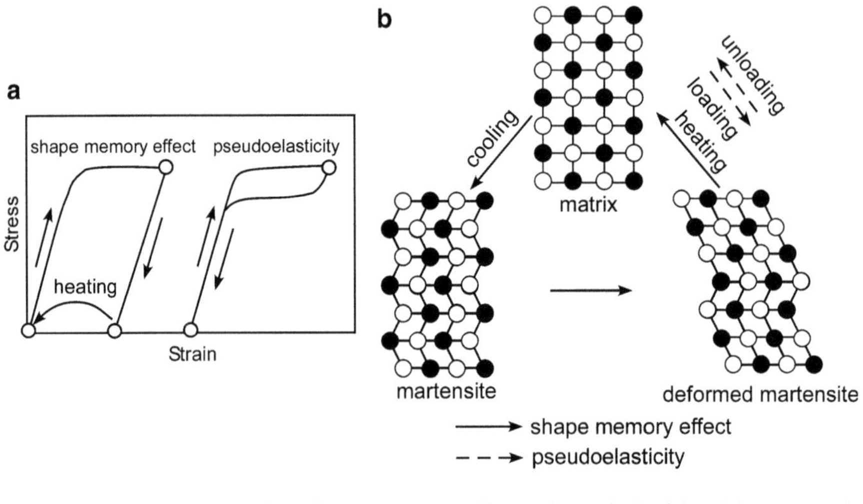

Fig. 15.1 Schematic illustration of shape memory effect and pseudoelasticity; (**a**) stress–strain curves, (**b**) mechanism of shape memory effect and pseudoelasticity based on thermoelastic martensitic transformation

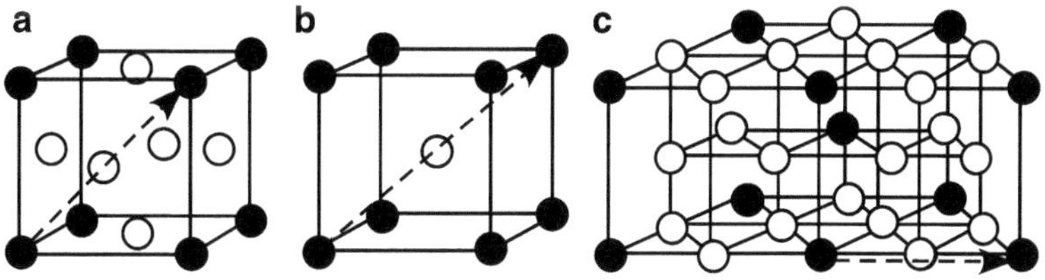

Fig. 15.2 Unit cells of the $L1_2$ (**a**), B2 (**b**) and $D0_{19}$ (**c**) superlattice structures based on f.c.c., b.c. c. and h.c.p. lattices, respectively. The Burgers vectors of the structures are indicated by a *dashed arrow*

dragging an antiphase boundary (APB) is responsible for the pseudoelasticity in Fe_3Al [9, 10, 13]. Thus, this phenomenon is called "APB pseudoelasticity". Moreover, control of the ordered domain structure is an effective method for improving the pseudoelastic properties of Fe_3Al alloys [9]. In the following sections, the dislocation configurations and ordered domain structures of intermetallic compounds are described. Then, the mechanism of pseudoelasticity in Fe_3Al alloys and the method for improving their pseudoelastic properties via an advanced microstructural control are explained.

15.2.1 Dislocation Structure of Intermetallic Compounds

An intermetallic compound is composed of regularly arranged two or more types of metal atoms [14]. The strong bond between the different metal atoms sometimes leads to a high melting point and high strength. Thus, some intermetallic compounds have been considered as potential candidates for high temperature structural materials. In the 1980s, extensive efforts were devoted to understanding the deformation behaviour of intermetallic compounds [14]. In particular, dislocations in intermetallic compounds, which are carriers of plastic deformation, have been studied either through a theoretical approach or by direct observation using a transmission electron microscope (TEM), especially for the compounds with the superlattice structure based on the f. c. c., b. c. c. and h. c. p. structures. Figure 15.2 shows the unit cells of the $L1_2$, B2 and $D0_{19}$ superstructures based on f. c. c., b. c. c. and h. c. p. structures, respectively. The Burgers vector of a dislocation is a translation vector of a crystal lattice representing the displacement of the material that creates the dislocation. The Burgers vectors of superlattice dislocations in the $L1_2$, B2 and $D0_{19}$superlattice structures are $\langle 1\ 1\ 0\rangle$, $\langle 1\ 1\ 1\rangle$ and 1/3 $\langle 11\bar{2}0\rangle$, two times larger than those of the f. c. c., b. c. c. and h. c. p. structures, respectively, owing to the ordered arrangements of the different metal atoms. The elastic energy around a dislocation is nearly proportional to the square of the Burgers vector. Therefore, in order to decrease the elastic energy, a superdislocation is generally dissociated into superpartial dislocations bound by an APB. The characteristic dislocation dissociation with the APB sometimes induces

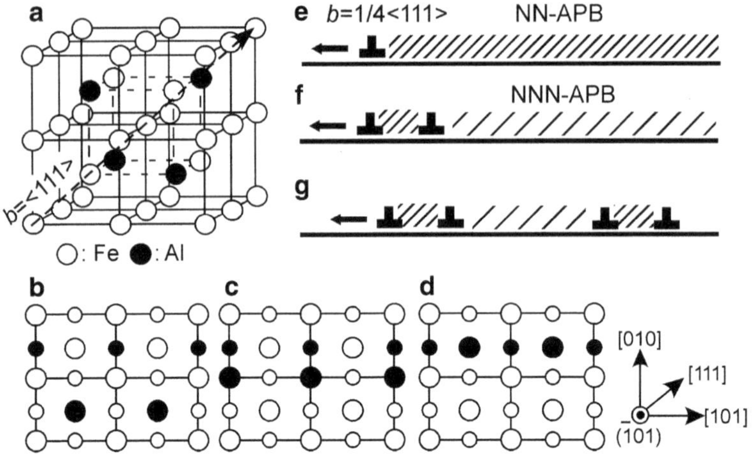

Fig. 15.3 Unit cell (**a**), atomic arrangement on (1 0 1) plane (**b–d**) and three types of dislocation dissociation (**e–g**) in $D0_3$-ordered Fe_3Al; (**b**) the perfect atomic arrangement, (**c**) NN-APB and (**d**) NNN-APB

peculiar material properties. For instance, the yield stress of Ni_3Al alloys with the $L1_2$ structure are known to demonstrate a positive temperature dependence, which is closely related to the difference in the APB energy between {1 1 1} and {0 0 1} planes [15]. As a consequence, Ni-based superalloys containing the Ni_3Al phase has been used for a turbine blade in aircraft engines.

Fe_3Al is an intermetallic compound with the $D0_3$ structure based on the b. c. c. lattice as shown in Fig. 15.3 [16]. The Burgers vector of a superdislocation is $\langle 1\ 1\ 1 \rangle$, which is four times larger than that in b. c. c. metals (Fig. 15.3a). In general, the superdislocation is dissociated into four 1/4 $\langle 1\ 1\ 1 \rangle$ superpartial dislocations bound by two types of APBs (Fig. 15.3g): nearest-neighbour (NN)-APB (Fig. 15.3c) and next-nearest-neighbour (NNN)-APB (Fig. 15.3d). In Fe-rich Fe_3Al single crystals, however, 1/4 $\langle 1\ 1\ 1 \rangle$ superpartial dislocations move independently dragging the NN-APB as shown in Fig. 15.3e, which leads to large pseudoelasticity in the alloys, as described in 15.2.3 [9, 10, 13]. Moreover, the dislocation configuration is closely related to the ordered domain structure in the $D0_3$ phase as described in Sects 15.2.2 and 15.2.4.

15.2.2 *Ordered Domain Structure*

An ordered domain structure is generally observed in weakly ordered alloys such as Cu_3Au ($L1_2$) [17], CuZn (B2) [18], Fe_3Al ($D0_3$) [16] and Ti_3Al ($D0_{19}$) [19]. In general, an ordered phase nucleates from the disordered region and the nuclei impinge on each other, resulting in the formation of an ordered domain structure.

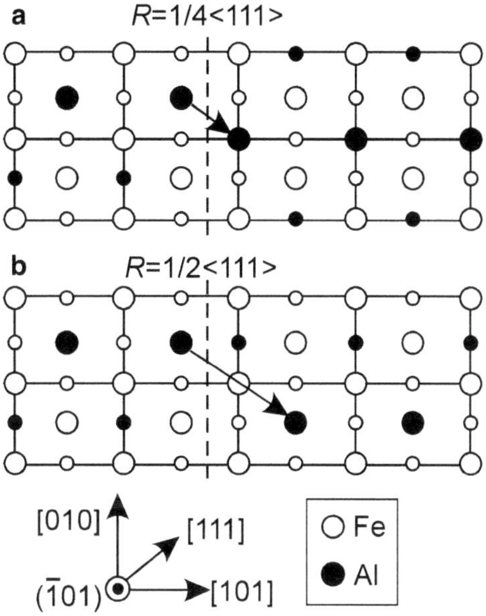

Fig. 15.4 Atomic arrangement near ordered domain boundaries in the $D0_3$ phase; (**a**) $R = 1/4\ \langle 1\ 1\ 1\rangle$ and (**b**) $R = 1/2\ \langle 1\ 1\ 1\rangle$

Figure 15.4 shows a schematic drawing of the atomic arrangement near the ordered domain boundaries in the $D0_3$-ordered Fe_3Al phase. The atomic arrangement is characterized by a displacement vector (R). The $D0_3$ phase has two types of ordered domain boundaries: $R = 1/4\ \langle 1\ 1\ 1\rangle$ (Fig. 15.4a) and $1/2\ \langle 1\ 1\ 1\rangle$ (Fig. 15.4b). It is also noted that the ordered domains and their boundaries (i.e. the ordered domain boundaries) can be observed using the TEM with a superlattice reflection (g). The domain boundaries with $R = 1/4\ \langle 1\ 1\ 1\rangle$ are visible with both $g = 111$ and $g = 020$ while those with $R = 1/2\ \langle 1\ 1\ 1\rangle$ are out of contrast with $g = 020$. In some ordered alloys such as Cu_3Au [17] and Ti_3Al [19], ordered domain boundaries can be a barrier to the dislocation motion, which leads to extreme hardening.

15.2.3 Pseudoelasticity in Fe_3Al Single Crystals

As mentioned above, Fe-rich Fe_3Al single crystals with the $D0_3$ structure demonstrate significant pseudoelasticity though martensitic transformation never occurs in the crystals [9, 10, 13]. Figure 15.5a shows a shear stress–strain curve of Fe–23.0 at. % Al single crystals deformed at room temperature. A plastic strain of 5.0 % is fully recovered during unloading, which is comparable with that of Ti–Ni shape memory alloys. The pseudoelasticity in Fe_3Al single crystals is based on the motion of $1/4\ \langle 1\ 1\ 1\rangle$ superpartial dislocation dragging the NN-APB. Let us consider the stress acting on $1/4\ \langle 1\ 1\ 1\rangle$ superpartial dislocations in the course of

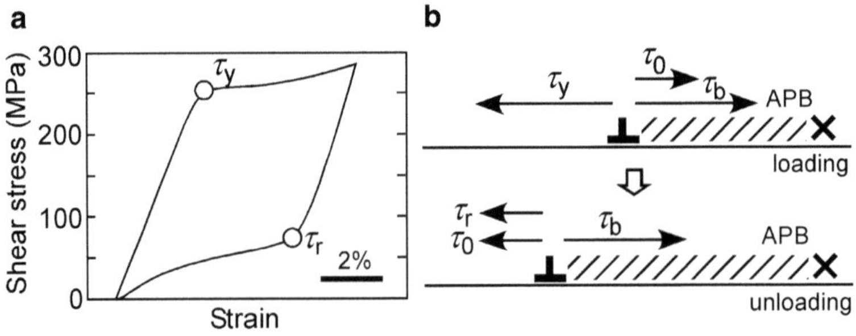

Fig. 15.5 (**a**) A shear stress–strain curve of Fe–23.0 at.% Al single crystals compressed with ⟨1 4 9⟩ orientation at room temperature, (**b**) stress acting on 1/4 ⟨1 1 1⟩ superpartial dislocations during loading and unloading

pseudoelasticity. Three types of stresses act on the dislocations: external stresses (τ_y and τ_r shown in Fig. 15.5a), a frictional stress of 1/4 ⟨1 1 1⟩ superpartial dislocation (τ_0) and an APB back stress (τ_{APB}) [9, 10, 13]. The stress balance during loading and unloading is shown in Fig. 15.5b. The following simultaneous equations hold true during loading and unloading:

$$\tau_y = \tau_0 + \tau_b, \quad \tau_r + \tau_0 = \tau_b \tag{15.1}$$

τ_y and τ_r can be obtained from the curve shown in Fig. 15.5a and therefore, τ_0 and τ_b can be calculated by solving Eq. (15.1). At 23.0 at.% Al, τ_0 and τ_b are calculated to be 73 MPa and 177 MPa, respectively [9]. Since τ_b is much higher than τ_0, 1/4 ⟨1 1 1⟩ superpartial dislocations are likely to be pulled back by the NN-APB during unloading. τ_b can also be given by [20],

$$\tau_b = \frac{\gamma_{NN}}{b} \tag{15.2}$$

where γ_{NN} is the energy of the NN-APB and b is the magnitude of 1/4 ⟨1 1 1⟩. τ_b obtained from Eq. (15.1) is similar to that from Eq. (15.2). This strongly suggests that the motion of 1/4 ⟨1 1 1⟩ superpartial dislocations dragging the NN-APB is responsible for the pseudoelasticity. It should also be noted that Fe_3Ga single crystals with the $D0_3$ structure also exhibit the APB pseudoelasticity [21].

The pseudoelastic behaviour of Fe_3Al single crystals depends strongly on Al concentration as shown in Fig. 15.6 [10]. The recovery ratio, r is a ratio of recovery strain to maximum plastic strain. In general, a parameter characterizing intermetallic compounds shows a maximum or a minimum around the stoichiometric composition [14]. However, the r shows a maximum at 23.0 at.% Al and decreases with increasing deviation from the Al concentration. The dependence of r on Al concentration is closely related to the ordered domain structure developed in the $D0_3$ phase as described in the next section.

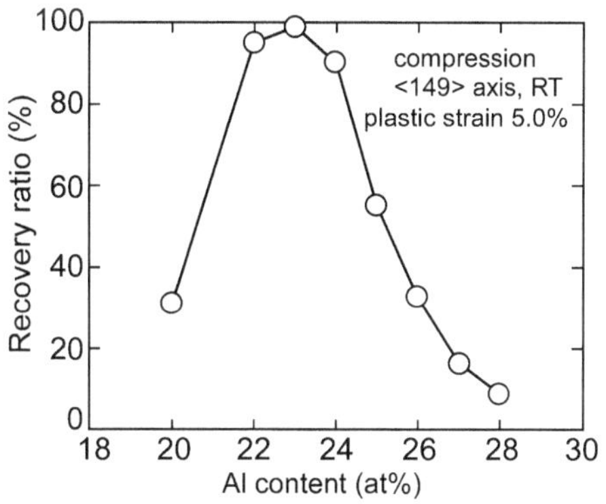

Fig. 15.6 Variation in recovery ratio with Al concentration in Fe_3Al single crystals compressed with $\langle 1\ 4\ 9 \rangle$ orientation to a plastic strain of 5.0 % at room temperature

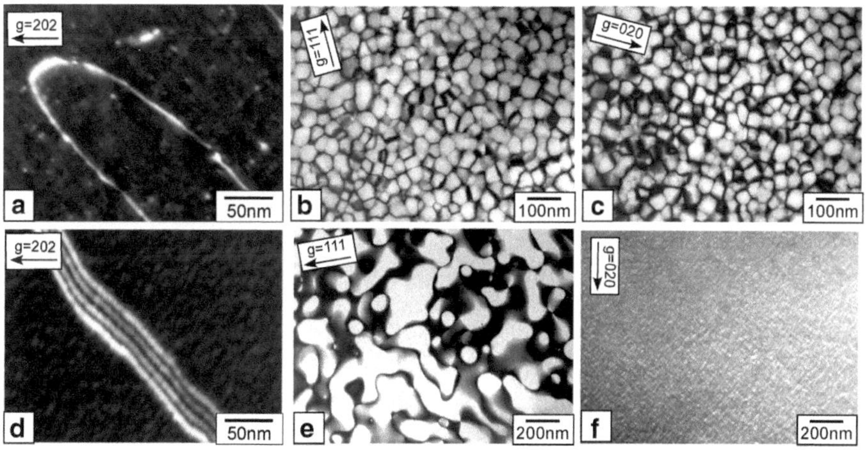

Fig. 15.7 Relationship between dislocation configuration (**a**), (**d**) and ordered domain structure (**b**), (**c**), (**e**), (**f**) in Fe_3Al single crystals compressed with $\langle 1\ 4\ 9 \rangle$ orientation to a plastic strain of 5.0 % at room temperature. (**a–c**) Fe–23.0 at.% Al, (**d–f**) Fe–28.0 at.% Al. (**b**), (**e**) $g = 111$, (**c**), (**f**) $g = 020$. Note that the domain boundaries with $R = 1/2 \langle 1\ 1\ 1 \rangle$ are invisible in (**c**), (**f**)

15.2.4 Controlling Ordered Domain Structure for Pseudoelasticity

The pseudoelastic behaviour of Fe_3Al single crystals depends strongly on Al concentration [10]. This is because the dislocation structure and the ordered domain structure vary with Al concentration. Figure 15.7 shows the relationship between the dislocation configuration and the ordered domain structure in Fe–23.0 at.% Al

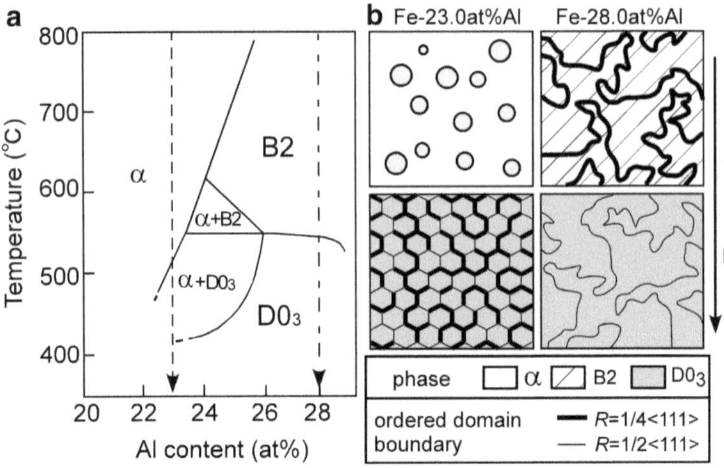

Fig. 15.8 Fe–Al phase diagram (**a**) and ordering process of Fe_3Al alloys (**b**)

and Fe–28.0 at.% Al single crystals. At 23.0 at.% Al, 1/4 $\langle 1\ 1\ 1\rangle$ superpartial dislocations move individually dragging the NN-APB, as shown in Fig. 15.7a. On the other hand, during unloading, the NN-APB pulls back 1/4 $\langle 1\ 1\ 1\rangle$ superpartial dislocations due to its tension (τ_b in Eq. (15.1)), resulting in the pseudoelasticity. In contrast, four 1/4 $\langle 1\ 1\ 1\rangle$ superpartial dislocations bound by the NN-APB and NNN-APB move in a group in Fe–28.0 at.% Al single crystals (Fig. 15.7d). In this case, no APB is left behind the dislocations and therefore, the pseudoelasticity never takes place at 28.0 at.% Al. The dislocation configuration reflects the ordered domain structure. At 23.0 at.% Al, a fine ordered domain structure develops in the $D0_3$ phase while the domain boundaries with $R = 1/4$ $\langle 1\ 1\ 1\rangle$ and 1/2 $\langle 1\ 1\ 1\rangle$ can be densely observed (Fig. 15.7b, c). In contrast, there exists coarse domain structure and the domain boundaries with $R = 1/4\ \langle 1\ 1\ 1\rangle$ are rarely observed at 28.0 at.% Al, as shown in Fig. 15.7e, f. The difference in the ordered domain structure between Fe–23.0 at.% Al and Fe–28.0 at.% Al arise from the ordering process, as shown in Fig. 15.8. At 23.0 at.% Al, the $D0_3$ phase nucleates from the disordered α matrix and the nuclei impinge on each other resulting in the formation of the domain boundaries with $R = 1/4\ \langle 1\ 1\ 1\rangle$ and 1/2 $\langle 1\ 1\ 1\rangle$. On the other hand, at 28.0 at.% Al, the formation of the B2 phase occurs prior to that of the $D0_3$ phase. Since the B2 ordering occurs at high temperatures, the ordered domains surrounded by the boundaries with $R = 1/4\ \langle 1\ 1\ 1\rangle$ become coarse. During the B2-$D0_3$ phase transition, the domain boundaries with $R = 1/4$ $\langle 1\ 1\ 1\rangle$ in the $D0_3$ phase are inherited from the B2 phase. Therefore, the number of boundaries with $R = 1/4\ \langle 1\ 1\ 1\rangle$ is small at 28.0 at.% Al.

The ordered domain structure strongly affects the dislocation motion in Fe_3Al single crystals [9, 10]. Figure 15.9a shows 1/4 $\langle 1\ 1\ 1\rangle$ superpartial dislocations

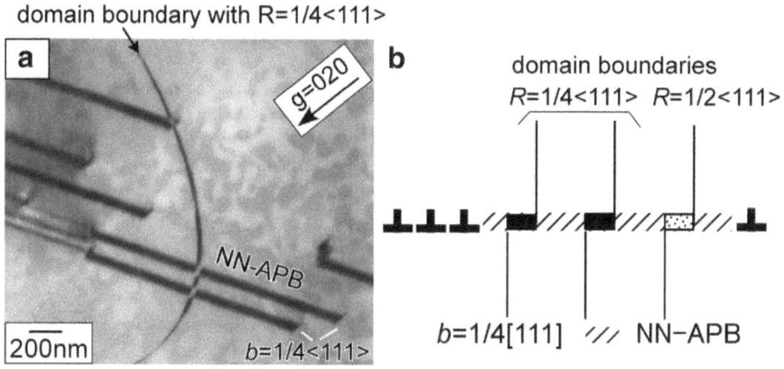

Fig. 15.9 (**a**) A TEM micrograph showing 1/4 ⟨1 1 1⟩ superpartial dislocation passing through an ordered domain boundary with $R = 1/4\ \langle 1\ 1\ 1\rangle$. (**b**) A schematic drawing of intersection between 1/4 ⟨1 1 1⟩ superpartial dislocation and the ordered domain boundaries

passing through the ordered domain boundary with $R = 1/4\ \langle 1\ 1\ 1\rangle$. The leading 1/4 ⟨1 1 1⟩ superpartial dislocations can pass through the boundary but the trailing superpartial dislocations are blocked by the boundary. When 1/4 ⟨1 1 1⟩ superpartial dislocation dragging the NN-APB cut the domain boundaries, a step-like APB is created at the intersection, as shown in Fig. 15.9b. This step-like APB has high energy because of its complicated atomic arrangement [9]. Thus, in order to decrease the total energy, the passage of the trailing superpartials is suppressed by the domain boundaries with $R = 1/4\ \langle 1\ 1\ 1\rangle$, which leads to the individual motion of 1/4 ⟨1 1 1⟩ superpartial dislocations dragging the NN-APB and the resultant pseudoelasticity. At 23.0 at.% Al, there are numerous domain boundaries with $R = 1/4\ \langle 1\ 1\ 1\rangle$, which is favourable for inducing the pseudoelasticity. In contrast, at 28.0 at.% Al, the domain boundaries with $R = 1/4\ \langle 1\ 1\ 1\rangle$ are hardly formed during the ordering process and consequently, the four superpartial dislocations move in a group. Thus, the dislocation configuration and the pseudoelastic behaviour in Fe_3Al single crystals depend strongly on Al concentration and the ordered domain structure.

Further improvement of the pseudoelasticity of Fe_3Al single crystals can be realized by controlling the ordered domain structure in the $D0_3$ phase [9]. If Fe–23.0 at.% Al alloys are cooled slowly from 1,073 K at a cooling rate of 1 K/h, a bimodal ordered domain structure composed of tiny and coarse domains is formed as shown in Fig. 15.10. In this case, the Fe atoms are separated from the $D0_3$ phase at an early stage of slow cooling and consequently, coarse $D0_3$ domains are surrounded by the disordered α phase. Furthermore, at the late stage of cooling, a tiny $D0_3$ phase precipitates from the disordered α region along the coarse domains. The fine $D0_3$-ordered domain structure around the coarse domains accelerates the individual motion of 1/4 ⟨1 1 1⟩ superpartial dislocations, which is favourable for the pseudoelasticity [9].

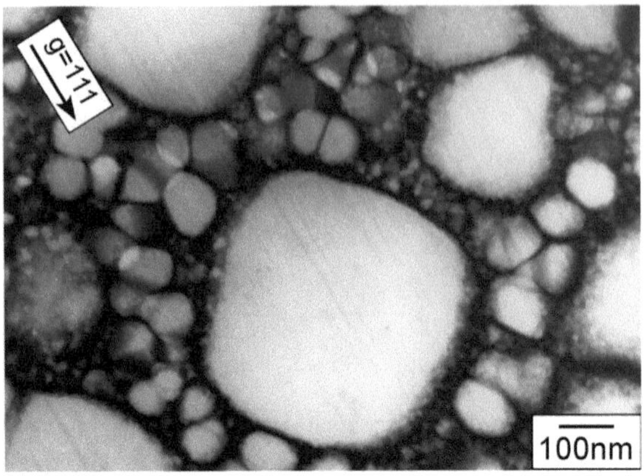

Fig. 15.10 A bimodal ordered domain structure developed in Fe–23.0 at.% Al alloys cooled from 1,073 K at a cooling rate of 1 K/h

15.3 Summary

This chapter highlights a new approach to microstructural control in crystalline materials. In particular, pseudoelasticity can be realized in Fe-based intermetallic compounds by controlling their nano-scale ordered domain structure. The mechanism of the pseudoelasticity in Fe_3Al alloys is rather different from that in conventional shape memory alloys; the peculiar dislocation motion induced by the microstructure is responsible for the pseudoelasticity in the crystals. Thus, the advanced microstructural control provides a new method for producing crystalline materials with fascinating properties.

Acknowledgments This work was supported by a Grant-in Aid for Scientific Research from the Ministry of Education, Culture, Sports, Science and Technology (MEXT), Japan. This study was supported by the Priority Assistance for the Formation of Worldwide Renowned Centers of Research—The Global COE Program (Project: Center of Excellence for Advanced Structural and Functional Materials Design) from the MEXT, Japan. The author is grateful to the support and collaboration with Y. Umakoshi (Osaka University, Japan), J. Th. M. De Hosson, P. M. Bronsveld (University of Groningen, the Netherlands), Y. Adachi (Kagoshima University, Japan), and S. Harjo (Japan Proton Accelerator Research Complex, Japan).

References

1. Bhadeshia HKDH, Honeycombe R (2006) Steels: microstructure and properties, 3rd edn. Butterworth-Heinemann, Oxford
2. Hall EO (1951) The deformation and ageing of mild steel: III. Discussion and results. Proc Phys Soc Lond 64:747–753
3. Petch NJ (1953) The cleavage strength of polycrystals. J Iron Steel Inst 174:25–28
4. Harase J, Shimizu R (1990) Texture evolution by grain growth in the presence of MnS and AIN precipitates in Fe-3% Si alloy. Acta Metall Mater 38:1395–1403

5. Hirosawa S (2004) Development of industrial nanocomposite permanent magnets: a review. Trans Magn Soc Jpn 4:101–112
6. Gleiter H (2001) Nanostructured materials: basic concepts and microstructure. Acta Mater 48:1–29
7. Yoshimi K, Kobayashi T, Yamauchi A, Haraguchi T, Hanada S (2005) Surface mesostructure change of B2-type FeAl single crystals by condensation of supersaturated thermal vacancies. Philos Mag 85:331–344
8. Nakamura A, Matsunaga K, Tohma J, Yamamoto T, Ikuhara Y (2003) Conducting nanowires in insulating ceramics. Nat Mater 2:453–456
9. Yasuda HY, Nakano K, Nakajima T, Ueda M, Umakoshi Y (2003) Effect of ordering process on giant pseudoelasticity in Fe_3Al single crystals. Acta Mater 51:5101–5112
10. Yasuda HY, Nakajima T, Nakano K, Yamaoka K, Ueda M, Umakoshi Y (2005) Effect of Al concentration on giant pseudoelasticity in Fe_3Al single crystals. Acta Mater 53:5343–5351
11. Yasuda HY, Murakami S, Umakoshi Y (2006) Effect of heat treatment on pseudoelasticity in Fe–25.0 at.% Al single crystals. Intermetallics 14:1221–1225
12. Otsuka K, Wayman CM (1998) Shape memory materials. Cambridge University Press, Cambridge
13. Kubin LP, Fourdeux A, Guedou JY, Rieu J (1982) Pseudoelasticity and slip reversibility in $D0_3$-ordered Fe–Al single crystals by in situ experiments. Philos Mag A 46:357–378
14. Yamaguchi M, Umakoshi Y (1990) The deformation behaviour of intermetallic superlattice compounds. Prog Mater Sci 34:1–148
15. Paidar V, Pope DP, Vitek V (1984) A theory of the anomalous yield behavior in $L1_2$ ordered alloys. Acta Metall 32:435–448
16. Marcinkowski MJ, Brown N (1961) Theory and direct observation of dislocations in the Fe_3Al superlattices. Acta Metall 9:764–786
17. Ardley GW (1954) On the effect of ordering upon the strength of Cu_3Au. Acta Metall 3:525–532
18. Brown N (1959) The cause of the strengthening in quenched beta brass. Acta Metall 7:210–215
19. Koizumi Y, Minamino Y, Nakano T, Umakoshi Y (2008) Effects of antiphase domains on dislocation motion in Ti_3Al single crystals deformed by prism slip. Philos Mag 88:465–488
20. Leamy HJ, Kayser FX (1969) The compressive deformation behavior of long range ordered polycrystalline iron-aluminium alloys. Phys Status Solidi 34:765–780
21. Yasuda HY, Aoki M, Umakoshi Y (2007) Effect of ordering process on pseudoelasticity in Fe_3Ga single crystals. Acta Mater 55:2407–2415

Part III
Advanced Materials Research Project for Functional Applications

Chapter 16
Fabrication of Photonic Crystals by Stereolithography Technique

Soshu Kirihara

Abstract Photonic crystals are periodically arranged structures of dielectric media. These structures have photonic band gaps that do not permit the propagation of electromagnetic waves through them. Localized modes appear in the photonic band gap when the periodicity of photonic crystals is varied locally by introducing a defect. Such localization of electromagnetic waves can be employed in various novel devices, e.g., resonators, waveguides, and antennas. Three-dimensional (3D) photonic crystals with a diamond structure are regarded as ideal because they can prohibit the propagation of electromagnetic waves in all directions in the band gap. This chapter presents a novel technique for fabricating microphotonic crystals. Micrometer-order diamond structures were fabricated successfully by stereolithography, a computer aided designing and manufacturing (CAD/CAM) process, to demonstrate electromagnetic wave control in terahertz frequency ranges. Terahertz waves have received considerable attention and have been investigated widely owing to their interesting features applicable to various fields such as materials, communication, medicine, and biology.

Keywords Photonic crystal • Electromagnetic band gap • Micro stereolithography

16.1 Photonic Crystal

Photonic crystals with periodically arranged dielectric structures can show forbidden gaps in the transmission spectra of electromagnetic waves propagating through them [1, 2]. By Bragg diffraction, these artificial crystals can completely reflect light or microwaves incident at wavelengths comparable to lattice spacings, as shown in Fig. 16.1. Two different standing waves oscillating in the air and in the

S. Kirihara (✉)
Joining and Welding Research Institute, Osaka University, 11-1 Mihogaoka, Ibaraki, Osaka 567-0047, Japan
e-mail: kirihara@jwri.osaka-u.ac.jp

T. Kakeshita (ed.), *Progress in Advanced Structural and Functional Materials Design*, DOI 10.1007/978-4-431-54064-9_16, © Springer Japan 2013

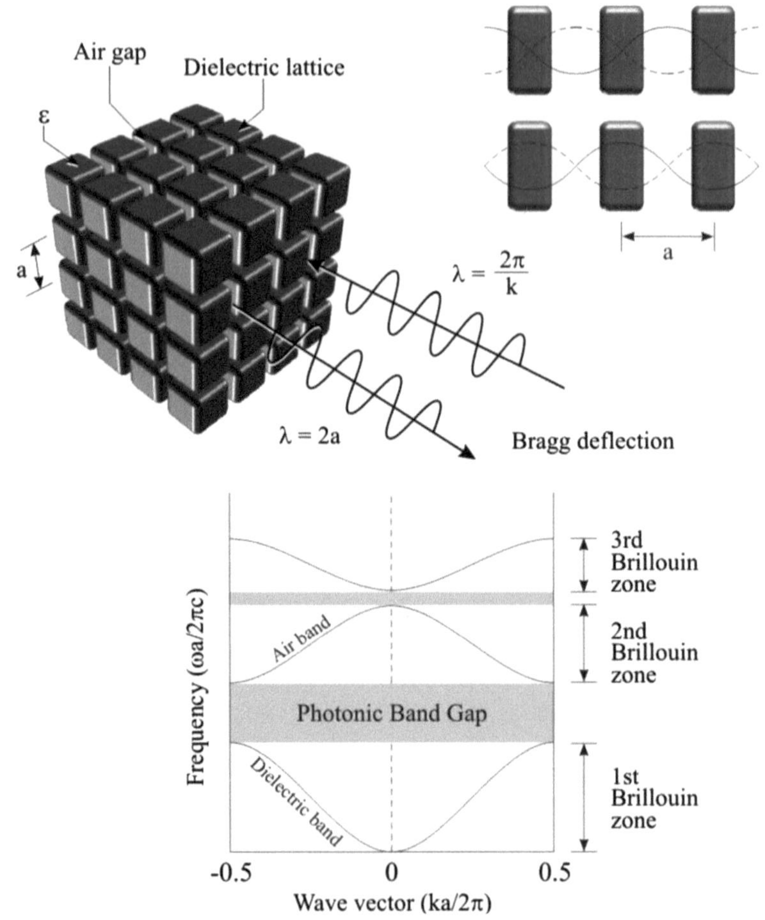

Fig. 16.1 Photonic band gap formations in periodic structures of dielectric materials. Two standing waves with high and low frequencies are formed in a photonic crystal, and a forbidden gap is formed between these frequencies

dielectric matrices form high- and low-frequency band edges in the first and second Brillouin zones, respectively. The band gap can be increased by optimizing the structure, filling ratio, and dielectric constant of the crystal lattice. Structural modifications carried out by introducing a defect in the crystal structure can control electromagnetic wave propagation through the structure, as shown in Fig. 16.2. The incident wave can resonate strongly if the defect is introduced at a wavelength comparable to the cavity size, and the amplified wave can propagate through the crystal [3, 4]. A localized mode corresponding to the transmission peak is observed in the photonic band gap.

Typical photonic crystal geometries are schematically illustrated in Fig. 16.3. A woodpile structure (a) having a simple pattern of stacked rods can provide a band gap suitable for prohibiting light wave propagation in all directions. Photonic crystals of GaAs or InP have been fabricated by semiconductor processes [5].

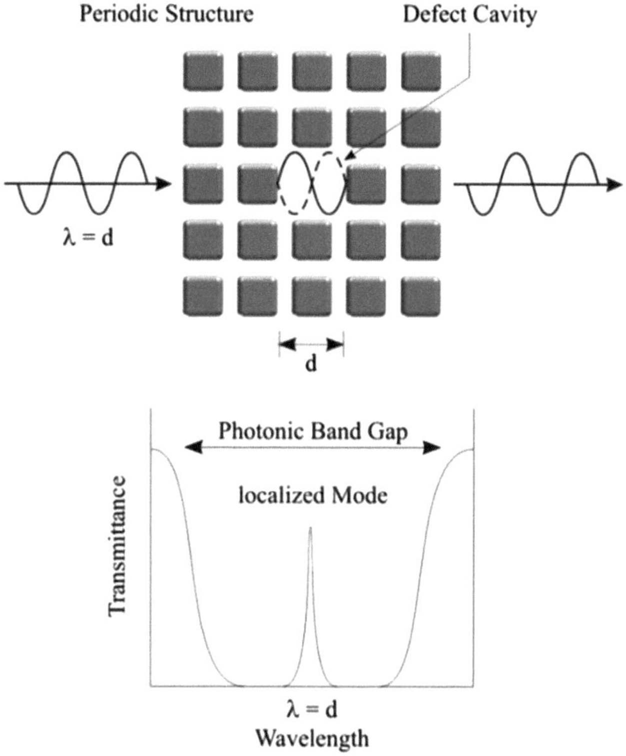

Fig. 16.2 Electromagnetic wave resonance in structural defect introduced in periodic structure. A localized mode of a transmission peak forms in the photonic band gap according to the defect size

A layered structure (b) composed of Si and SiO_2 having different dielectric constants enables light wave polarization and exhibits superprism effects [6]. These layers are stacked by self-organized growth involving alternate sputtering and etching. An inverse opal structure (c) is composed of air spheres with a TiO_2, Si, Ge, or CdS matrix having a face-centered cubic structure [7]. In this type of structure, polystyrene spheres are initially arranged by self-organization in colloidal solutions. Then, the slurry of these dielectric media is infiltrated into the periodic structure and sintered. An optical fiber (d) with a photonic crystal structure can efficiently guide light along the central core [8]. Silica fibers and glass capillaries are bundled together by drawing wires at high temperatures.

16.2 Terahertz Wave

Photonic crystals used for controlling light and microwave propagation in various wavelength ranges are shown in Fig. 16.4 [9]. Air cavities formed in a photonic crystal of nanometer order can serve as lightwave circuits in an optimally reflective

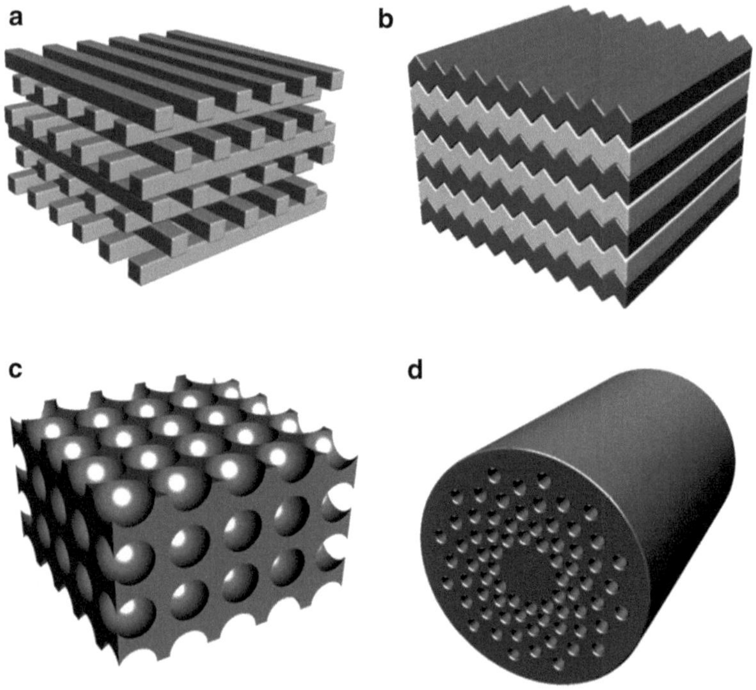

Fig. 16.3 Typical periodic structures of the photonic crystals with woodpile structure (**a**), stacked layer (**b**), inverse opal structure (**c**) and bundled fiber (**d**)

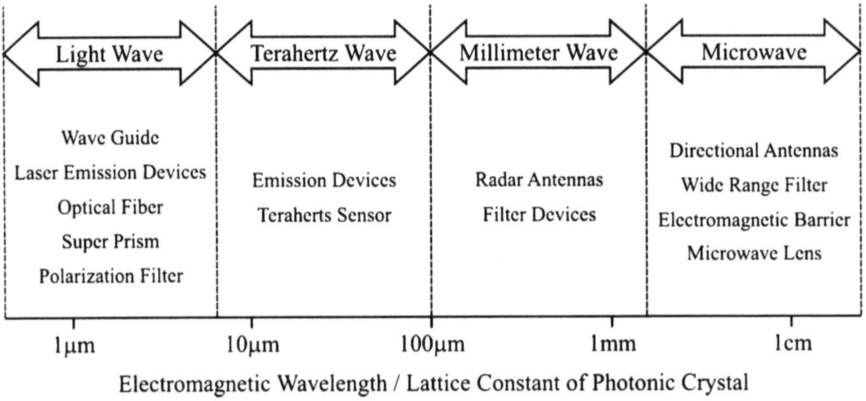

Fig. 16.4 Expected applications of the photonic crystals according to various electromagnetic wavelengths and the lattice constants

structure. When a light emitting diode is placed in an air cavity formed in a photonic crystal, efficient laser emission can be obtained because of highly coherent resonance in the microcavity. As millimeter-order periodic structures can control microwaves effectively, directional antennas and filters composed of photonic crystals can be used in millimeter-wave radar devices for intelligent traffic management and wireless communication. The perfect reflection of millimeter-order waves by photonic crystals will be useful for overcoming barriers that prevent wave interference. Terahertz waves with micrometer-order wavelengths can be used in various types of sensors for the analysis of various chemical and biological materials. Micrometer-order photonic crystals can be used in terahertz wave cavities, filters, and antennas.

Terahertz waves with micrometer-order wavelengths and far-infrared frequencies have generated much interest and have been investigated extensively owing to their many interesting features applicable in various fields such as materials, communication, medicine, and biology [10, 11]. It is possible to detect gun powder and ceramic blades hidden in bags, clothes, and envelopes by using terahertz waves because they can penetrate plastic, paper, and clothes without causing radiation damage to living cells. Using terahertz waves, toxic drugs can also be identified from their spectral fingerprints or absorption spectra. Moreover, terahertz waves have been studied widely as novel analytical light sources. Because electromagnetic wave frequencies ranging from 0.1 to 10 THz can be synchronized with collective vibration modes of saccharide or protein molecules, terahertz wave spectroscopy can be applied in various types of sensors for detecting harmful substances in human blood, cancer cells in the skin, and microbacteria in vegetables. The terahertz sensing technologies for aqueous phase environments in nature fields to detecting dissolved matters are extremely interesting topics.

16.3 Diamond Structure

The band diagram of a photonic crystal is drawn theoretically along the symmetry lines in the Brillouin zone. Maxwell's equations (16.1) and (16.2) can be solved by the plane wave expansion method [12], where ω and c denote the frequency and light velocity, respectively.

$$\nabla \times \left\{ \frac{1}{\varepsilon(r)} \nabla \times H\bar{\omega}(r) \right\} = \left(\frac{\bar{\omega}}{c} \right)^2 H\bar{\omega}(r) \tag{16.1}$$

$$\frac{1}{\varepsilon(r)} \nabla \times \{ \nabla \times E\bar{\omega}(r) \} = \left(\frac{\bar{\omega}}{c} \right)^2 E\bar{\omega}(r) \tag{16.2}$$

The electric and magnetic fields Eω(r) and Hω(r) are described using the following plane wave equations (16.3) and (16.4), respectively.

$$H_{k,n}(r) = \sum_G H_{k,n}(G) e^{e(k+G)\cdot r} \tag{16.3}$$

$$E_{k,n}(r) = \sum_G E_{k,n}(G) e^{e(k+G)\cdot r} \tag{16.4}$$

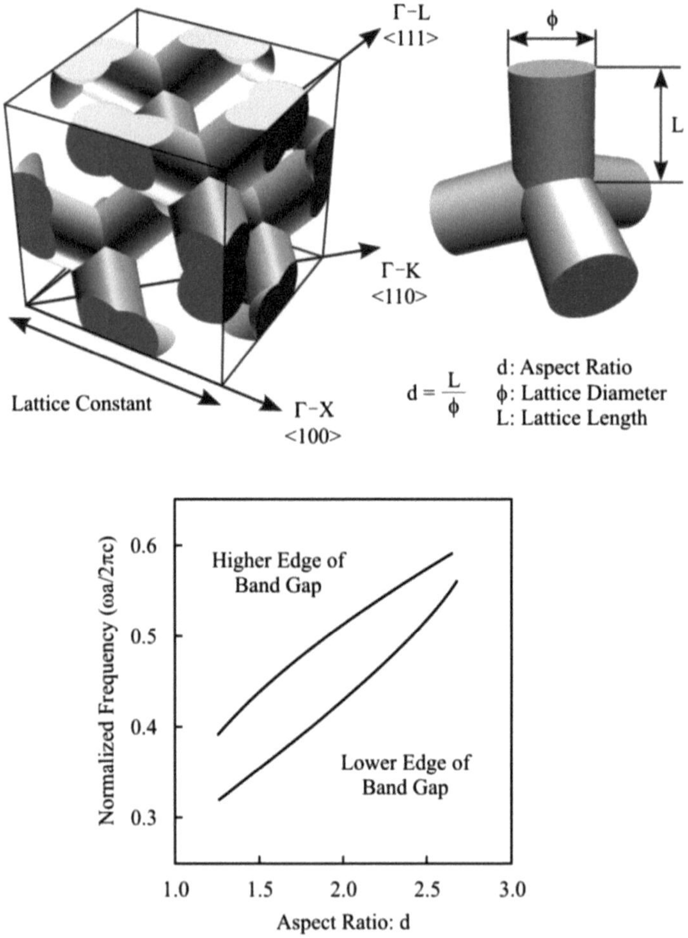

Fig. 16.5 Computer graphics model of unit cell of diamond structure, definition of aspect ratio, and variations in band gap width as a function of aspect ratio

The dielectric constant ε(r) of the periodically arranged crystal structure can be expressed by Eq. (16.5). G and k are the reciprocal and the wave vectors, respectively.

$$\frac{1}{\varepsilon(r)} = \sum_{G} \frac{1}{\varepsilon(G)} e^{iG \cdot r} \tag{16.5}$$

Photonic crystal having a diamond structure can allow band gaps to transmit waves in all directions in similar frequency ranges [13, 14]. The wave propagation should be prohibited adequately in the overlapping regions of band gaps. The electromagnetic band diagrams of the diamond structures were calculated to determine the geometric parameters of the structures. The dielectric constant of alumina lattice used in the calculation was 10. Figure 16.5 shows a unit cell of the diamond

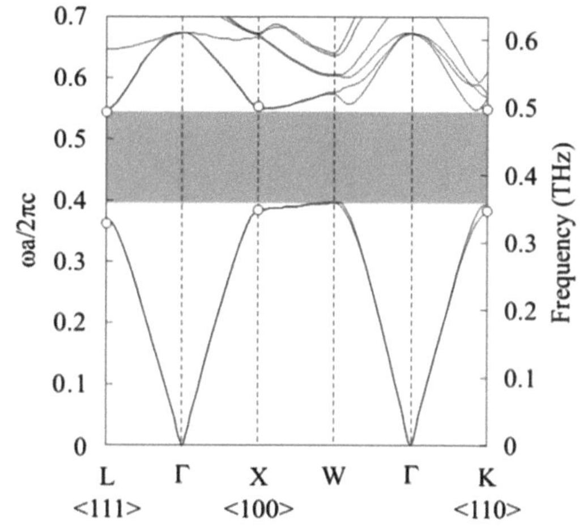

Fig. 16.6 Photonic band diagram calculated by plane wave expansion method. Open circles indicate the measured edge frequencies of photonic band gaps. The dielectric constant of the lattice was 10. The frequency range indicated in gray color depicts the optimum band gap in all the directions

structure, the definition of the aspect ratio of the diamond structure, and a plot of the calculated band gap width as a function of the aspect ratio. The aspect ratio of the diamond structure was designed to be 1.5. The lattice dielectric constant was 500 μm. The diamond structure was 4 × 4 × 2 mm in size, and it consisted of 8 × 8 × 4 unit cells. Figure 16.6 shows the calculated band diagram of an optimized diamond lattice. Solid lines indicate the transmission modes of the electromagnetic waves. Thus, the blank region indicates band gap formation. The optimum band gap opening for the propagation of waves in all crystal directions is seen clearly in the terahertz wave frequency range.

16.4 Stereolithography

A photonic crystal having a diamond structure was modeled using a computer graphics application (Toyota Caelum Co. Ltd., Thinkdesign ver. 7.0). The graphic data of the crystal was subsequently converted into a stereolithography file format. The three-dimensional (3D) model designed using the application was sliced into a series of two-dimensional (2D) cross-sectional patterns. This numerical data file was then transferred to a micro-stereolithography system (D-MEC Co. Ltd., Japan, SI-C1000). Figure 16.7 shows a schematic illustration of the micro stereolithography technique. During actual processing, photosensitive acrylic resin dispersed with alumina particles of 170 nm diameter at 40 vol.% was dispensed onto a substrate from a nozzle. The highly viscous paste of resin and alumina particles was dispensed at controlled air pressure. The paste was then spread uniformly over the substrate by the edge of a knife. The thickness of each layer of the paste was maintained at 10 μm. A 2D pattern was observed by transmitting a visible illuminating laser beam of 405 nm wavelength on the resin surface. High-resolution images were captured using a digital micromirror device and an objective lens. This optical device consisted of an assembly of mirrors with 14 μm edge length. The tilt of each

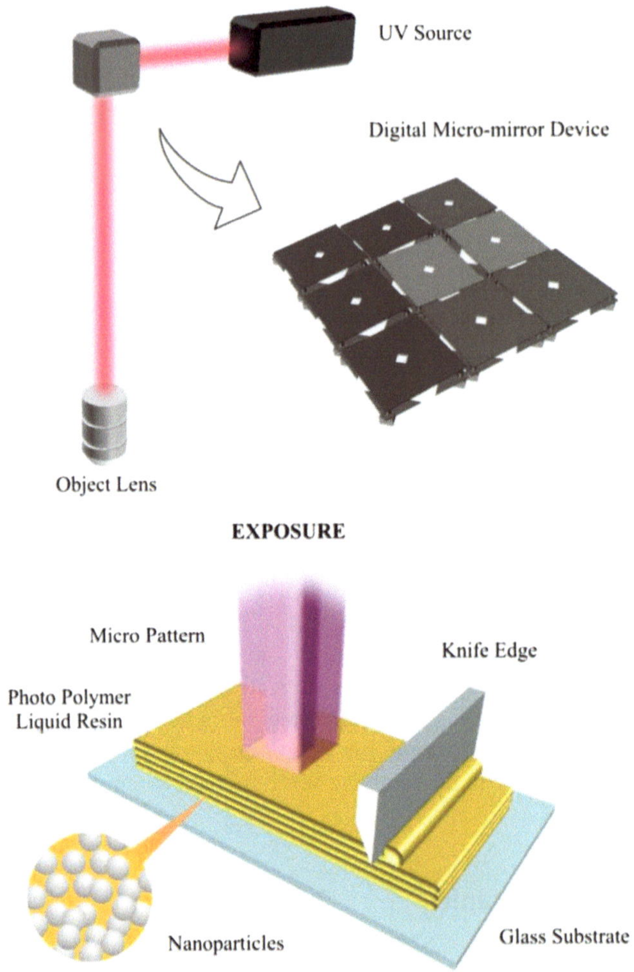

Fig. 16.7 Schematic of micropatterning stereolithography system based on computer aided design and manufacturing processes (CAD/CAM) to create resin components including ceramic or metal nanoparticles

micromirror was adjusted according to the 2D cross-sectional data obtained from the computer. A 3D structure was built by stacking these 2D micro patterns layer by layer. The entire fabrication system is shown in Fig. 16.8.

The alumina-dispersed resin precursor fabricated by the micro stereolithography technique is shown in Fig. 16.9. The lattice constant of the fabricated diamond structure was 500 μm. The spatial resolution was approximately 0.5%. In order to avoid deformation and the formation of cracks during dewaxing, dewaxing was carried out carefully. The precursors with diamond structures were heated at various temperatures from 100°C to 600°C, and the heating rate was maintained at 1.0°C/min. The precursor color changed to black at 400°C because of the

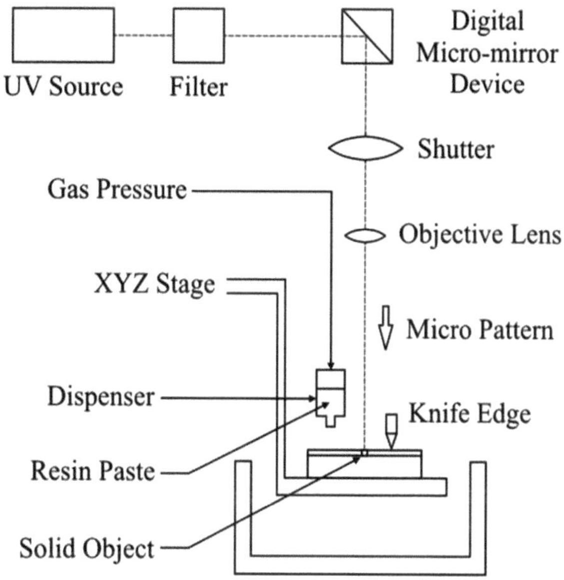

Fig. 16.8 Schematic of free-forming system for micro stereolithography. Three-dimensional structures can be fabricated automatically through stacking processes of cross-sectional two-dimensional layers

carbonization of resin. The precursor then turned white at 600°C, suggesting the burning out of resin. Thus, the dewaxing process was assumed to start at 200°C and finish at 600°C. The optimal dewaxing temperature was 600°C. Next, alumina particles were sintered at 1,500°C at a heating rate of 8.0°C/min. After dewaxing and sintering processes, ceramic diamond structures were obtained.

Figure 16.10 shows the (1 1 1), (1 0 0), and (1 1 0) planes of the sintered diamond structures having micro alumina lattices with four coordination numbers [15]. The lattice constant was estimated as 375 μm. Deformation or cracks were not observed in optical microscopic observations. The linear shrinkage along the horizontal axis was 23.8% and that along the vertical axis was 24.6%. A uniform shrinkage can be obtained by designing the diamond structure to be appropriately elongated in the vertical direction in order to compensate for the gravitational effect. The density of the sintered structure was measured by the Archimedes method. The maximum relative density was found to be 97.5%. Translucent ceramic lattices were obtained. The microstructures of the lattices were observed by scanning electron microscopy (SEM); results showed the formation of dense alumina microstructures with an average grain size of approximately 2 μm.

16.5 Optimum Band Gap

The attenuation of terahertz transmission waves through the diamond photonic crystals was measured by using a time-domain spectrometer (Advanced Infrared Spectroscopy Co. Ltd., Japan, Pulse-IRS 1000). Figure 16.11 shows a schematic of the spectroscopic measurement system. Femtosecond laser beams were irradiated on a micro-antenna fabricated on a semiconductor substrate to generate terahertz

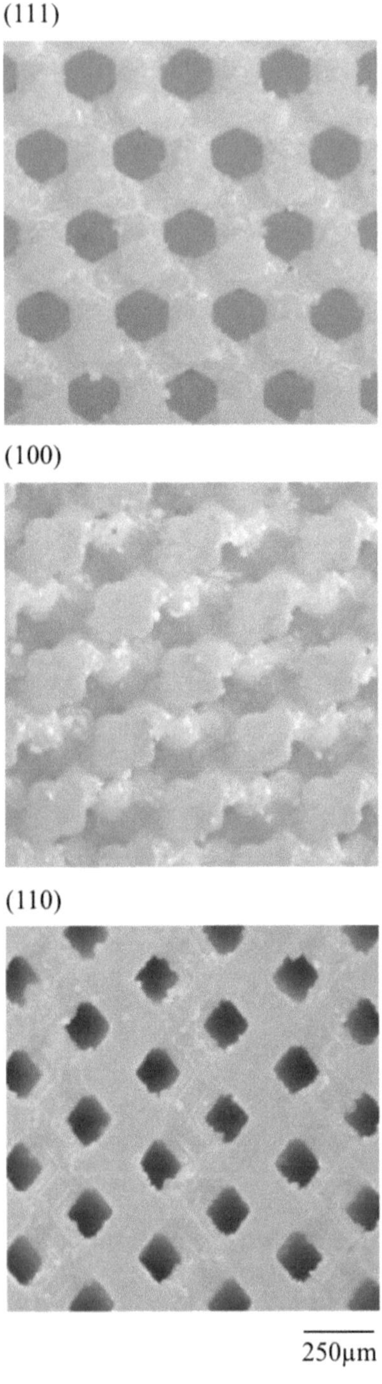

Fig. 16.9 Fabricated photonic crystals with diamond structures composed of acrylic lattices with alumina nanoparticles formed by using micro stereolithography process

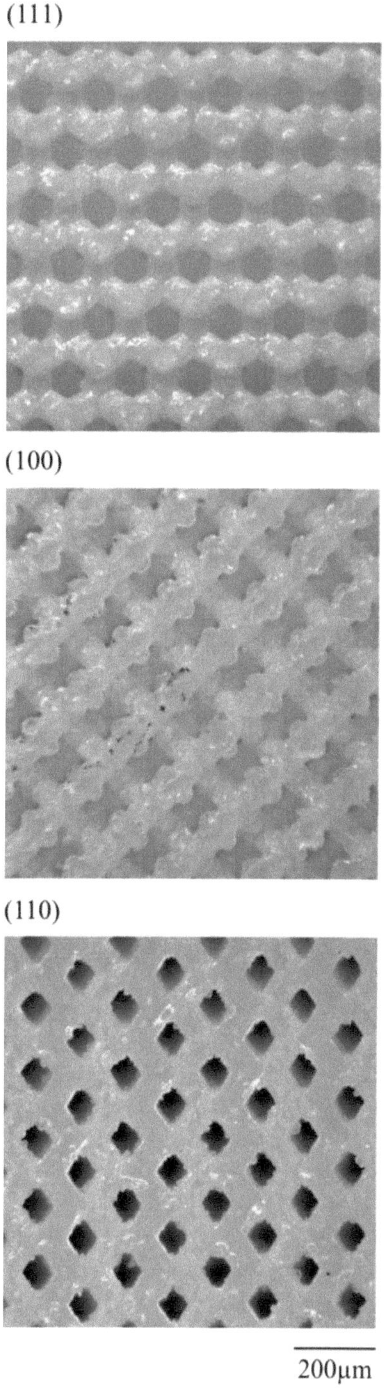

Fig. 16.10 Formed crystal planes in alumina photonic crystals having diamond structures. Sintering density of the lattices is 98.5%. Dielectric constant of the lattice is 10

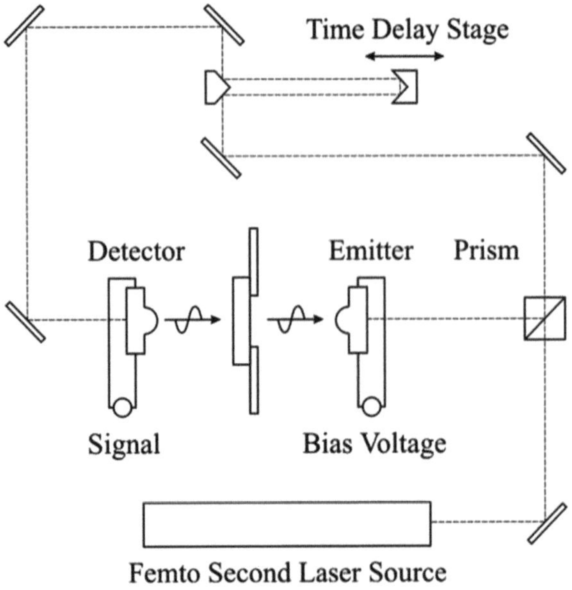

Fig. 16.11 Schematic of measuring system of terahertz wave analyzer by time-domain spectroscopic detection method

wave pulses. The terahertz waves were transmitted perpendicularly through the samples, and signals were detected by another micro-antenna. The transmission amplitudes of the terahertz waves were estimated by Fourier transform. The dielectric constants of the bulk samples were measured by calculating the phase shift. The measured dielectric constant of the sintered alumina was about 10.

The attenuation of the terahertz waves transmitted through the alumina diamond structure in the Γ–L ⟨1 1 1⟩, Γ–X ⟨1 0 0⟩, and Γ–K ⟨1 1 0⟩ crystal directions are shown in Fig. 16.12 [16]. Forbidden gaps were formed in the frequency ranges of 0.32–0.49, 0.35–0.53, and 0.35–0.52 THz in the transmission spectra for the Γ–L ⟨1 1 1⟩, Γ–X ⟨1 0 0⟩, and Γ–K ⟨1 1 0⟩ directions, respectively. An overlapping band gap was observed in all the directions in the frequency range of 0.35–0.50 THz; this observation implied that the electromagnetic waves were not transmitted through the crystal and were totally reflected in all the directions. The measured band gap frequencies were compared with those estimated by the plane wave expansion method, as shown in Fig. 16.6. The open circles indicate the high and low edges of the measured band gaps. The measured frequency ranges of opaque regions corresponded to the calculated frequency ranges.

16.6 Localized Mode

A cubic air defect having the same dimensions as the unit cell of the diamond structure was introduced in the diamond structure, as shown in Fig. 16.13 [17]. The transmission spectrum of the electromagnetic waves in the Γ–X ⟨1 0 0⟩

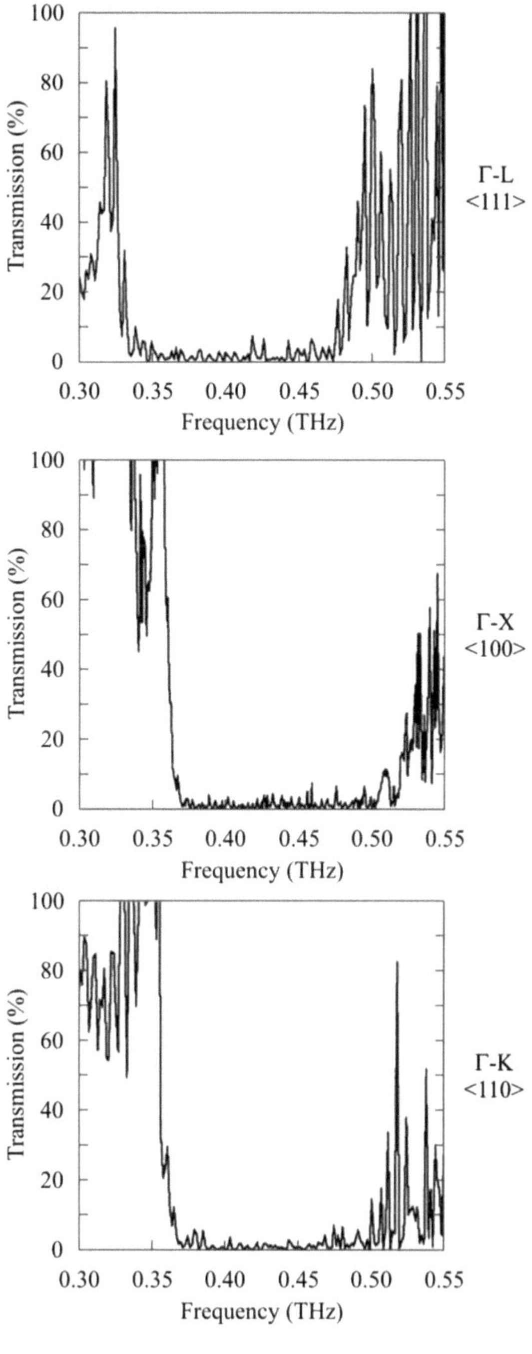

Fig. 16.12 Attenuation of terahertz transmission waves in Γ–L ⟨1 1 1⟩, Γ–X ⟨1 0 0⟩, and Γ–K ⟨1 1 0⟩ directions in alumina photonic crystal with diamond structures by terahertz time-domain spectroscopy

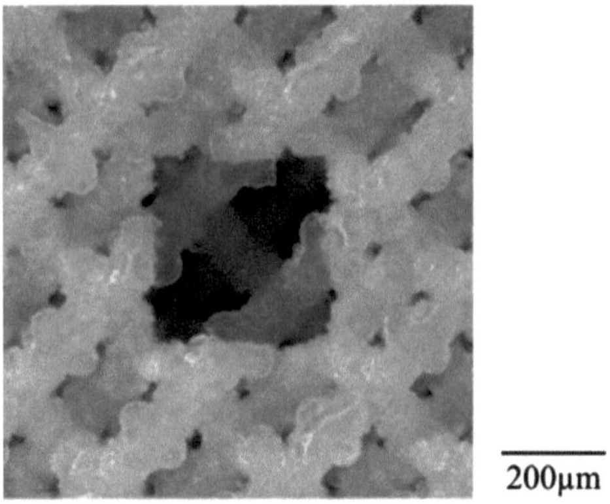

Fig. 16.13 Defect introduced in alumina lattice with diamond structures. The edge length of the air cavity is equal to the lattice constant

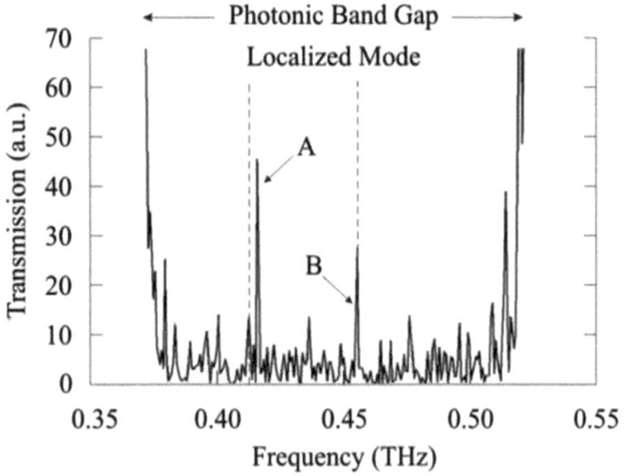

Fig. 16.14 Transmission spectrum of structure with defect. Localized modes appear in the band gap. *Dashed lines* indicate the estimated localized frequencies

direction is shown in Fig. 16.14. Two localized modes of the transmission peaks were observed in the band gap at frequencies of 0.42 and 0.46 THz. The crystal structure with the periodic arrangement can exhibit the photonic band gap, and the introduced defects can the localized mode. Diffraction and resonance behaviors in the dielectric pattern of the crystal structure were simulated theoretically by the finite-difference time-domain method using a transmission line simulator (Flomerics, UK, Microstripes Ver. 7.5). The measured peak frequencies were compared with the simulated ones, as shown in Fig. 16.14. It was observed that the measured peak frequencies were in good agreement with the simulated ones. The first and second peaks are denoted as modes A and B, respectively. The electric field distributions of these modes were simulated by the same method. Figure 16.15a, b shows cross-sectional images of the electric field distributions. The red region in the images indicates a high electric field intensity, whereas the blue and green regions indicate a low electric field intensity. Thus, it was considered that the mode A concentrated the oscillation energy of a half wavelength with an antinode in the cube. Also, mode B concentrated the energy of a half wavelength on the sides of the cube with a node in the cube.

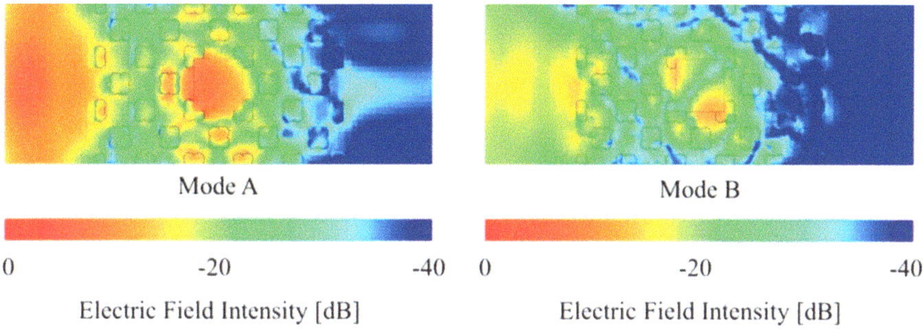

Fig. 16.15 Electric field distributions of localized modes A (**a**) and B (**b**) simulated by modeling transmission line using finite-difference time-domain method

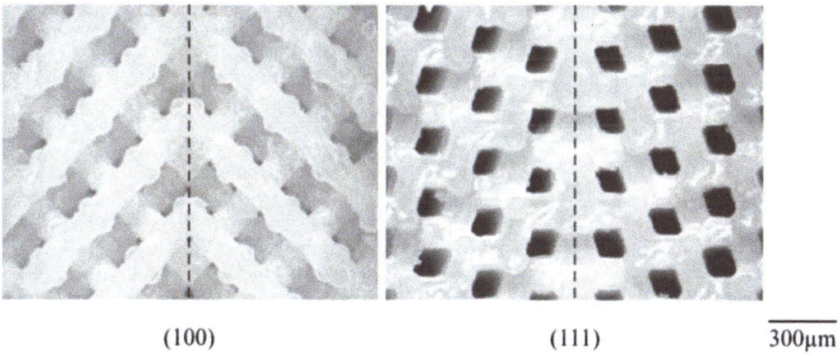

Fig. 16.16 Modified photonic crystals composed of alumina lattices. Plane defects were introduced parallel to (1 0 0) and (1 1 1) layers between twinned diamond lattices with mirror symmetries

Figure 16.16 shows the alumina photonic crystals with twinned diamond lattices. The spatial tolerances of the diamond lattices were within 10 μm. Figure 16.17 shows the measured transmission spectra of the twinned diamond structures. The defect interfaces parallel to the (1 0 0) and (1 1 1) planes were sandwiched between the mirror symmetric diamond lattice blocks composed of four and three periods, respectively. These structural periods were optimized to obtain clear localized modes with the sharp resonation peaks in the band gaps. These localized modes of 22% and 38% of the transmission intensity were formed at frequencies of 0.414 and 0.409 THz, respectively. The localized mode frequencies were included in the perfect band gap. Figure 16.18 shows the cross-sectional images of the electric field intensity distributions simulated at the localized frequencies. The electromagnetic waves propagated from left to right. The red and blue regions indicate high and low electric field intensities, respectively. The incident waves were resonated, and they localized strongly through the multiple reflections in the twinned defect interfaces between the mirror symmetric diffraction lattices. The amplified electromagnetic waves propagated, and transmission peaks were observed in the band gaps. Moreover, the transmitted waves exhibited clear beam

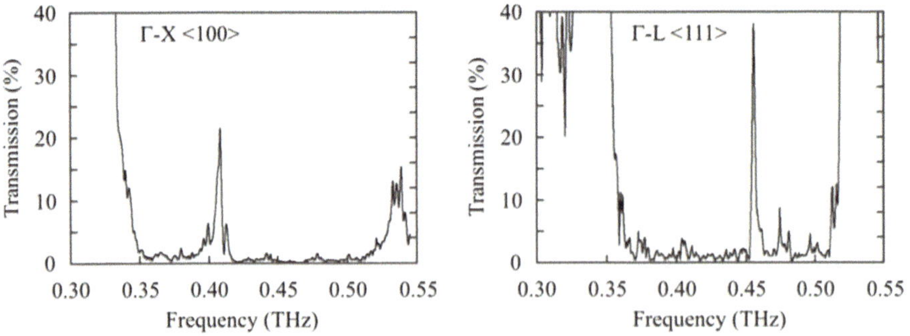

Fig. 16.17 Localized modes of transmission peaks in photonic band gaps formed by twinned diamond lattice structures

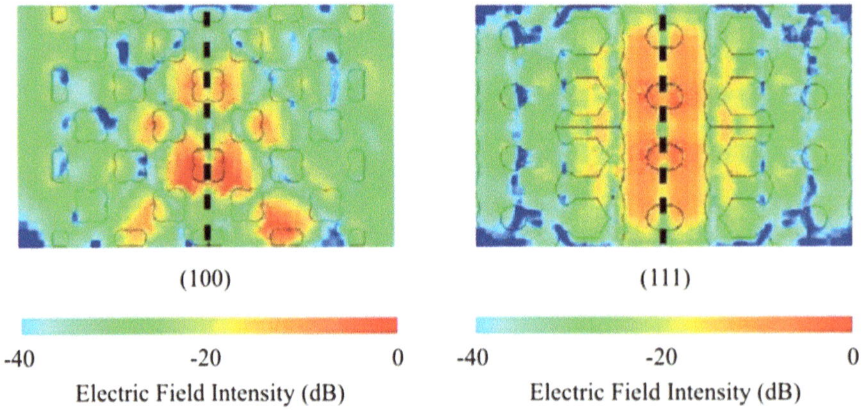

Fig. 16.18 Electric field intensity in twinned diamond structures. Localized modes are formed along the plane defects

profiles of plane wave propagations, because multiple resonances with coherent modes were realized in the twinned defects. The localization observed in the plane defect parallel to the (1 1 1) plane was stronger than that observed in the case of (1 0 0), as shown in Fig. 16.18. These results agree with the disparity in the peak intensities of the localized modes, as shown in Fig. 16.17.

References

1. Ohtaka K (1979) Energy bang of photons and low energy photon diffraction. Phys Rev B 19(10):5057–5067
2. Yablonovitch E (1987) Inhabited spontaneous emission in solid-state physics and electronics. Phys Rev Lett 58(20):2059–2062

3. Noda S, Yamamoto N, Kobayashi H, Okano M, Tomoda K (1999) Optical properties of three-dimensional photonic crystals based on III-V semiconductors at infrared to near-infrared wavelengths. Appl Phys Lett 75(16):905–907
4. Kanehira S, Kirihara S, Miyamoto Y (2005) Fabrication of TiO_2–SiO_2 photonic crystals with diamond structure. J Am Ceram Soc 88(6):1461–1464
5. Noda S (2000) Three-dimensional photonic crystals operating at optical wavelength region. Physica B 279(1):142–149
6. Kosaka H, Kawashima T, Tomita A, Notomi M, Tamamura T, Sato T, Kawakami S (1999) Photonic crystals for micro wave circuits using wavelength-dependent angular beam steering. Appl Phys Lett 74(8):1370–1378
7. Cregan R, Mangan B, Night J, Birks T, Russell S, Roberts P, Allan D (1999) Singlemode photonic bandgap guidance of light in air. Science 285:1537–1539
8. Vos W, Sprik R, Blaaderen A, Imhof A, Lagendijk A, Wegdam G (1996) Strong effects of photonic band structures on the diffusion of colloidal crystals. Phys Rev B 53(24): 16231–16235
9. Kawakami S (2002) Photonic crystals. CMC, Tokyo
10. Clery D (2002) Brainstorming their way to an imaging revolution. Science 297:761–763
11. Kawase K, Ogawa Y, Watanabe Y, Inoue H (2003) Non-destructive terahertz imaging of illicit drugs using spectral fingerprints. Opt Express 11(20):2549–2554
12. Haus J (1994) A brief review of theoretical results for photonic band structures. J Mod Opt 41(2):195–207
13. Ho K, Chan C, Soukoulis C (1990) Existence of a photonic gap in periodic dielectric structures. Phys Rev Lett 65(25):3152–3165
14. Kirihara S, Miyamoto Y, Takenaga K, Takeda M, Kajiyama K (2002) Fabrication of electromagnetic crystals with a complete diamond structure by stereolithography. Solid State Commun 121(8):435–439
15. Chen W, Kirihara S, Miyamoto Y (2007) Fabrication and measurement of micro three-dimensional photonic crystals of SiO_2 ceramic for terahertz wave applications. J Am Ceram Soc 90(7):2078–2081
16. Kanaoka H, Kirihara S, Miyamoto Y (2008) Terahertz wave properties of alumina microphotonic crystals with a diamond structure. J Mater Res 23(4):1036–1041
17. Kirihara S, Miyamoto Y (2009) Terahertz wave control using ceramic photonic crystals with diamond structure including plane defects fabricated by micro-stereolithography. Int J Appl Ceram Technol 6(1):41–44

Chapter 17
Design, Fabrication, and Properties of Nanomaterials Using Ultrathin Film Techniques

Yu Shiratsuchi

Abstract The nanostructure of an ultrathin film is determined by the initial stage of the thin film growth. In addition, the physical properties of ultrathin films are sometimes dominated by the surface/interface properties because of the large surface-to-volume ratio. Focusing on a magnetic ultrathin film, this chapter describes the fabrication techniques for ultrathin films, the magnetic properties of two-dimensionally aligned nanoparticles, and the surface/interface magnetic properties of ultrathin films.

Keywords Exchange bias • Interface • Molecular beam epitaxy • Perpendicular magnetic anisotropy • Superparamagnetism • Surface • Ultrathin film

17.1 Introduction

As materials become smaller and approach characteristic lengths, various unique phenomena appear. As examples of the magnetic characteristic lengths, the magnetic domain wall is on the order of 10 nm and the exchange length is several nanometers, as shown in Fig. 17.1. In this size regime, the finite size effects and surface/interface properties play important roles in the physical properties. The effects caused by geometric confinement have been predicted theoretically since the late 1940s [1]. However, only recently have they been verified experimentally, as a result of advances in fabricating and characterizing nanostructures.

Ultrathin films provide opportunities to fabricate various types of nano-sized materials [2]. This is partly because the nanostructure of an ultrathin film is closely related to the growth mode of the film. In particular, in the thickness regime below

Y. Shiratsuchi (✉)
Division of Materials and Manufacturing Science, Graduate School of Engineering, Osaka University, 2-1 Yamadaoka, Suita, Osaka 565-0871, Japan
e-mail: shiratsuchi@mat.eng.osaka-u.ac.jp

T. Kakeshita (ed.), *Progress in Advanced Structural and Functional Materials Design*, DOI 10.1007/978-4-431-54064-9_17, © Springer Japan 2013

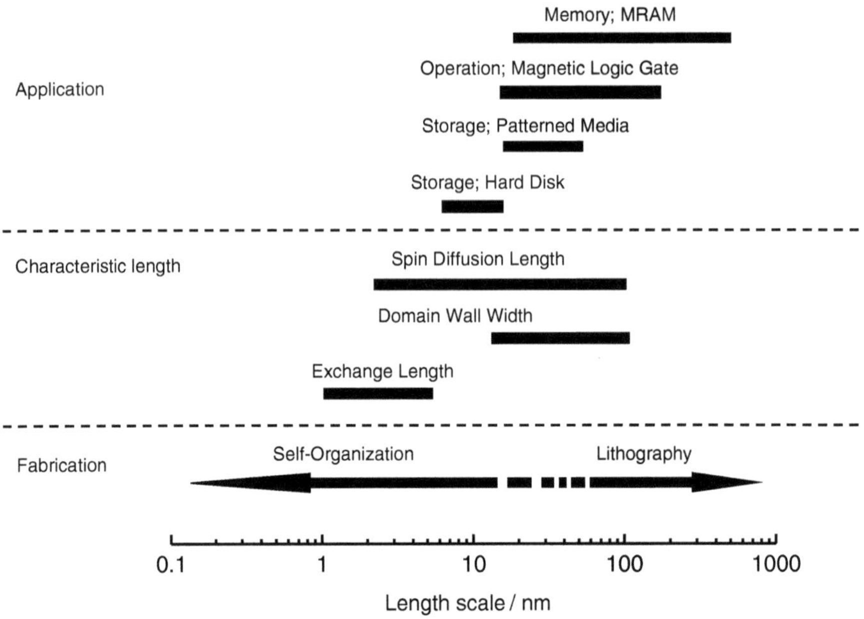

Fig. 17.1 Magnetic characteristic lengths for various length scales. The expected magnetic devices and fabrication techniques for each length scale are also shown

several nanometers, geometric confinements occur in both the growth and the lateral directions, which make it possible for low-dimensional nanostructures to be formed. In this chapter, we first review the fabrication techniques for ultrathin films and the growth mechanism in the ultrathin regime. We then describe experimental results, mainly for the magnetism of some low-dimensional systems.

17.2 Fabrication and Growth of Ultrathin Film

Preparing a high quality ultrathin film requires several experimental environments. Even under vacuum, evaporated atoms may meet other species at a given distance, known as the mean free path, while travelling from the evaporator to the substrate. Because the mean free path is inversely proportional to the pressure, a high vacuum below 10^{-6} Pa is necessary. In addition, the nanostructure is sensitive to the residual gas in the vacuum, and the impurities on the substrate alter the structure of an ultrathin film. In order to reduce these extrinsic influences, an ultrahigh vacuum (UHV) below 10^{-8} Pa is required. A UHV condition offers other advantages when preparing a high quality thin film. For example, when a substrate surface is cleaned in a UHV chamber, it remains clean for a long time. A clean substrate surface is essential for a high quality ultrathin film because the initial stage of thin film growth is very sensitive to the surface structure of the substrate.

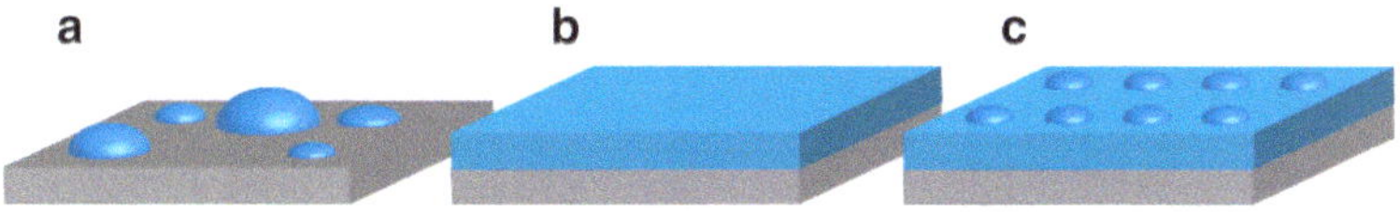

Fig. 17.2 Growth modes for thin film: (**a**) island growth or Volmer–Weber growth, (**b**) layer-by-layer growth or Frank van Merwe growth, and (**c**) Stranski–Krastanov growth

The growth modes of a thin film are schematically shown in Fig. 17.2: (a) island growth or Volmer–Weber (V–W) growth, (b) layer-by-layer growth or Frank van Merwe growth, and (c) Stranski–Krastanov (S–K) growth. In V–W growth, nanoparticles with typical in-plane diameters of less than 10 nm are formed, and their shape is often disk-like [2]. This type of growth occurs easily when the substrate/underlayer has a higher surface energy than the thin film or when the interface energy between the substrate/underlayer and the thin film is high. The layer-by-layer growth produces a two-dimensional ultrathin film. In general, this growth mode requires several conditions, including a small lattice mismatch between the thin film and the substrate. The layer-by-layer growth is characterized through the intensity oscillation of reflection high-energy electron diffraction (RHEED) during the thin film growth [3]. In particular, when the absorbed atoms nucleate at the surface step and grow along the step edge, e.g., step flow growth, one-dimensional atomic wires are formed. As examples, such one-dimensional atomic wires have been observed in Ag on Pt(9 9 7) [4], Fe on W(1 1 0) [5], and Fe on Cu(1 1 1) [6]. In the S–K growth, the film forms a continuous layer structure in the first few monolayers, after which islands form on the underlying continuous layer. This characteristic growth is explained by the following scenario for the relaxation of the lattice strain in the film. When the lattice mismatch between the film and the substrate is not very large, the thin film can form a continuous layer at the very initial stage of growth. However, this continuous layer stores strain energy. The stored strain energy is released by increasing the surface area. Consequently, several islands are formed. S–K growth is often observed in some semiconductor systems, and quantum dots are successfully formed [7].

The deposition method is also important for controlling the abovementioned growth mode. Molecular beam epitaxy (MBE) is one of the ideal techniques for fabricating low dimensional structures [3]. In MBE, thermally-evaporated atoms or molecules are deposited on the substrate from an effusion cell (K-cell) or e-beam heating (Fig. 17.3). The growth rate is generally a few monolayers/minute. A slow growth rate is essential to control the nanostructure at an atomic scale. In addition, as a result of the slow growth rate, varying the growth temperature alters the film structure and changes the growth mode because the growth temperature changes the kinetics of the absorbed atoms. An MBE chamber is generally used to maintain the UHV condition during growth. Thus, real-time observation of the thin film growth is possible through an in situ RHEED observation.

Other deposition methods such as pulsed layer deposition (PLD), in which atoms are ablated from the target by LASER irradiation, and a sputtering technique are also available to fabricate ultrathin films. The atoms evaporated using these techniques

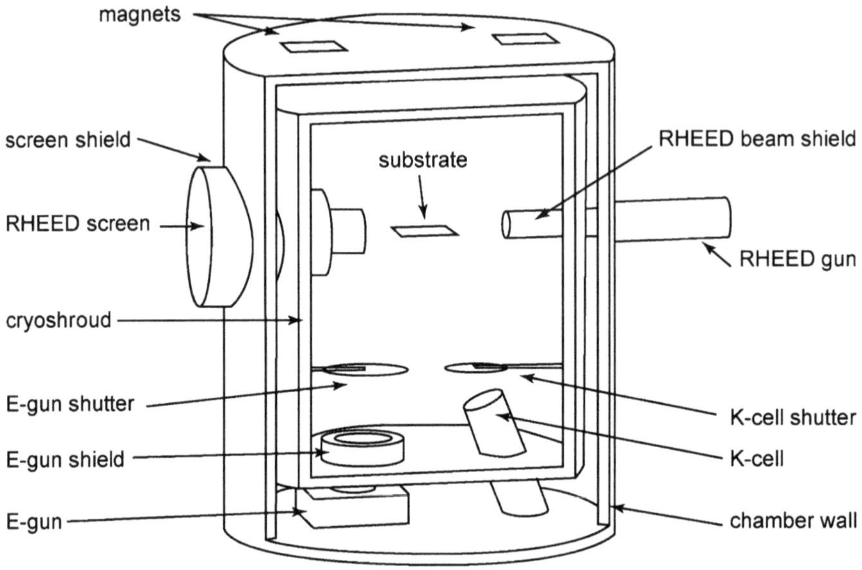

Fig. 17.3 Schematic drawing of MBE chamber

have a high kinetic energy. In addition, these methods can be used to fabricate compound films such as those containing an oxide, nitride, and fluoride because a reactive gas can be introduced into the chamber during the thin film growth.

17.3 Magnetic Nanoparticles Fabricated by Volmer–Weber Growth

V–W growth provides an opportunity to fabricate nanoparticles smaller than several nanometers. The nanoparticles formed by the V–W growth have some structural advantages compared to those fabricated using chemical methods. The crystalline orientation of the nanoparticles is controllable by the epitaxial relationship with the underlying substrate. The arrangement of the nanoparticles is also controllable through the growth condition. In this section, we describe an example of the influence of the growth condition on the physical properties by using the superparamagnetism of Fe nanoparticles grown on an α-Al_2O_3(0 0 0 1) substrate [8–10].

Figure 17.4 shows atomic force microscope images of Fe nanoparticles. The nominal thickness of the Fe is 1.0 nm, and the growth temperatures are (a) 473 K, (b) 573 K, and (c) 773 K. This figure also shows the diameter distributions and cross-sectional views corresponding to the arrows. Nanoparticles with a diameter of about 4 nm are clearly observed. The shape of these nanoparticles is altered by

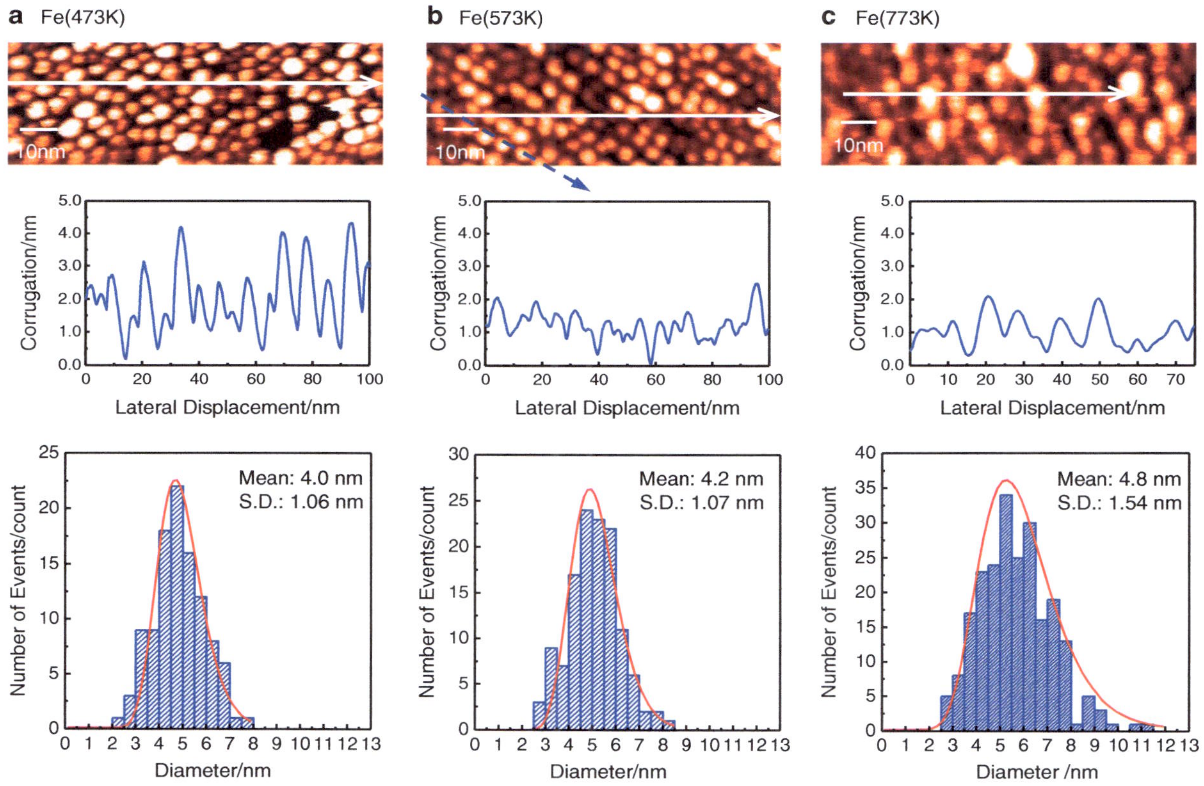

Fig. 17.4 Atomic force microscope image, corresponding cross-sectional view, and diameter distribution of Fe nanoparticles fabricated by V–W growth with growth temperatures of (**a**) 473 K, (**b**) 573 K, and (**c**) 773 K

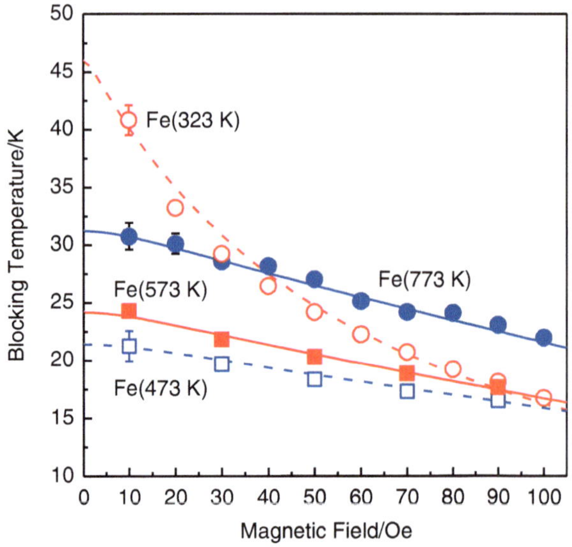

Fig. 17.5 Measured magnetic field dependence of blocking temperature for Fe nanoparticles [10]

altering the growth temperature. At 473 K, the nanoparticles are almost spherical, whereas at 573–773 K, they are disk-like. The diameter of the Fe nanoparticles increases with an increase in temperature; however, the size is, at most, 12 nm. In addition, at 573 K, it seems that the Fe nanoparticles align regularly, as indicated by the broken blue arrow. The reason for this regular alignment is unclear, but it may be correlated with the epitaxial growth of Fe. In fact, the crystalline orientation of the Fe nanoparticles normal to the surface is aligned with bcc (1 1 0) below the growth temperature of 473 K, while it becomes random above 573 K [9].

The fabricated Fe nanoparticles are superparamagnetic at room temperature. Superparamagnetism is characterized by a blocking temperature that depends on the energy barrier to reverse the magnetization direction [11]. This "blocking" refers to the competition between the energy barrier of a magnetization reversal and the thermal energy. Although the blocking temperature is sometimes defined as the peak temperature of zero-field-cooled magnetization (ZFCM), the ZFC magnetization includes, not only the thermally-activated magnetization, but also the magnetization in a state of thermal equilibrium [10]. Thus, in an actual system, the mean blocking temperature should be estimated from the following relationship [12]

$$f(T_B) = -\frac{\mathrm{d}(\mathrm{FCM}(T) - \mathrm{ZFCM}(T))}{\mathrm{d}T} \tag{17.1}$$

where *FCM* is the field-cooled magnetization and T is the absolute temperature. The blocking temperature estimated under a finite field includes various contributions such as the Zeeman energy and interparticle magnetic interactions. Thus, the details of the superparamagnetic behavior can be obtained through the blocking

Growth Temperature (K)		323	373	473	573	673	773
Structure	Morphology	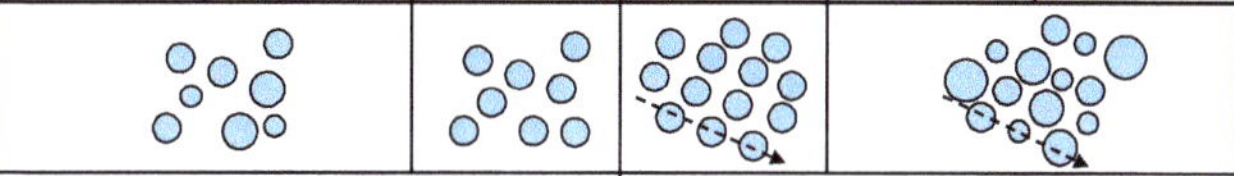					
	Alignment	Random			One directional (dotted arrow)		
	Shape	Sphere			Disk		
	Crystallinity*	Single-crystalline				Poly-crystalline	
Magnetism	Dominant factor of ZFC magnetization	Thermal activation			Langevin behavior		
	Difference between V_{MAG} and V_{AFM}	Large ←→ Small					
Size Uniformity (structural and magnetic)		Uniform ←→ Disperse					

Fig. 17.6 Correlation between structural and magnetic parameters [10]

temperature. As an example, the magnetic field dependence of the blocking temperature is shown in Fig. 17.5 [10]. The theoretically calculated curves are also shown by the lines. Although the blocking temperature of Fe nanoparticles grown at 323 K is reproduced by assuming the interparticle interactions, those of the other studied Fe nanoparticles do not require the interparticle interaction. This is explained by the changes in the particle size and crystalline orientation (Fig. 17.6 [10]). The Fe nanoparticles are larger for the higher growth temperature, and this increase in size indicates that the distance between the nanoparticles increases because the total amount of deposited Fe is the same. Assuming that the dipole interaction is an origin of the interparticle interaction, the dipole interaction is proportional to r^{-3} and M^2, where r is the distance between Fe nanoparticles and M is the magnetization of a single Fe nanoparticle. Hence, a decrease in r should rapidly enhance the interparticle interactions. In addition, the aligned crystalline orientation of the Fe nanoparticles below 473 K may promote the enhancement of the dipole interparticle interaction through the alignment of the easy magnetic direction of magneto-crystalline anisotropy.

17.4 Interfacial Phenomenon in Magnetic Superlattice/Multilayer

At a surface or at an interface, the chemical bonds between atoms are broken or the chemical bonds with different species exist. These broken or different chemical bonds generate a unique electronic state at the surface/interface. At the surface/ interface, the density of states (DOS) at the Fermi energy is narrowed, and this narrowed DOS causes unique magnetic properties such as an enhanced magnetic moment and surface/interface magnetic anisotropy [13]. These properties have

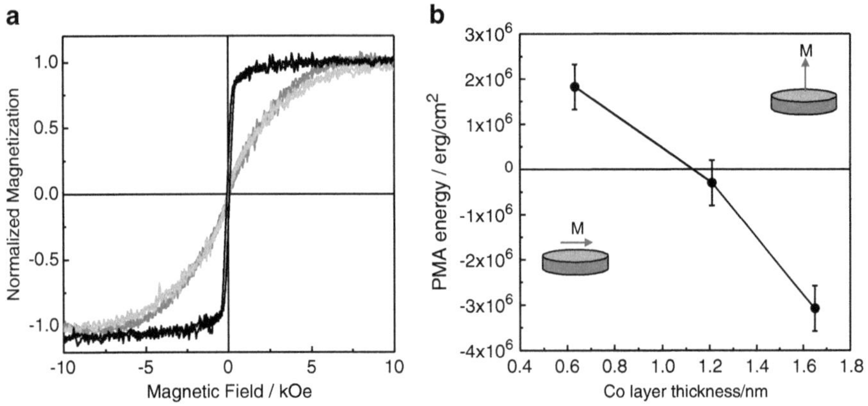

Fig. 17.7 (**a**) Magnetization curves of [Co (0.63 nm)/Cr (5.0 nm)]^{10} superlattice showing PMA. *Black* and *gray lines* represent the curves in the direction perpendicular and parallel to the film, respectively. (**b**) Changes of PMA energy with the Co layer thickness

attracted attention from both the fundamental research and the engineering viewpoints. For example, surface/interface magnetic anisotropy has been utilized in magnetic devices such as a hard disk drive (HDD) and magnetic random access memory (MRAM). In this section, we present perpendicular magnetic anisotropy and exchange anisotropy as representative surface/interface magnetic anisotropies.

17.4.1 Perpendicular Magnetic Anisotropy

In a normal thin film, the magnetization lies in the film plane because of the high demagnetization field. However, in some cases, interface magnetic anisotropy, for which the easy magnetic direction is normal to the film, overcomes the demagnetization field. In this case, the direction of magnetization rises upwards and orients normal to the film. This type of interface magnetic anisotropy is called perpendicular magnetic anisotropy (PMA). PMA was first observed in Co/Pt and Co/Pd multilayers [14]. Since the discovery of PMA, it has been found in various systems such as Co/Au [15], Fe/Au [16], and Co/Ni [17]. The microscopic origin of PMA is essentially the same as that for magneto-crystalline anisotropy, e.g., the spin–orbit interaction [18]. The aforementioned band narrowing at the Fermi energy generates a unique spin–orbit interaction at the interface and induces an additional orbital magnetic moment at the interface. This unique spin–orbit interaction and the induced orbital magnetic moment generate PMA. Because the band narrowing originates with the chemical bonds between the different species at the interface, the sign and magnitude of PMA are roughly determined by the 3d electron occupation at the Fermi level, e.g., band filling [18].

Figure 17.7a shows the representative magnetization curves of a Co/Cr superlattice showing perpendicular magnetic anisotropy. It is clearly seen that both the remanent magnetization and coercivity are higher in the direction perpendicular to the film compared to those in the direction parallel to the film. These are a clear signature of PMA. Considering the fact that PMA is an interface effect, the effective PMA energy per unit volume, K_{eff}, is phenomenologically expressed as

$$K_{\mathrm{eff}} = K_V - 2\pi M_S^2 + 2\frac{K_S}{t_{\mathrm{FM}}} \qquad (17.2)$$

where K_{V} is the bulk-term of magnetic anisotropy such as magneto-crystalline anisotropy; M_{S} is the saturation magnetization; K_{S} is interface magnetic anisotropy constant; and t_{FM} is the ferromagnetic layer thickness. In this formula, a positive (negative) K_{eff} represents PMA (in-plane anisotropy). According to Eq. (17.2), PMA should be linearly weakened with an increase in the ferromagnetic layer thickness. In fact, the K_{eff} estimated from the magnetization curves decreases with an increase in t_{FM}, as shown in Fig. 17.7b.

PMA is not only of scientific interest but also offers engineering advantages, especially for magnetic memory and storage applications. The perpendicularly oriented magnetization contributes to the high integration and low power consumption of such devices. Because of this, huge efforts have been devoted to developing systems with suitable PMA [19].

17.4.2 Exchange Anisotropy

Exchange anisotropy is another representative of interface magnetic anisotropy and is widely utilized in spin electronic devices such as MRAM. Exchange anisotropy is interface magnetic anisotropy between a ferromagnet (FM) and an antiferromagnet (AFM) [20–22]. Exchange anisotropy is referred to as a shift in the magnetization curve along the magnetic-field axis, and this shift is called the exchange bias. Because of this exchange bias, the remanent magnetization direction of the FM layer attached to the AFM layer, unlike the bi-stability of the usual FM, is defined in one direction. The defined magnetization direction is utilized as the reference direction of magnetization in magneto-resistive devices such as spin valves. In the present devices, the Mn–Ir alloy is used as the AFM to induce the exchange bias. However, high-integration, low-power consumption devices require a change in the magnetization direction from in-plane to out-of-plane. This condition requires a perpendicularly oriented exchange bias, e.g., perpendicular exchange bias. In principle, a high perpendicular exchange bias requires (1) perpendicularly oriented interfacial AFM spins, (2) PMA at the FM layer, and (3) PMA at the FM/AMF interface. In the intensively studied Co(−Fe)/Mn–Ir system, the interfacial

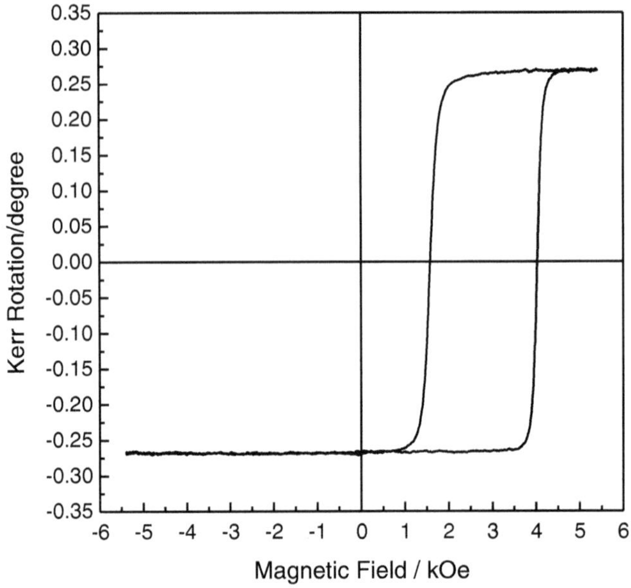

Fig. 17.8 Magneto-optic Kerr effect loop of Pt/Co/α-Cr_2O_3 thin film showing the high perpendicular exchange bias. Measurement temperature is 80 K. Applied field direction is perpendicular to the film

Mn spins that lie in the film plane [23] and Co(−Fe)/Mn–Ir interface induce in-plane magnetic anisotropy [24]. Thus, in order to realize a high perpendicular exchange bias, new AFM materials are desired. In this section, we describe a high perpendicular exchange bias using an α-Cr_2O_3 layer as an AFM [25–27].

Figure 17.8 shows the magnetic hysteresis loop of the Pt/Co/α-Cr_2O_3 system measured using the magneto-optic Kerr effect (MOKE). MOKE measurements were carried out in the polar configuration, which gives perpendicular magnetization. The loop shift along the magnetic-field axis is clearly seen, and an exchange bias field of about 3 kOe is obtained. Using the saturation magnetization value, the exchange anisotropy energy is estimated to be about 0.3 erg/cm^2. This is the highest value reported for a perpendicular exchange bias. The high value obtained is explained by the spin configuration of Cr and Co.

Recently, methods for controlling the exchange bias using an external field such as an electric field have attracted considerable attention [28]. α-Cr_2O_3 is a promising candidate because of its magnetoelectric ability through an magnetoelectric effect [29]. In principle, this concept does not require an electric current. Thus, magnetic devices with very low power consumption can be realized. In this sense, although the exchange bias has been known since the middle 1950s, its new functionality opens a new window on spin electronics.

17.5 Summary

In this chapter, we reviewed the basics for designing and fabricating nano-materials using ultrathin film techniques. In particular, the fabrication and growth of ultrathin films, the superparamagnetic properties of the Fe nanoparticles formed by V–W growth, and the representative interfacial magnetism in two-dimensional magnetic thin films were highlighted. In the nanometer regime, the initial stage of thin film growth determines the nanostructure, and the surface/interface properties dominate its physical properties. Thus, controlling these factors is essential for fabricating suitable nano-materials.

Acknowledgments This study was partly supported by the Encouragement of Young Scientists (B), Priority Assistance for the Formation of Worldwide Renowned Centers of Research—The Global COE Program (Project: Center of Excellence for Advanced Structural and Functional Materials Design) from the Ministry of Education, Culture, Sports, Science and Technology (MEXT), Japan. It was also supported by the Murata Science Foundation.

References

1. Néel L (1949) C R Acad Sci (Paris) 228:664
2. Shiratsuchi Y, Yamamoto M, Bader SD (2007) Prog Surf Sci 82:121
3. Herman MA, Sitter H (1989) Molecular beam epitaxy. Springer, Berlin
4. Gamberdella P, Blamc M, Bruke H, Kuhnke ad K, Kern K (2000) Phys Rev B 61:2254
5. Elmers HJ, Hauschild J, Gradmann U (1999) Phys Rev B 59:3688
6. Shen J, Skomski R, Klaua M, Jenniches H, Mohoharan SS, Kischner J (1997) Phys Rev B 56:2340
7. Temmyo J, Kuramochi E, Kamada H, Tamamura T (1998) J Cryst Growth 195:516
8. Shiratsuchi Y, Endo Y, Yamamoto M, Li D, Bader SD (2003) J Appl Phys 94:7675
9. Shiratsuchi Y, Endo Y, Yamamoto M (2004) Thin Sold Films 465:141
10. Shiratsuchi Y, Yamamoto M (2007) Phys Rev B 76:114432
11. Dormann J, Fiorani D, Tronc E (1997) Adv Chem Phys XCVIII:283
12. Chantrell RW, Eil-Hilo M, O'Grady K (1991) IEEE Trans Magn 27:3570
13. Bruno P, Renard J-P (1989) Appl Phys A 49:499
14. Carcia PF, Meinhaldt AD, Suna A (1985) Appl Phys Lett 47:178
15. Chappert C, Bruno P (1988) J Appl Phys 64:5736
16. Takanashi K, Mitani S, Himi K, Fujimori H (1998) Appl Phys Lett 72:737
17. Girod S, Gottwald M, Andrieu S, Mangin S, McCord J, Fullerton EE, Beaujour J-ML, Krishnatreya BJ, Kent AD (2009) Appl Phys Lett 94:262504
18. Kyuno K, Ham J-G, Yamamoto R, Asano S (1996) J Appl Phys 79:7084
19. Ikeda S, Miura K, Yamamoto H, Mizunuma K, Gan HD, Endo M, Kanai S, Hayakawa J, Matsukura F, Ohno H (2010) Nat Mater 9:721
20. Meiklejohn WH, Bean CP (1956) Phys Rev 102:1413
21. Meiklejohn WH, Bean CP (1957) Phys Rev 105:904
22. Nogués J, Shuller IK (1999) J Magn Magn Mater 192:203
23. Mitsumata C, Sakuma A, Fukamichi K, Tsunoda M, Takahashi M (2008) J Phys Soc Jpn 77:044602
24. van Dijken S, Besnier M, Moritz J, Coey JMD (2005) J Appl Phys 97:10K114

25. Shiratsuchi Y, Fujita T, Oikawa H, Noutomi H, Nakatani R (2010) Appl Phys Express 3:113001
26. Shiratsuchi Y, Noutomi H, Oikawa H, Fujita T, Nakatani R (2011) J Appl Phys 109:07C101
27. Shiratsuchi Y, Fujita T, Noutomi H, Oikawa H, Nakatani R (2011) IEEE Trans Magn 47:3909
28. He X, Wang Y, Wu N, Caruso AN, Vescovo E, Belashchenko KD, Dowben PA, Binek C (2010) Nat Mater 9(579)
29. Astrov DN (1961) Sov Phys JETP 13:729

Chapter 18
Advanced Materials Design via Low-Damage Plasma Processes

Yuichi Setsuhara

Abstract Low-damage plasma processing of materials is strongly desired for development of a variety of advanced devices with inorganic/organic hybrid materials structure (formation of inorganic functional layers on soft-materials substrate and/or stack layer formation with inorganic functional layers and organic functional layers), especially for development of flexible electronics, flat-panel displays, thin-film photovoltaic cells, biomaterials and microelectronics. For successful development of the organic/inorganic hybrid devices, low-temperature formation of high-quality inorganic functional layers (inorganic semiconductors and/or transparent conductive oxides) on soft materials and ultra-fine control of interface structure are required to avoid considerable degradation of soft materials. In this chapter, low-damage plasma processes have been described on the basis of plasma production with low-inductance antenna (LIA) modules to sustain radio-frequency inductively coupled discharges, which can provide one of the solutions to realize high-density and low-damage plasma production and active control of power deposition profiles over large area.

Keywords Flexible device • Inductively-coupled plasma • Inorganic/organic device • Low inductance antenna • Low-damage process

18.1 Introduction

For more than three decades since last century, plasma processes have been intensively developed and have made outstanding progress as one of the key technologies for leading development of a variety of industrial applications [1]

Y. Setsuhara (✉)
Joining and Welding Research Institute, Osaka University, 11-1 Mihogaoka, Ibaraki, Osaka 567-0047, Japan
e-mail: setsuhara@jwri.osaka-u.ac.jp

T. Kakeshita (ed.), *Progress in Advanced Structural and Functional Materials Design*, DOI 10.1007/978-4-431-54064-9_18, © Springer Japan 2013

ranging from surface modification of materials [2, 3], protective coatings [4, 5] to advanced technologies including flat-panel displays (FPDs) [6], thin-film photovoltaic cells [7], biomaterials [8] and microelectronics [9, 10].

Challenges in development of the new plasma processes are continuously in progress in accordance with developments in novel applications including nanostructure materials formation toward new materials synthesis in future. In other words, it may not be exaggerated to say that the plasma-process technologies have been developed and are to be developed as key technologies for a variety of innovations on a background of economical and social trends on a global scale. Especially, large-area processes are required for enhancement of production efficiency and/or cost reduction [5, 6].

Furthermore, low-damage processing of soft-materials (polymers, biomaterials) [7] attract great attentions for development of next-generation devices in inorganic/organic hybrid materials, which are expected to offer a wide range of applications including flexible electronic devices [11] and advanced ULSIs [12]. As a means of low-temperature processes and nano-structure formation, plasma processes are considered as one of the most promising technologies.

For successful development of the inorganic/organic hybrid devices, low-temperature formation of high-quality inorganic functional layers (including semiconductors and transparent conductive electrodes) on soft materials and ultra-fine control of interface are required for avoiding considerable degradation of soft materials. For ultra-fine control of interface between soft materials and inorganic functional films, low-damage plasma-process technologies must be developed via basic understandings of plasma interactions with soft materials during plasma processes.

Moreover, technology development to form the inorganic/organic hybrid structures, which consist of inorganic functional layer (inorganic semiconductors and/or transparent electrode) stacked on an organic functional layer (organic semiconductor and/or electrode), may provide advanced flexible devices with new functions. However, the conventional technologies are constrained to utilize vacuum evaporation for the formation of the inorganic layer on the organic functional layer because plasma-induced damages are strongly anticipated.

For successful development of plasma processing technologies applicable to fabrications of organic/inorganic hybrid devices, it is of great significance to avoid unwanted degradation of organic molecules due to exposure with ions [13, 14], radicals [15], photons [16] and electrons [17] during plasma processes because the bond-dissociation energies of soft materials are comparatively lower than those of inorganic materials. In the plasma processes, these fundamental processes may contribute to modification and/or degradation of the soft materials in complex synergetic manners.

Among these processes, the plasma-process damage due to ion bombardment is closely related to bond-dissociation energies in soft materials via nuclear collision process of ions impinging onto the surface of the soft materials. The bond-dissociation energies are, in general, about 4eV for the C–CH_3 bond, about 5eV for the O–C(=O) bond and about 8eV for C=O bond [18]. Considering elastic collision of an Ar^+ ion with a carbon atom incorporated in an organic molecule of soft materials, it is required to lower the average ion energy below ~7eV in order to avoid bond dissociation of the O–C(=O) bond assuming head-on collision of the Ar^+ ion with the carbon atom as a collision event for maximum energy transfer to the recoiled carbon atom [19]. Thus it is significant to develop plasma-process technologies, which can lower ion energy impinging onto the surface during the process. However, the methods to reduce irradiation flux of ions generally require processing of materials in lowered plasma-density condition, in which processing throughput should also be degraded. Therefore, it is considered that the plasma-processing technologies with reduced ion-damage are attractive from the practical point of view.

In order to meet above-mentioned requirements, low-damage plasma-process technologies have been developed via employing low-inductance antenna (LIA) modules [20] to sustain inductively coupled plasma (ICP), which can provide one of the solutions to realize high-density plasma production with lowered sheath-edge potential and active control of power deposition profiles over large area. [19–29] Ion energy distributions measured with a mass-separated ion energy analyzer showed significantly lowered ion energy at the sheath edge as low as 5eV [27].

In this chapter, low-damage plasma-process technologies are described on the basis of plasma production with the LIA modules to sustain radio-frequency inductively coupled discharges, which can provide one of the solutions to realize high-density and low-damage plasma production and active control of power deposition profiles over large area.

18.2 Designs of ICP Sources

Inductively coupled plasmas (ICP) can be sustained by applying radio-frequency (RF) current at frequencies of 1–100 MHz to inductive antenna conductor [1, 10, 30]. Electrons are accelerated by inductive electric field $\boldsymbol{E}_{\mathrm{ind}}$, which is induced by sinusoidal temporal variation of RF magnetic field $\boldsymbol{B}_{\mathrm{rf}}$ via RF current, following the Faraday's law of induction; i.e., rot $\boldsymbol{E}_{\mathrm{ind}} = -\partial \boldsymbol{B}_{\mathrm{rf}}/\partial t$. The vector differential equation implies that (a) the direction of the induced electric field is the rotational direction of the temporal variation of the magnetic field, and (b) the strength of the induced electric field is in proportion to the temporal differential of the magnetic field strength. In other words, (a) the electric field induced by the RF antenna conductor is in parallel along the antenna conductor and (b) the strength of the induced electric field is in proportion to the amplitude of the RF current and the frequency of the RF current.

Typical plasma density (electron density or ion density) of ICP is in the range of 10^{10}–10^{12} cm^{-3}, which is one or two orders of magnitude higher than that in capacitively coupled RF plasmas (CCP), in gas pressures in the range of 10^{-1} to 10^3 Pa. In these typical discharge conditions, electron temperature (1–10eV) is much higher than gas temperature, and thus the ICPs generated in low pressure

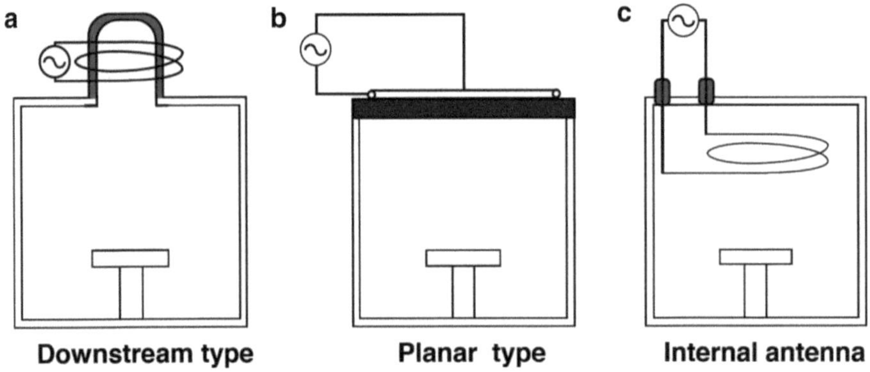

Fig. 18.1 Schematic illustration of antenna configurations for ICP production; (**a**) downstream type, (**b**) planar-antenna configuration and (**c**) internal antenna configuration

regions are in non-equillibrium state. Whereas, the ICPs sustained at higher pressures tend to be thermalized to approach thermal equilibrium with increasing pressure. Also, in most of the discharge conditions, the electron plasma frequency (in proportion to square-root of the plasma density) is of the order of 1–10 GHz, which is much higher than the frequency of the RF power source (1–100 MHz). This implies that the induced electric field cannot penetrate deeply into plasma region due to skin effect. Thus RF power is absorbed only in the skin sheath region by plasmas.

Variations of ICP reactors with different antenna configurations are schematically shown in Fig. 18.1. The downstream type shown in Fig. 18.1a employs the helical coil, which is wound around a dielectric tube. In the planar antenna geometry shown in Fig. 18.1b, helical coil wound on a plane is employed for enlargement of processing areas. In these antenna configurations, the RF antenna is located in air and the induction electric field is applied to the skin sheath region through a dielectric window (external antenna configuration). Here one of the major problems associated with the dielectric window in these ICP configurations is degradation of the source efficiency because the field strength for sustaining the discharge tends to be reduced by the thick dielectric window [20].

From this viewpoint, an internal-antenna configuration, as shown in Fig. 18.1c to produce ICP has attracted great interests as a promising candidate as an efficient high-density source, as well as an alternative to avoid problems associated with dielectric windows in the external antenna configurations. In the internal antenna configurations, however, it is essential to minimize the electrostatic coupling of RF antenna voltages to the plasma, which may cause anomalous rise of plasma potential [20, 31, 32].

An electrical circuit representation of ICP antenna and schematic illustrations of RF voltage distribution along the antenna are shown in Fig. 18.2. When a sinusoidal RF current I_{rf} is applied to the ICP antenna with an inductance L, the RF voltage arising at the power-end of the antenna V_1 is given by $V_1 = \omega L I_{rf}$, where ω is an

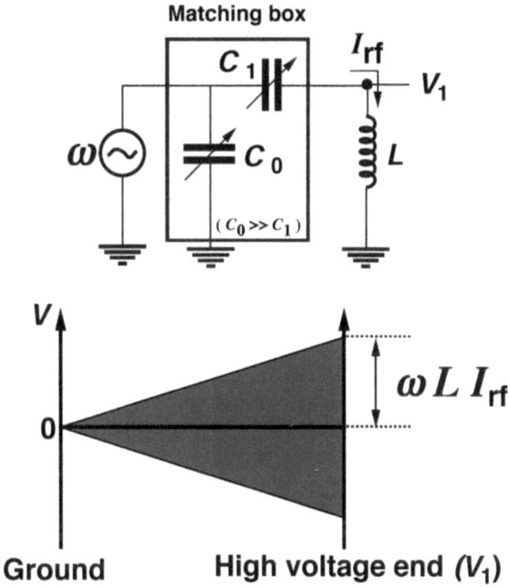

Fig. 18.2 Electrical circuit representation of ICP antenna and RF voltage distribution along the antenna

angular frequency of the RF current. Assuming that the RF current leakage to the plasma is neglected, the RF voltage may be linearly distributed along the antenna electrode as schematically illustrated in Fig. 18.2. Here it is pointed out that the RF voltage is always present at the powered end of the antenna, and thus the electrostatic coupling of the RF voltage to the plasma is always present in generation of ICPs.

Reduction of the electrostatic coupling of RF antenna voltages to the plasma is of great importance for ICP generation with lowered plasma potential, which is significant for low-damage high-quality processing of materials. Furthermore, considering the plasma-source designs to satisfy the requirement for enlargement of plasma sources toward a meter scale, increase of an antenna inductance and hence increase of an RF-voltage amplitude arising at the antenna terminals cannot be avoided with increasing source size, when the source employs a large loop-shaped antenna.

Feasibility of high-density plasma production with suppressed electrostatic coupling by lowering the RF voltage of the internal antenna has been demonstrated via (a) the employment of antenna configurations with lowered antenna inductance, which is roughly proportional to the square of turn numbers and the area size of the loop, (b) lowering of the RF-voltage amplitude by the antenna termination with a blocking capacitor and (c) dielectric isolation of the antenna conductor from plasma [20]. As a novel technology to achieve low-voltage operation of ICPs suitable for producing large-area source with low-damage process capability, an internal-antenna configuration with multiple "low-inductance antenna (LIA) module," as schematically shown in Fig. 18.3, has been proposed [20]. The ICP production using the LIA modules has exhibited stable production of plasmas at RF input powers of 3 kW to attain densities approaching as high as 1×10^{12} cm^{-3} at argon

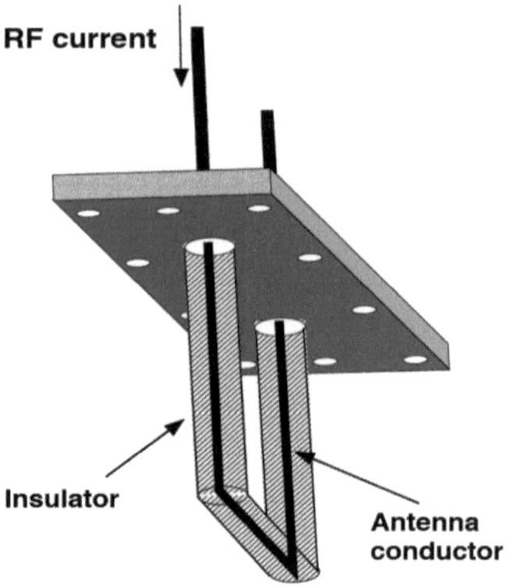

Fig. 18.3 Schematic of low-inductance antenna

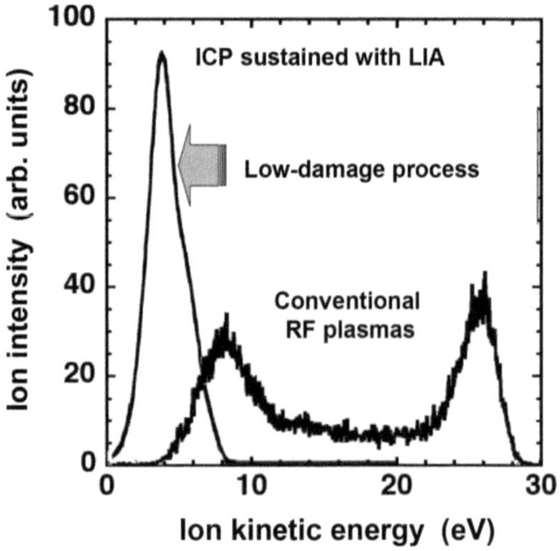

Fig. 18.4 Ion energy distribution function (IEDF) measured in an ICP sustained with LIA modules in Ar gas at a pressure of 13 Pa and with 13.56-MHz RF power of 1 kW with typical IEDF for conventional RF plasma source (CCP mode with large potential fluctuation) for comparison

pressures around 1 Pa with simultaneous achievement of the suppression of the electrostatic coupling [20].

Furthermore the lowering of the electrostatic RF voltage via reduction in the antenna inductance for sustaining ICPs has exhibited additional favorable features for low-damage plasma processes via low-voltage operations of ICPs. The ion energy distribution function (IEDF) attained in an ICP sustained with LIA at Ar at a pressure of 13 Pa and with 13.56-MHz RF power of 1 kW is shown in Fig. 18.4, together with a typical IEDF for conventional RF plasma source (CCP mode with larger potential fluctuation) for comparison. The peak ion energy in the IEDF for the ICP sustained with the LIAs shows significantly lowered as being equivalent to or less than 5eV as compared with conventional RF plasma sources. Moreover, the IEDF for the ICP sustained with the LIA showed a very narrow energy width of about 2eV, which is significantly narrower than that for the conventional RF plasma sources.

18.3 Plasma Interactions with Soft Materials

In this section, effects of argon plasma exposure onto the surface of soft materials are described on the basis of chemical bonding states analysis via conventional X-ray photoelectron spectroscopy (XPS) [19]. Polyethylene terephthalate (PET) film has been selected as a test material for investigations in the present study not because of its specific applications, such as a substrate material, but because PET is one of the well defined organic materials containing a variety of major components in a variety of functional soft materials; C–C main chain, CH bond, oxygen functionalities (O=C–O bond and C–O bond) and phenyl group. Especially, changes in the phenyl group due to argon plasma exposures have been investigated in the present article in order to examine plasma interactions with π-conjugated component, which is in charge of electronic functions in many of the π-conjugated electronic organic materials to be utilized as functional layer for advanced flexible device applications.

Argon plasmas for this investigation were generated in a plasma chamber with 500-mm inner diameter and 200-mm height, which was connected to a diffusion chamber with a 500 mm inner diameter and a 400 mm height, as previously reported elsewhere [19–21]. The LIA modules consisted of a U-shaped antenna conductor, which was fully covered with dielectric tubing for complete isolation from the plasma. Eight LIA modules with a 70 mm width and a 160 mm height were mounted on the top flange of the chamber and were coupled to an RF power generator at 13.56 MHz via a matching network. A water-cooled substrate holder was placed at a distance of 297 mm from the top flange. The base pressure of the chamber evacuated with a turbo-molecular pump was 3×10^{-4} Pa.

Ion energy distribution function (IEDF) of the ions impinging onto the ground potential from the plasmas was measured using a mass-separated ion-energy analyzer (Hiden, EQP500), which was mounted beside the substrate holder [27].

For investigations of the plasma-polymer interactions, PET films (0.1 mm thick) were exposed to argon plasmas sustained at an RF power of 1,000 W at Ar pressures of 0.67–26 Pa. Here it is noted that the PET films were set on water-cooled substrate holder when they were exposed to the plasmas.

Chemical bonding states at nano-surface layer of the PET films exposed to argon plasmas were analyzed using conventional XPS. The XPS analysis was performed using AXIS-165x spectrometer (Shimadzu Corp., JAPAN) with non-monochromatized MgKa radiation (photon energy of 1253.6eV). The conventional XPS analyses were carried out directly after plasma exposure without formation of any additional conductive coating on the sample surface due to

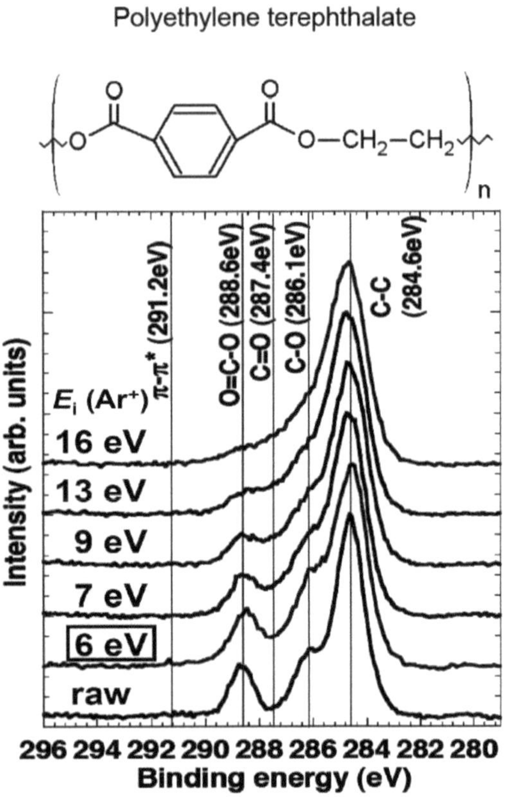

Fig. 18.5 Photoelectron C1s spectra for PET films before and after exposure to argon plasmas with a variation of argon pressures (or ion bombardment energy)

charging-suppression function of the spectrometer. Here it is also noted that the PET samples were taken out to the air after the plasma exposure before the XPS measurements.

Before the plasma exposure experiment, the IEDF of the argon ions impinging to the ground potential through the sheath edge of the argon plasmas were measured using the mass-separated ion-energy analyzer. Peak values of ion energy distributions decreased from 15 to 6eV with increasing Ar pressure from 0.67 to 26.6 Pa (15eV at 0.67 Pa, 13eV at 1.3 Pa, 9eV at 6.5 Pa, 7eV at 13 Pa, and 6eV at 26 Pa) [29]. Furthermore, the ion-bombardment energy onto non-conductive substrate (the PET film in the present investigation) is almost equivalent to potential drop from plasma potential to floating potential. As reported in the previous work, the potential drop of argon plasma was in the range of 3–15eV for Ar pressures of 0.26–13 Pa (15eV at 0.26 Pa, 8eV at 1.3 Pa, and 3eV at 13 Pa) [29].

Chemical bonding states of the PET films exposed to argon plasmas were examined via conventional XPS. The PET films were exposed to argon plasmas sustained at an RF power of 1,000 W and argon pressures of 0.67–26 Pa with an ion dose of 4.3×10^{18} ions/cm^2. The photoelectron C1s spectra for PET films without and with exposure to argon plasmas with a variation of argon pressures are shown in

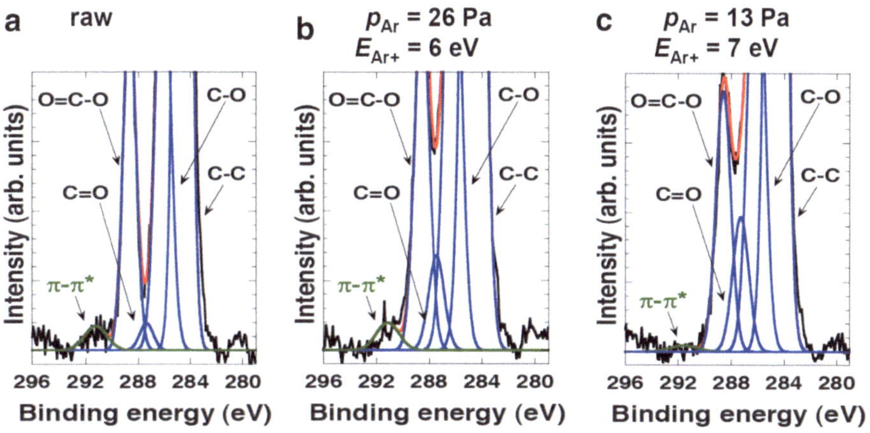

Fig. 18.6 XPS C1s spectra to highlight the phenyl group for PET films; (**a**) without plasma exposure and with exposure to argon plasmas sustained at an RF 1,000 W at argon pressure of (**b**) 26 Pa and (**c**) 13 Pa

Fig. 18.5. The C1s spectra of the PET samples can be deconvoluted into following components; C–C bond at 284.6eV, C–O bond at 286.1eV, C=O bond at 287.4eV, O=C–O bond at 288.6eV and π–π* shake-up satellite at 291.2eV [33, 34].

The C1s XPS spectra show that the exposure with the argon plasmas tended to degrade the O=C–O bond and the C–O bond with slight increase of the C=O bond with decreasing argon pressure (i.e., increasing ion energy) [19, 29]. These tendencies of the variation of the chemical bonding states indicate that the scissions of the O=C–O bond and the C–O bond are significantly enhanced by increasing energy of the ion bombardment and the scission of the O=C–O bond may result in formation of the C=O bond. Here it is noted that the raw PET sample before the plasma exposure shows that the photoelectron component corresponding to the C=O bond is insignificant because the carbon atom with an oxygen double bond (C=O) is bonded also with another neighbor oxygen atom via single bond and a carbon atom in the pristine molecule of the PET material, thus the photoelectron corresponding to the C=O bond is not present in the pristine PET. Thus the sight increase in the C=O bond component with increasing ion energy is considered to be due to the bond scission of O=C–O structure to form the C=O bond with a dangling bond.

Additionally, it is remarkable to stress here that the degradation of the oxygen functionalities (the O=C–O bond and the C–O bond) during the plasma exposure at 26 Pa was insignificant, indicating that the suppression of the plasma process damage may be feasible via controlling the ion bombardment energy below ~ 6eV during plasma processing of polymers as previously reported elsewhere [19, 29].

Furthermore, in order to examine the effect of the argon plasma exposure on the phenyl group, which is considered to be one of the essential components in a variety of functional organic molecules especially for electronic functions, the C1s XPS spectra to highlight the phenyl group (π → π* shake-up satellite peak) are shown in

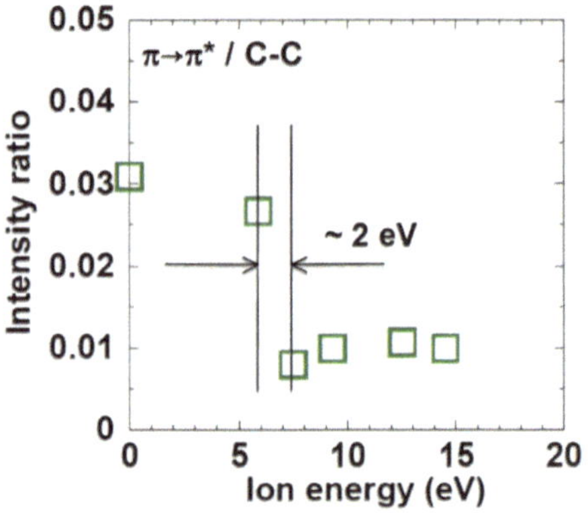

Fig. 18.7 Variation of the peak-area ratio of π → π* shake-up satellite peak to C–C bond ($I_{\pi\rightarrow\pi^*}/I_{C\text{–}C}$) evaluated from the XPS C1s spectra

Fig. 18.6, in which the spectra in Fig. 18.5 are expanded vertically in the intensities with the C–C bond intensity normalized. Peak-area ratio of π → π* shake-up satellite peak to C–C bond ($I_{\pi\rightarrow\pi^*}/I_{C\text{–}C}$) evaluated from the XPS C1s spectra are summarized in Fig. 18.7 as a function of the peak ion energy measured with the mass-separated ion-energy analyzer. The π → π* shake-up satellite peak intensity clearly decreased after the plasma exposure with ion bombardment energy above 6–7eV.

These results indicate that it is possible to prevent the degradation of C–O bond, O=C–O bond and phenyl group via controlling argon pressure to suppress the ion energy less than 6eV as previously reported elsewhere [19, 29]. Furthermore, it should be stressed that exhibition of the remarkable variation in the peak-area ratio of π → π* shake-up satellite peak to C–C bond as shown in Fig. 18.7 is considered to be due to extremely narrow energy width in the IEDF of approximately 2eV in the present plasmas sustained with the LIAs. This means that significantly fine control of bond dissociation can be feasible with the present plasma technology, which can control the IEDF with very narrow width due to low-voltage operation of ICPs.

These findings described above indicate that it is significant to control the ion bombardment energy or the ion energy distributions sufficiently below the threshold value, which may provide advanced process technology to realize "bond engineering" of the organic molecules of interest for development of advanced flexible devices.

18.4 Summary

In this chapter, plasma-process technologies for low-damage processing of materials were described on the basis of plasma production with low-inductance antenna (LIA) modules to sustain ICPs. The design issues and basic background involved in the ICP sources were briefly reviewed and feasibility of low-damage plasma sources were shown for the ICPs sustained with the LIAs. The interactions between argon plasmas and the PET films were examined for investigations of physical damages induced by plasma exposures to the organic material via chemical bonding-structure analyses via conventional XPS. The results indicate that it is significant to control the ion bombardment energy or the ion energy distributions sufficiently below the threshold value of interest, for development of successful processing of soft materials, especially for development of advanced flexible devices via formation of the structure with inorganic functional layers and/or electrodes to be stacked on organic functional materials as functional layers.

Acknowledgments This work was supported partly by The Global COE Program "Center of Excellence for Advanced Structural and Functional Materials Design" from the Ministry of Education, Culture, Sports, Science and Technology (MEXT), Japan.

References

1. Conrads H, Schmidt M (2000) Plasma Sources Sci Technol 9:441
2. Czerwiec T, Renevier N, Michel H (2000) Surf Coatings Technol 131:267
3. Mayrhofer PH, Mitterer C, Hultman L, Clemens H (2006) Prog Mater Sci 51:1032
4. Robertson J (1992) Surf Coatings Technol 50:185
5. Bhushan B (1999) Diamond Relat Mater 8:1985
6. Kuo Y (1995) J Electrochem Soc 142:2486
7. Goetzbergera A, Heblinga C, Schock H-W (2003) Mat Sci Eng R 40:1
8. Chua PK, Chena JY, Wanga LP, Huang N (2002) Mat Sci Eng R 36:143
9. Mogab CJ, Adams AC, Flamm DL (1978) J Appl Phys 49:3796
10. Lieberman MA, Lichtenberg AJ (1994) Principles of plasma discharges and materials processing. Wiley, New York
11. Choi M-C, Kim Y, Ha C-S (2008) Prog Polym Sci 33:581
12. International Technology Roadmap for Semiconductors, 2007 edition, Executive Summary
13. Gancarz I, Pozniak G, Bryjak M (1999) Eur Polym J 35:1419
14. Setsuhara Y, Cho K, Shiratani M, Sekine M, Hori M, Ikenaga E, Zaima S (2010) Thin Solid Films 518:3555
15. Steckenreiter T, Balanzat E, Fuess H, Trautmann C (1997) Nucl Instrum Methods Phys Res B 131:159
16. Day M, Willes DM (1972) J Appl Polymer Sci 16:203
17. Masseya S, Cloutierb P, Sancheb L, Roy D (2008) Rad Phys Chem 77:889
18. Stoliarov SI, Westmoreland PR, Nyden MR, Forney GP (2003) Polym 44:883
19. Setsuhara Y, Cho K, Takenaka K, Shiratani M, Sekine M, Hori M (2011) Thin Solid Films 519:6721
20. Setsuhara Y, Shoji T, Ebe A, Baba S, Yamamoto N, Takahashi K, Ono K, Miyake S (2003) Surf CoatTechnol 174–175:33
21. Takenaka K, Setsuhara Y, Nishisaka K, Ebe A (2006) Jpn J Appl Phys 45:8046
22. Tsuda O, Ishihara M, Koga Y, Fujiwara S, Setsuhara Y, Sato N (2005) J Phys Chem B 109:4917
23. Deguchi H, Yoneda H, Kato K, Kubota K, Hayashi T, Ogata K, Ebe A, Takenaka K, Setsuhara Y (2006) Jpn J Appl Phys 45:8042
24. Setsuhara Y, Takenaka K, Ebe A, Nishisaka K (2007) Solid State Phenomena 127:239
25. Setsuhara Y, Takenaka K, Ebe A, Nishisaka K (2007) Plasma Process Polym 4:S628

26. Setsuhara Y, Takenaka K, Ebe A, Han JG (2008) Surf CoatTechnol 202:5230
27. Takenaka K, Setsuhara Y, Nishisaka K, Ebe A (2008) Jpn J Appl Phys 47:6900
28. Takahashi E, Nishigami Y, Tomyo A, Fujiwara M, Kaki H, Kubota K, Hayashi T, Ogata K, Ebe A, Setsuhara Y (2007) Jpn J Appl Phys 46:1280
29. Setsuhara Y, Cho K, Shiratani M, Sekine M, Hori M (2010) Thin Solid Films 518:6492
30. Hopwood J (1992) Plasma Sources Sci Technol 1:109
31. Setsuhara Y, Kamai M, Miyake S, Musil J (1997) Jpn J Appl Phys 36:4568
32. Yamashita M, Setsuhara Y, Miyake S, Kumagai M, Shoji T, Musil J (1999) Jpn J Appl Phys 38:4291
33. Miyayama T, Sanada N, Iida S-I, Hammondb JS, Suzuki M (2008) Appl Surf Sci 255:951
34. Cui N-Y, Upadhyay DJ, Anderson CA, Meenan BJ, Brown NMD (2007) Appl Surf Sci 253:3865

Chapter 19
Advanced Analysis of Magnetic Structure in Materials

Tomoyuki Terai and Tomoyuki Kakeshita

Abstract Magnetic materials in which the atoms (ions) have magnetic moments show arrangements of these magnetic moments (magnetic structures). Analyzing these magnetic structures is very important to understand the magnetic properties of magnetic materials. There are many methods to determine the magnetic structures and the proper analysis method depends on the kind of magnetic structures. In this section, by using the typical spintronics materials, perovskite manganites and cobalt oxide, we show the analyses of (1) ferromagnetic structure (easy and hard axes of magnetization) by M–H curves of single crystal, (2) antiferromagnetic (canted-antiferromagnetic) structure by neutron diffraction and (3) spin glass by ac-susceptibility measurement.

Keywords Easy-axis • Hard-axis • Magnetic space groups • Magnetocrystalline anisotropy

19.1 Introduction

A word, "magnet," originated from magnesian stone in ancient Greece and a nature that a magnet attracts the other one or irons has attracted much interest. This nature was used for a compass in ancient and it is used nowadays for motive power and magnetic record media such as a motor, a HDD (Hard Disk Drive), etc. Recently, a technology, so-called "spintronics," in which not only the "sum" of spins of electrons in solids but also the "direction (up or down)" of each electron is utilized have been investigated extensively.

T. Terai (✉) • T. Kakeshita
Division of Materials and Manufacturing Science, Graduate School of Engineering, Osaka University, 2-1 Yamadaoka, Suita, Osaka 565-0871, Japan
e-mail: terai@mat.eng.osaka-u.ac.jp

T. Kakeshita (ed.), *Progress in Advanced Structural and Functional Materials Design*, DOI 10.1007/978-4-431-54064-9_19, © Springer Japan 2013

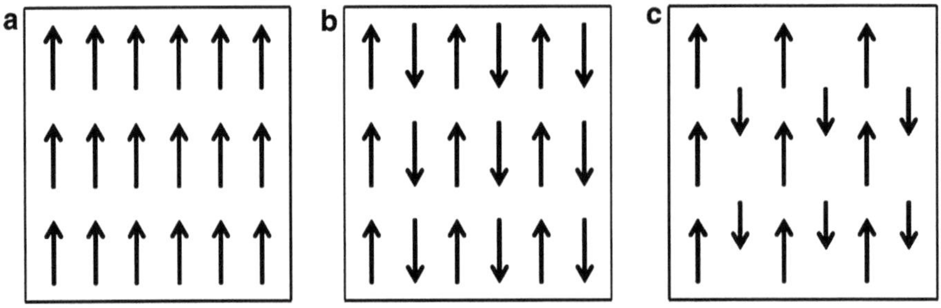

Fig. 19.1 Magnetic structures of (**a**) ferromagnetism, (**b**) antiferromagnetism and (**c**) ferrimagnetism

All materials show some response by applying external magnetic field because of the electrons in them. Especially, when unpaired electrons exist in atoms (ions) of solid materials, each atom (ion) has a magnetic moment and the solid materials show a large response to the external magnetic field. The magnetisms of them are classified into three types, "ferromagnetism, antiferromagnetism and ferrimagnetism" as shown in Fig. 19.1.[1] These arrangements of magnetic moments in the unit cell are called, "magnetic structure." As the crystal structure is classified into 230 space groups by the containing symmetry operations, the magnetic structure is able to be classified into 1,651 magnetic space groups [1].

To determine the value and arrangement of magnetic moments in materials is essential for the researches of magnetic materials and there are several ways for the determination. In this section, we will show the recent researches about the magnetic structures (and magnetism) in the typical spintronics materials, perovskite manganites and cobalt oxide and also show the method of analysis.

19.2 Magnetic Structures in Ferromagnets

As mentioned above, all magnetic moments of materials showing ferromagnetism (ferromagnet) are aligned in the grand state. With increasing temperature, the spontaneous magnetization decreases by thermal fluctuation and then becomes zero at Curie temperature, T_C. This temperature dependence is well expressed by a classical molecular field approximation [2] as shown in the following:

[1] In addition to these magnetic structures, the magnetic structures exist that magnetic moments rotate along an axis, so-called "helimagnetism" or the magnetic moments in Fig. 1b cant from the vertical direction and a small ferromagnetic component appears, so-called "canted-antiferromagnetism." They are explained by the competition between ferromagnetic and antiferromagnetic molecular fields and Dzyaloshinski–Moriya interaction ($E = D[\mathbf{S}_i \times \mathbf{S}_j]$) derived from the spin-orbital interaction and the symmetry of crystal.

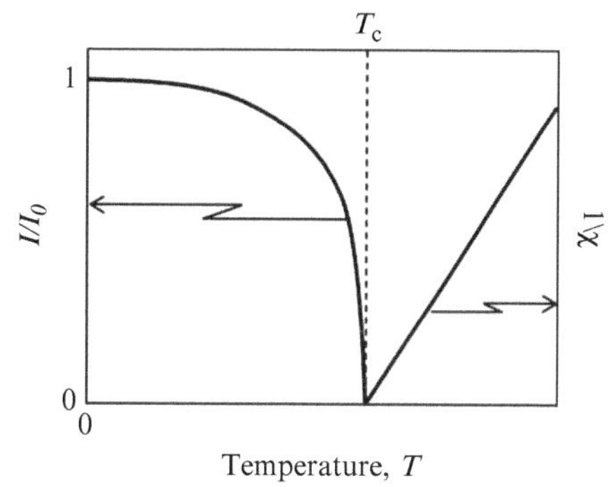

Fig. 19.2 Temperature dependences of spontaneous magnetization and magnetic susceptibility

$$I = \frac{C}{T}(H + \omega I), \tag{19.1}$$

$$\chi = \frac{I}{H} = \frac{C}{T - C\omega} = \frac{C}{T - \Theta}, \tag{19.2}$$

where I is magnetization, T is temperature, H is external magnetic field, ω is molecular field coefficient, χ is magnetic susceptibility and C is a constant. The temperature dependences of I and χ are schematically shown in Fig. 19.2. As known from the figure, $1/\chi$ is proportional to temperature above T_C. These values are able to be measured by the instruments such as magnetic balance, VSM (vibrating sample magnetometer) and SQUID (superconducting quantum interference device).[2]

Perovskite manganite, $R_{1-x}A_xMnO_3$ (R: rare earth ions, A: alkaline earth ions), and layered perovskite manganite, $R_{2-2x}A_{1+2x}Mn_2O_7$, show interesting phenomena such as metal-insulator transition, colossal magnetoresistance and charge ordering transition. Therefore, they have been extensively in the last two decades [3]. A characteristic feature of these oxides is that they show various magnetisms such as ferromagnetism, antiferromagnetism, canted-antiferromagnetism and spin-glass, and the magnetism is able to be tuned by the substitution of alkaline earth ions for rare earth ions. One of them, $(La_{1-x}Dy_x)_{0.7}Ca_{0.3}MnO_3$ ($x = 0.143$), show a typical ferromagnetism [4] and the temperature dependence of magnetization curve of a sintered polycrystalline specimen is shown in Fig. 19.3a.

As known from the figure, magnetic moment per Mn ion is $3.9\mu_B$ in the grand state. Considering the average ion valence of manganese ions, we can find that orbital angular momentum is almost quenched and spin quantum number is a good quantum number. With increasing temperature, the saturated magnetization

[2] When a ferromagnet is magnetized, a magnetic field being anitparallel to the external magnetic field occurs in the inside of ferromagnet by the magnetization of itself. This is named as demagnetization field and then, the effective magnetic field, H_{eff}, in the ferromagnet is $H_{eff} = H_{ex}\text{-}NI/\mu_0$. The demagnetization coefficient, N, depends on the shape of the ferromagnet (if the shape is sphere, N is 1/3).

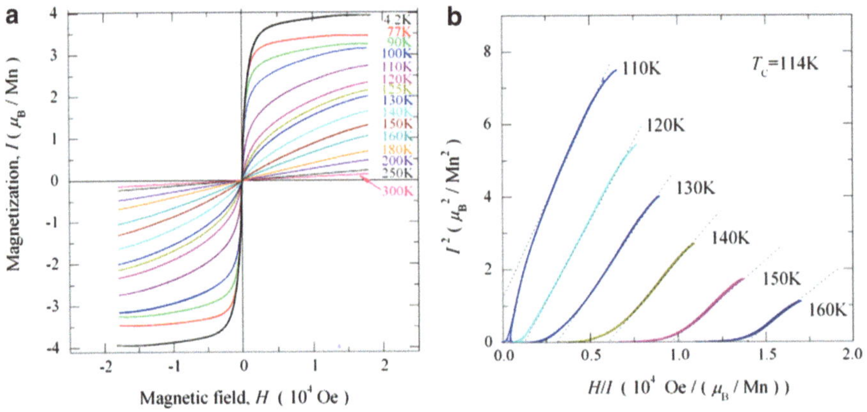

Fig. 19.3 (**a**) Magnetization curves and (**b**) Arrott-plots of $(La_{1-x}Dy_x)_{0.7}Ca_{0.3}MnO_3$ ($x = 0.143$)

decreases and then the magnetization is almost proportional to the external magnetic field at around room temperature and does not saturate in the range of applied external magnetic field. The Arrott-plot of the magnetization is shown in Fig. 19.3b. In molecular field approximation,[3] a temperature where I^2 is equal to zero at $H/I = 0$ is the Curie temperature and it is 114 K.

To determine the direction of magnetic moments in a ferromagnet, the magnetization curve for each direction of the single crystal should be measured and it should be estimated which direction is easy to saturate the magnetization by applying external magnetic field. As an earliest study, there has been a study about the magnetocrystalline anisotropy of Fe, Ni and Co single crystals by Honda et al. [5, 6] and they reported that the easy direction of magnetization of them are [1 0 0], [1 1 1] and *c*-axis, that is, the magnetic moments are aligned in these directions preferably. Incidentally, pure iron (and other metals) has a band structure of orbitals and the electrons itinerate in crystal. Therefore, the description that they have localized magnetic moments as shown in Fig. 19.1a is not correct. However, the result of neutron diffraction shows that 3d electrons generating its magnetism are relatively localized around Fe atoms and behave as Fe atoms have localized moments. The itinerant ferromagnetism in metals is explained by Stoner model [7].

Layered perovskite manganites, $La_{2-2x}Sr_{1+2x}Mn_2O_7$, consisting the stacking of MnO_2 conducting and (La, Sr)O insulating layers along *c*-axis show anisotropic magnetic behavior. Figure 19.4 shows the magnetization curves of $La_{2-2x}Sr_{1+2x}Mn_2O_7$ ($0.315 \leq x \leq 0.350$) in the grand state ($T = 4$ K) [8]. As know from

[3] Ferromagnets are composed of many magnetic domains in which magnetic moments are aligned to an easy direction of magnetization and the boundaries between magnetic domains are named domain wall. When magnetic field is applied, firstly the domain walls move and then, the magnetic moments thermally fluctuated rotate. The Arrott-plot indicates the relation between thermal fluctuation and rotation by magnetic field at around T_C.

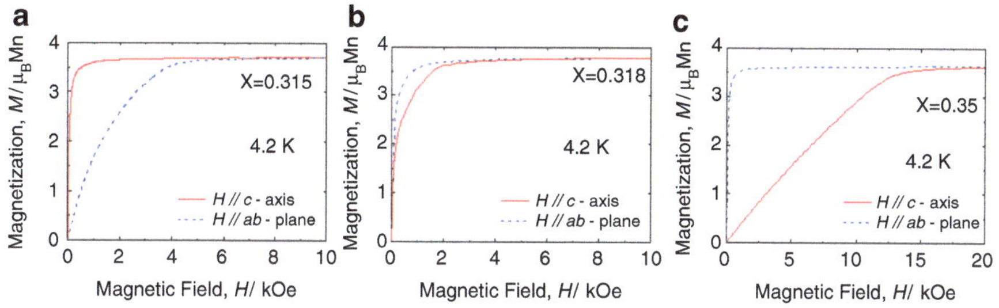

Fig. 19.4 Magnetization curves of $La_{2-2x}Sr_{1+2x}Mn_2O_7$ ($0.315 \leq x \leq 0.350$)

the figure, with increasing hole doping x, the easy direction of magnetization also changes from parallel into vertical to c-axis. The reason has not been clear yet. However, it is considered that it is closely related to the change of crystal field due to the distortion of MnO_6 octahedron. The area enclosed with two magnetization curves in each figure corresponds to magnetocrystalline anisotropy energy, K_a, and depends on the hole doping x ($-0.7 \times 10^6 \leq K_a \leq 2.5 \times 10^6$ erg/cm^3). The value of K_a is an important index showing the potential of permanent magnet and $Nd_2Fe_{14}B$ in Nd–Fe–B permanent magnet shows a large value of K_a (4.4×10^7 erg/cm^3).

19.3 Magnetic Structures in Antiferromagnets and Ferrimagnets

As mentioned in introduction, long range magnetic ordering in materials contains antiferromagnetism and ferrimagnetism (Fig. 19.1b, c) other than ferromagnetism (Fig. 19.1a). When magnetic field is applied, the magnetic susceptibility of the direction parallel to magnetic moments differs from that of the vertical direction. Figure 19.5 shows the magnetic susceptibility of CoO single crystal [9]. As known from the figure, in antiferromagnetic phase ($T \leq 293$ K), the values of χ along c-axis are lower than those along a-axis. From the molecular field theory for antiferromagnets, this result suggests that the magnetic moments are aligned along c-axis.[4] However, when a complicated magnetic structure has to be determined, neutron diffraction measurements are need. Neutron is an elementary particle and has spin of 1/2. Therefore, when neutrons are irradiated into materials, they are scattered by the magnetic moments of electrons (and nucleus). By using these scattering, the magnetic structure is able to be determined.

[4] Recent synchrotron and neutron diffraction measurements have shown that CoO has a monoclinic structure (β~90.3°) and a complicated magnetic structure. However, for simplicity, the crystal and magnetic structures are dealt as a pseudo tetragonal structure and a structure whose magnetic moments are aligned along c-axis.

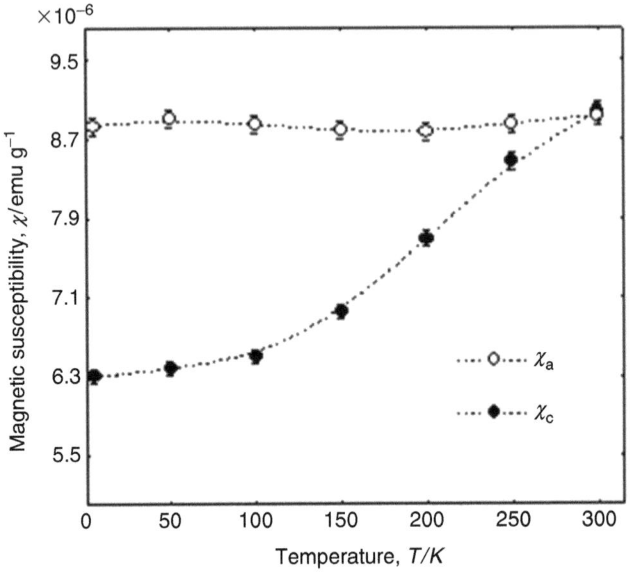

Fig. 19.5 Temperature dependence of magnetic susceptibility in CoO

Layered perovskite manganite, $La_{2-2x}Sr_{1+2x}Mn_2O_7$, has been reported to show antiferromagnetic structures at near $x = 0.3$ [10, 11], however the reported structures are different each other and the correct structure was not clear. Recently, it has been become clear by neutron diffraction using a good and large single crystal of $x = 0.307$ [12]. Figure 19.6 show the temperature dependences of $\{0\ 0\ l\}$ and $\{1\ 1\ l\}$ peaks $La_{2-2x}Sr_{1+2x}Mn_2O_7$ ($x = 0.307$) obtained by Tri-Axis Spectrometer (TAS-2) at JRR-3 in JAEA. Based on these data, magnetic structure was analyzed at each temperature. In the analysis, the magnetic diffraction intensities of $h + k + l = 2n$ are obtained by subtracting the nuclear diffraction intensity in paramagnetic structure at 160 K.

In the analysis, based on the reported electronic and magnetic properties of layered perovskite manganites ($x < 0.4$), we assume that magnetic structures satisfy the following:

1. The unit cell size of the magnetic structure is same as that of the crystal structure.
2. All magnetic moments of Mn sites in one MnO_2 conducting layer are parallel each other.
3. The magnetic moment lengths of Mn ions are constant.

Then, we calculate intensities based on the assumed structure and compare it with the observed ones. The theoretical integrated intensities are expressed as,

$$I_{\text{mag}} = A \cdot J \cdot L(\theta) \cdot \frac{d\sigma(\tau)}{d\Omega}, \quad (19.3)$$

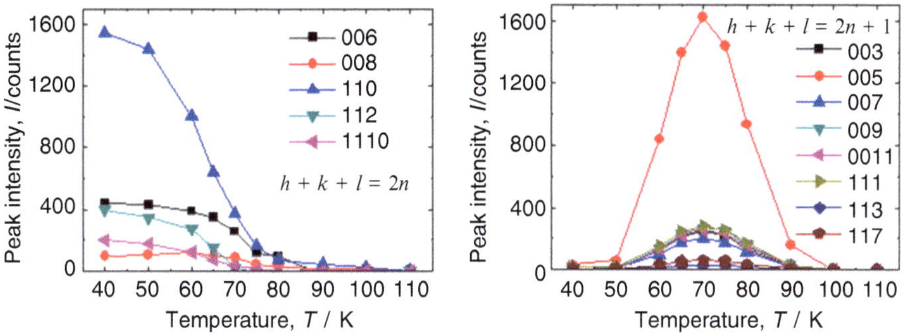

Fig. 19.6 Temperature dependences of integrated peak intensities of $La_{2-2x}Sr_{1+2x}Mn_2O_7$ ($x = 0.307$)

where A is proportion constant, J is correction factor of extinction effect. $L(\theta)$ is Lorenz factor, which is expressed as,

$$L(\theta) = \frac{1}{\sin(2\theta)}, \tag{19.4}$$

and $d\sigma(\boldsymbol{\tau})/d\Omega$ is magnetic scattering cross-sections on each magnetic structures, which are expressed as,

$$\frac{\mathrm{d}(\tau)}{\mathrm{d}\Omega} = \left| \sum_{j=0}^{\mathrm{n}} p_{\mathrm{j}} q_{\mathrm{j}} \exp(\mathrm{i}\tau \cdot r_{\mathrm{j}}) \right|^2, \tag{19.5}$$

where $\boldsymbol{\tau}$ is the diffraction vector, p_{j} is the average magnetic scattering amplitude of Mn sites and $\boldsymbol{q}_{\mathrm{j}}$ is the $\boldsymbol{q}$-factor of magnetic scattering. The value of p_{j} is expressed as,

$$p_{\mathrm{j}} = 0.269 \times 10^{12} |S_{\mathrm{j}}| f_{\mathrm{Mn}}(\tau), \tag{19.6}$$

$$S_{\mathrm{j}} = S_{\mathrm{F}} \exp(\mathrm{i} K_{\mathrm{F}} \cdot r_{\mathrm{j}}) + S_{\mathrm{AF}} \exp(\mathrm{i} K_{\mathrm{AF}} \cdot r_{\mathrm{j}}), \tag{19.7}$$

where $\boldsymbol{S}_{\mathrm{j}}$ is the magnetic moment of each Mn site, $f_{\mathrm{Mn}}(\boldsymbol{\tau})$ is the magnetic form factor, $\boldsymbol{S}_{\mathrm{F}}$ and $\boldsymbol{S}_{\mathrm{AF}}$ are the magnetic moments of ferromagnetic and antiferromagnetic components and $\boldsymbol{K}_{\mathrm{F}}$ and $\boldsymbol{K}_{\mathrm{AF}}$ are their propagation vectors, respectively. From the assumption 1 and 2, these vectors are

$$K_{\mathrm{F}} = 0, \tag{19.8}$$

and

$$K_{\mathrm{AF}} = 2\pi c^{*} \mathrm{Sq}(\mathrm{z}), \tag{19.9}$$

where $\boldsymbol{c}^*$ is a reciprocal lattice vector and Sq(z) is a square wave function which is expressed as,

$$\mathrm{Sq}(z) = \sum_{n=-\infty}^{\infty} 2\Pi(2z - 2n) - 1, \tag{19.10}$$

where $\Pi(z)$ is the rectangular function. From Eqs. (19.6) to (19.10), the magnetic scattering cross section of Eq. (19.5) is rewritten as,

$$\begin{aligned}\frac{d\sigma(\tau)}{d\Omega} &= 7.24 \times 10^{22} f_{\mathrm{Mn}}^2(\tau)\left|\sum_{j=0}^{n} |S_j| q_j \exp[i \cdot (\tau + K)] \cdot r_j\right|^2 \\ &= 7.24 \times 10^{22} f_{\mathrm{Mn}}^2(\tau)\big||S_F| q_F[\exp(2\pi i z_{\mathrm{Mn}} l) \\ &\quad + \exp(-2\pi i z_{\mathrm{Mn}} l)] \cdot \{1 + \exp[\pi i(h + k + l)]\} \\ &\quad + |S_{AF}| q_{AF}[\exp(2\pi i z_{\mathrm{Mn}} l) + \exp(-2\pi i z_{\mathrm{Mn}} l)] \cdot \{1 + \exp[\pi i(h + k + l)]\}\big|^2,\end{aligned} \tag{19.11}$$

where $\boldsymbol{q}_{\mathrm{F}}$ and $\boldsymbol{q}_{\mathrm{AF}}$ are the q-factor of ferromagnetic and antiferromagnetic components and z_{Mn} is the fractional coordinate of c-axis for Mn sites.

When the sum of $h + k + l$ is an even number, first term of Eq. (19.11) is zero. If each magnetic domain exists equivalently, Eq. (19.11) is expressed as,

$$\begin{aligned}\frac{d\sigma(\tau)}{d\Omega} &= 1.16 \times 10^{20} f_{\mathrm{Mn}}^2(\tau) S_{\mathrm{F}}^2 \langle q_{\mathrm{F}}^2\rangle \cos^2(2\pi z_{\mathrm{Mn}} l) \\ &= 1.16 \times 10^{20} f_{\mathrm{Mn}}^2(\tau) S_{\mathrm{F}}^2 \left[1 - \left(\frac{1}{2}\frac{h^2 + k^2}{a^2}\sin^2\theta_{\mathrm{F}} + \frac{l^2}{c^2}\cos^2\theta_{\mathrm{F}}\right) d_{hkl}^2\right] \cos^2(2\pi z_{\mathrm{Mn}} l),\end{aligned} \tag{19.12}$$

where $\langle \boldsymbol{q}_{\mathrm{F}}^2\rangle$ is the average of $\boldsymbol{q}_{\mathrm{F}}^2$ and θ_{F} is the angle between the c-axis and the magnetic moment of ferromagnetic component.

On the other hand, when the sum of $h + k + l$ is an odd number, second term of Eq. (19.11) is zero. If each magnetic domain exists equivalently, Eq. (19.11) is expressed as,

$$\begin{aligned}\frac{d\sigma(\tau)}{d\Omega} &= 1.16 \times 10^{20} f_{\mathrm{Mn}}^2(\tau) S_{\mathrm{AF}}^2 \langle q_{\mathrm{AF}}^2\rangle \cos^2(2\pi z_{\mathrm{Mn}} l) = 1.16 \times 10^{20} f_{\mathrm{Mn}}^2(\tau) S_{\mathrm{AF}}^2 \\ &\quad \times \left[1 - \left(\frac{1}{2}\frac{h^2 + k^2}{a^2}\sin^2\theta_{\mathrm{AF}} + \frac{l^2}{c^2}\cos^2\theta_{\mathrm{AF}}\right) d_{hkl}^2\right] \cos^2(2\pi z_{\mathrm{Mn}} l),\end{aligned} \tag{19.13}$$

where $\langle \boldsymbol{q}_{\mathrm{AF}}^2\rangle$ is the average of $\boldsymbol{q}_{\mathrm{AF}}^2$ and θ_{AF} is the angle between the c-axis and the magnetic moment of antiferromagnetic component.

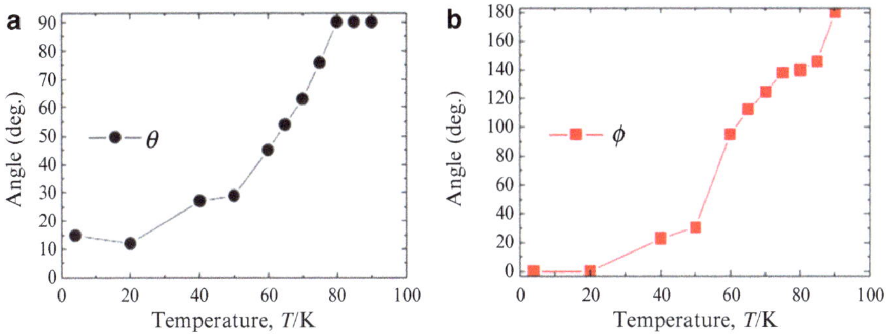

Fig. 19.7 Temperature dependence of (**a**) θ and (**b**) φ

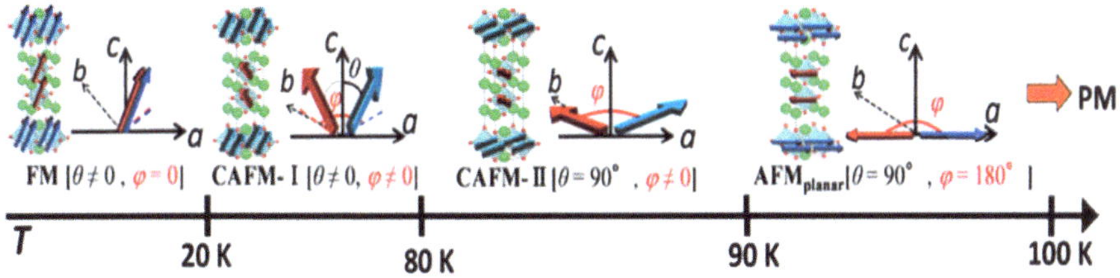

Fig. 19.8 Temperature dependence of magnetic structure. The *red* and *blue arrows* are magnetic moments of Mn ions in each MnO_2 conducting layer. The *a*, *b* and *c* are the crystal axes

We fit the observed intensities with calculated one obtained by using Eqs. (19.3)–(19.13) and determined the values of θ and φ which are the angle between the magnetic moments and *c*-axis and the angle between the projections of magnetic moments in a MnO_2 layers and a neighboring one on the *ab*-plane. The obtained values of θ and φ are shown in Fig. 19.7. As known from the figure, θ and φ increase with increasing temperature. The temperature dependence of magnetic structure of $La_{2-2x}Sr_{1+2x}Mn_2O_7$ ($x = 0.307$) is schematically shown in Fig. 19.8. The ground state has a ferromagnetic structure [$\theta \neq 0$]. At about 20 K, it changes to a canted-antiferromagnetic I (CAFM-I) structure [$\theta \neq 0$, $\phi \neq 0$]. At about 80 K, the CAFM-I structure changes to another canted-antiferromagnetic II (CAFM-II) structure [$\theta = 90°$, $\phi \neq 0$]. At about 90 K, the CAFM-II structure changes to AFM_{planar} structure [$\theta = 90°$, $\phi = 0$] and then changes to a paramagnetic structure at about 100 K.

19.4 The Other Magnetic Structures

All of magnetic structures mentioned above have long range magnetic orderings. However, some materials showing no long range ordering have a short range ordering. A typical example is spin glass [13] and magnetic moments in spin

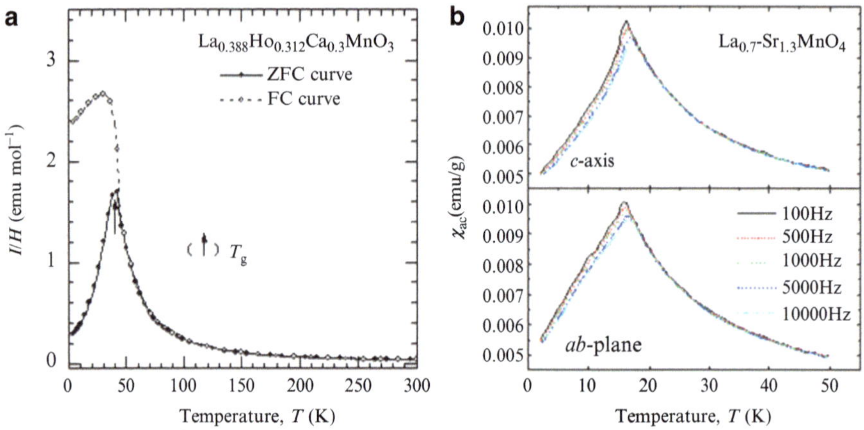

Fig. 19.9 (**a**) Temperature dependences of magnetic susceptibility for ZFC and FC runs of $La_{0.388}Ho_{0.312}Ca_{0.3}MnO_3$ and (**b**) temperature dependence of ac susceptibility of $La_{0.7}Sr_{1.3}MnO_4$

glass apparently have a random arrangement as atoms are frozen in glass. The freezing of magnetic moments are due to the competition of ferromagnetic and antiferromagnetic interactions and/or geometric frustration (triangle lattice, tetrahedron structure, etc.). Spin glasses show characteristic features such as huge thermal hysteresis and time dependence (frequency dependence). Figure 19.9a shows temperature dependence of magnetic susceptibility during heating process for a perovskite manganite, $La_{0.388}Ho_{0.312}Ca_{0.3}MnO_3$ [14]. A characteristic feature is that there is a large difference between the measured magnetic susceptibility after cooling under no magnetic field (ZFC run, zero field cooled run) and that after cooling under a finite magnetic field (FC run, field cooled run). This hysteresis is due to the response delay of spin to external magnetic field in the time range for measurement below spin glass transition temperature, T_g. Furthermore, ac susceptibility of spin glass shows the frequency dependence (Fig. 19.9b). The many of natures for spin glass have not been clear yet and they are actively discussed nowadays.[5]

References

1. Qpechowski W, Gucione R (1965) In: Suhl, Rado (eds) Magnetism, vol 2A. Academic, New York (Chap. 3)
2. Weiss P (1907) J Phys 6:661
3. Kuwahara H, Tomioka Y, Asamitsu A, Moritomo Y, Tokura Y (1995) Science 270:961

[5] Since Edward and Anderson had succeeded in a statistical treatment of spin glass, many studies have done. However, many things have been unknown and researchers dispute even whether spin glass has a phase transition or not.

4. Terai T, Kakeshita T, Fukuda T, Saburi T, Takamoto N, Kindo K, Honda M (1998) Phys Rev B 58:14908
5. Honda K, Kaya S (1926) Sci Rep Tohoku Univ 15:721
6. Honda K, Kaya S (1928) Sci Rep Tohoku Univ 17:1157
7. Stoner EC (1936) Proc R Soc A 154:656
8. Murata T, Terai T, Fukuda T, Kakeshita T (2006) J Magn Magn Mater 303:138
9. Yamamoto M, Terai T, Kakeshita T (2010) Philo Mag 90:2125
10. Kubota M, Fujioka H, Hirota K, Ohoyama K, Moritomo Y, Yoshizawa H, Endoh Y (2000) J Phys Soc Jpn 69:1606
11. Ling CD, Millburn JE, Mitchell JF, Argyriou DN, Linton J, Bordallo HN (2000) Phys Rev B 62:15096
12. Sonomura H, Terai T, Kakeshita T, Osakabe T, Kakurai K, Kuroiwa Y, Moriyoshi C, Okubo T, Kato K, Kim J, Takata M (2011) Solid State Phenomena 172–174:1301
13. Cannella V, Mydosh JA (1974) AIP Conf Proc 18:651
14. Terai T, Kakeshita T, Fukuda T, Kindo K, Honda M, Kishio K (2002) Philo Mag B 82:1099

Chapter 20
Advanced Materials Design by Lithography Technique

Ryoichi Nakatani

Abstract Magnetic materials have been known from at least BC seventh century. The oldest magnetic materials are thought to be magnetite. The word of "magnet" is thought to come from the name of the Magnesia district in ancient Greece. A lot of magnetite was produced in the Magnesia district. The magnetic materials have been applied to compass for voyages from fourteenth century in Europe. The scientific investigation on magnetism has started from sixteenth century. As mentioned above, the magnetic materials have a very long history. In modern world, the magnetic materials are widely applied to the permanent magnets, magnetic sensors, transformers, medical equipments, and so on. From the 1990s, the magnetic materials have been used for spin-electronics devices. The first application of the spin-electronics devices was the magnetic heads (Tsang et al., IEEE Trans Magn 30:3801–3806, 1994; Heim et al., IEEE Trans Magn 30:316–321, 1994) in hard disk drives. Recently, the spin-electronics devices have been widely investigated (Rippard et al., Phys Rev Lett 92:27201, 2004; Tulapurkar et al., Nature 438:339–342, 2005). In this chapter, magnetic memories, magnetic logic devices and lithography techniques that are utilized to fabricate the small spin-electronics devices are introduced.

Keywords Magnetic materials • Spin-electronics • Lithography • Magnetic memory • Logic devices

---

R. Nakatani (✉)
Division of Materials and Manufacturing Science, Graduate School of Engineering, Osaka University, 2-1 Yamadaoka, Suita, Osaka 565-0871, Japan
e-mail: nakatani@mat.eng.osaka-u.ac.jp

T. Kakeshita (ed.), *Progress in Advanced Structural and Functional Materials Design*, DOI 10.1007/978-4-431-54064-9_20,

20.1 Lithography Techniques for Fabrication of the Small Spin-Electronics Devices

The small spin-electronics devices [1–4] are generally fabricated by two methods, lift-off method and etching method. Figure 20.1 shows a process of the lift-off method [5, 6]. At first, the resist film is coated on the substrate. There are negative type resists and positive type resists. After the baking, the resist layer is exposed by a light or an electron beam. After the exposure, the development forms the resist pattern. The exposed area of the resist dissolves for positive type resists, and remains for the negative type resists, in the development process. After the development, the film is deposited on the substrate and resist pattern. The organic solvent removes the resist pattern, and thus the films on the resist pattern are also removed.

Figure 20.2 shows a process of an ion milling method [7] as a dry etching process. At first, the film is directly deposited on the substrate, and then the resist film is coated on the film. The exposure and the development are done as same as the lift-off method. The ion beam irradiates on the resist pattern. The parts of the film covered by the resist pattern are protected from the bombardment of the ion beam. On the other hand, the parts of the film, that are not covered by the resist pattern, are removed by the ion beam.

The optical lithography is generally used for the resist pattern with the size over 1 μm. For the resist pattern smaller than 1 μm, the electron beam lithography is utilized.

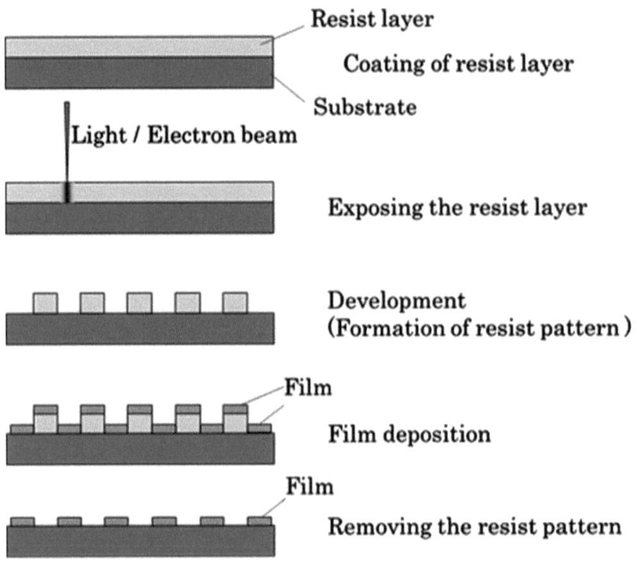

Fig. 20.1 Lift-off method

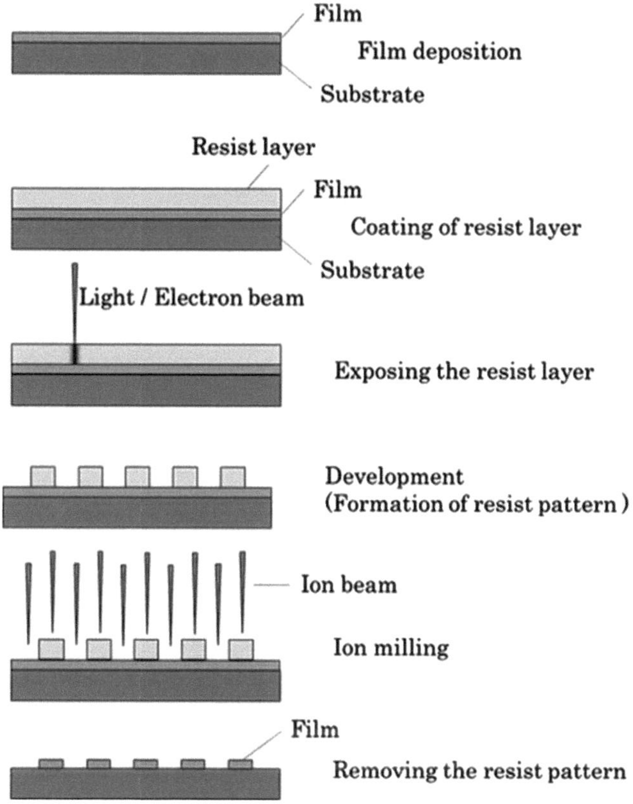

Fig. 20.2 Fabrication using ion milling method

20.2 Magnetic Memories

The development of the magnetic random access memory (MRAM) [8, 9] was started in 1990s. The MRAM is a promising memory device because the MRAM is non-volatile and displays high-speed potential. Figure 20.3 shows the simple stacking structure of the MRAMs. There are two magnetic layers which are magnetically separated by the non-magnetic spacer layer. The magnetization of the one of the magnetic layers is easily rotated by the external magnetic field, while another is fixed by the exchange coupling between the magnetic layer and the antiferromagnetic layer [10].

As shown in Fig. 20.4, the antiferromagnetic layer has the magnetic moments with the anti-parallel configuration. The magnetic moments of the antiferromagnetic layer are not rotated by the external magnetic field. Because of the exchange coupling at the interface between the antiferromagnetic layer and the ferromagnetic layer, the exchange bias field is caused and applied to the adjacent magnetic layer. And therefore, the magnetization of the ferromagnetic layer on the antiferromagnetic layer is fixed.

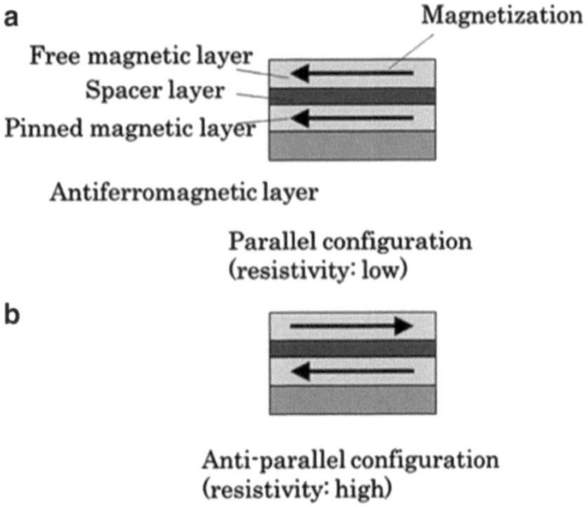

Fig. 20.3 Cross section of multilayers used for magnetic random access memories

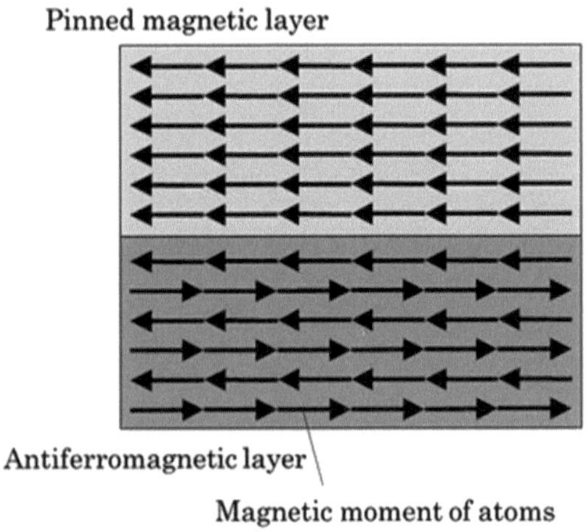

Fig. 20.4 Magnetic moments in pinned magnetic layer and antiferromagnetic layer

As shown in Fig. 20.3a, the parallel magnetization configuration is caused by the leftward external field. When the magnetizations are parallel, the resistivity of the stacking structure is relatively low. On the other hand, the anti-parallel configuration is caused by the rightward external field as shown in Fig. 20.3b. When the magnetizations are anti-parallel, the resistivity of the stacking structure is relatively high. One of the magnetization configuration is decided as the information of “0”, and another is decided as “1”. And therefore, the stored information can be detected by the measurement of the resistivity.

The memory cells are arranged as shown in Fig. 20.5. A pair of one word line and one bit line is selected and the electric currents are flowed along the lines in order to generate the magnetic fields to change the stored information of the memory cell at the intersection of the two lines. The information of other cells is not changed because of the low field.

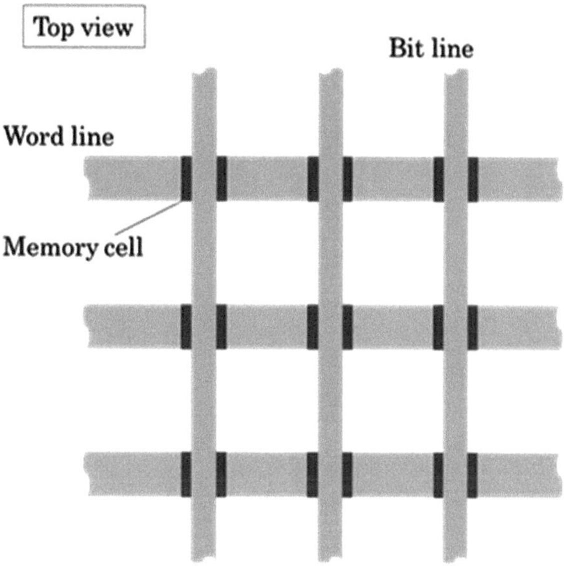

Fig. 20.5 *Top view* of the simple structure in magnetic random access memory

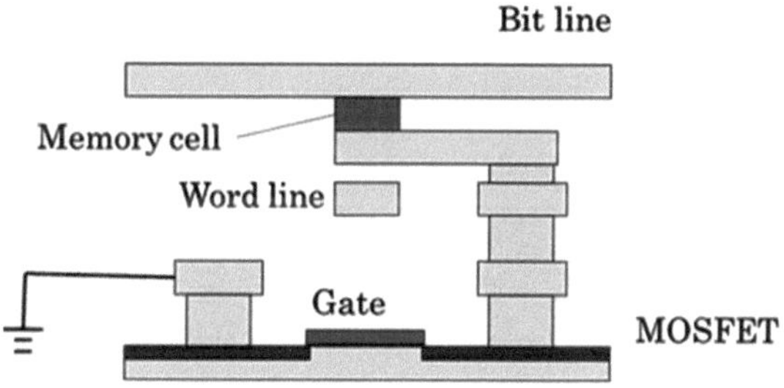

Fig. 20.6 Cross section of magnetic random access memory

Figure 20.6 shows the detail of the structure of one memory cell. The gate of the MOSFET (metal–oxide–semiconductor field–effect transistor) is the switch to read the information stored at the memory cell.

In order to increase the capacity of the memory, the ring memory cell has been investigated [11–15]. The ring memory cells do not cause the stray fields, and therefore, the memory cells can be arranged at a high density. The ring cells store information such as chirality of vortical magnetizations. However, in-plane magnetic fields cannot control the chirality of the ring cells, because of the symmetric structures. Asymmetric ring structures with partially-planed outer sides were proposed, and it was demonstrated that the chirality of the asymmetric ring memory cells can be controlled between clockwise and counterclockwise by the in-plane magnetic fields [11, 12].

The image observed by scanning electron microscopy (SEM) is shown in Fig. 20.7. The memory cell was micro-fabricated using ion beam sputtering, the electron beam lithography and lift-off method. As shown in Fig. 20.7, the cell is partially planed.

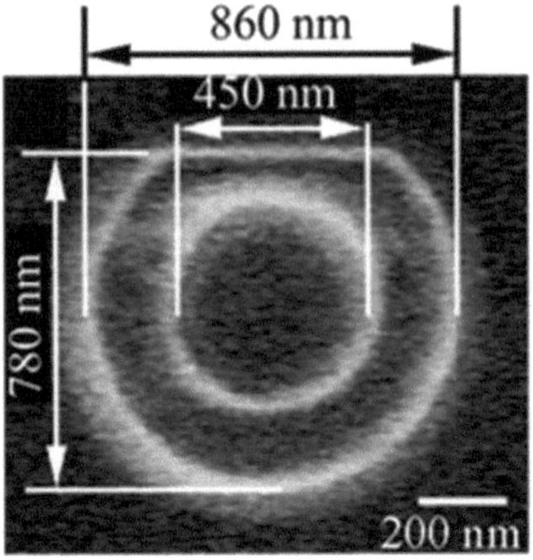

Fig. 20.7 SEM image of planed ring dot

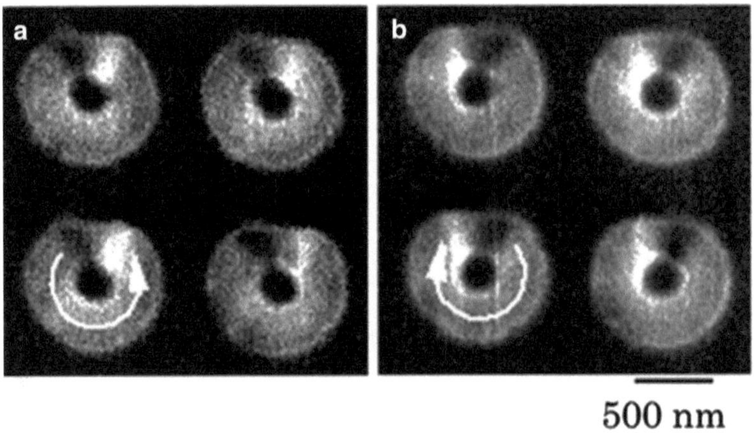

Fig. 20.8 MFM images at zero magnetic field after applying a field in (**a**) the right direction, (**b**) the left direction

The magnetic force microscopy (MFM) images of the asymmetric ring memory cells are shown in Fig. 20.8. Before the observations, a 1 kOe field was applied along the planed sides of the cells and then it was removed. Figure 20.8a shows the MFM images after positive saturation, where the field is applied in the right direction and then removed. A pair of black and white spots is seen near the planed side in each cell and the spots show stray fields from the planed sides. The white spots are located to the right of the black spots in Fig. 20.8a, which demonstrates that the chirality of the vortical magnetizations is counterclockwise.

On the other hand, as shown in Fig. 20.8b, the white spots are located to the left of the black spots after negative saturation, where the field is applied in the left direction and then removed, which shows that the chirality of the vortical magnetizations is clockwise.

From the results of the micromagnetics simulation [12], it is understood that the direction of the high magnetic field turns the magnetization of the circular arcs, which are opposite from the planed parts. The direction of the magnetizations of the circular arcs is preferentially maintained with the direction of the magnetizations of the parts near the planed side, which determines the chirality of the vortical magnetizations, either clockwise or counterclockwise, in asymmetric ring dots. Therefore, the in-plane magnetic field direction can control the chirality of the vortical magnetizations in the asymmetric ring dots.

On the other hand, the pinned magnetic layer with asymmetric ring structure can be obtained with using the antiferromagnetic layer that is adjacent to the magnetic layer [13–15]. The hybrid structure using free magnetic layer and pinned magnetic layer realize the MRAMs with asymmetric ring structures. The asymmetric ring memory cells can be arranged at a high density, and therefore, the asymmetric ring structure realizes the memory devices to store large amounts of information.

20.3 Magnetic Logic Devices

The magnetic logic devices have been investigated as future magnetic functional devices. The investigated structure of the magnetic logic devices is shown in Fig. 20.9 [17–19]. The magnetic logic devices consist of four elliptical permalloy dots. The magnetization directions of the magnetic cells correspond to digital information of "0" and "1". The three magnetic cells are for input of the information. Another magnetic cell is for output of the information. The magnetic cells are magnetically connected via magnetostatic interaction. The magnetostatic interaction operates the calculation.

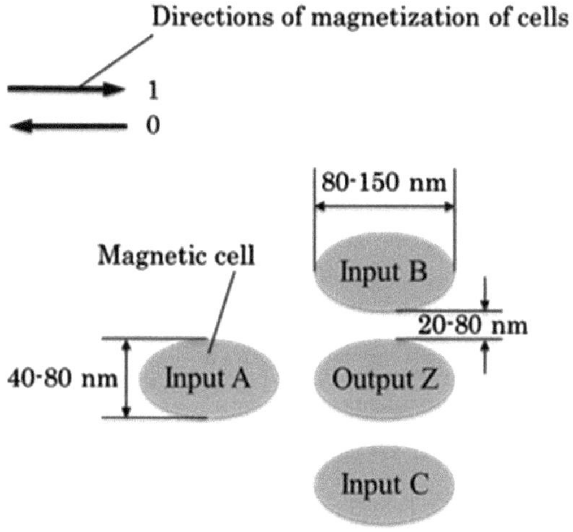

Fig. 20.9 Structure of magnetic logic devices. The thickness of cells is between 10 and 20 nm. The typical material is Ni–20 at.% Fe alloy

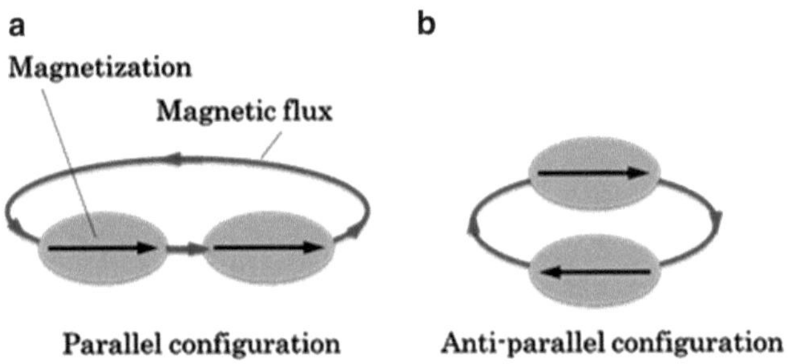

Fig. 20.10 Caused configuration due to magnetostatic interaction between two magnetic cells

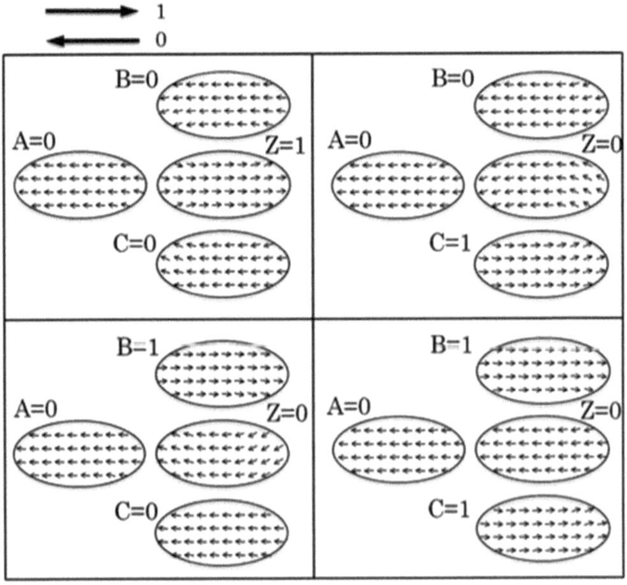

Fig. 20.11 Simulation results for A = 0

There are two sequences in the magnetic logic devices as shown in Fig. 20.10. As shown in Fig. 20.10a, the longitudinal sequence causes the parallel configuration of two magnetizations in the cells. On the other hand, as shown in Fig. 20.10b, the transverse sequence causes the anti-parallel configuration of two magnetizations in the cells. The total of the magnetic interactions in three sequences, "input A and output Z", "input B and output Z", and "input C and output Z", decides the magnetization direction of output Z which corresponds to digital information.

Figure 20.11 shows the results of the micromagnetics simulation for input A = 0. The length of long axis is 80 nm while that of short axis is 40 nm. The distance between the adjacent dots is 20 nm and thickness of permalloy cells

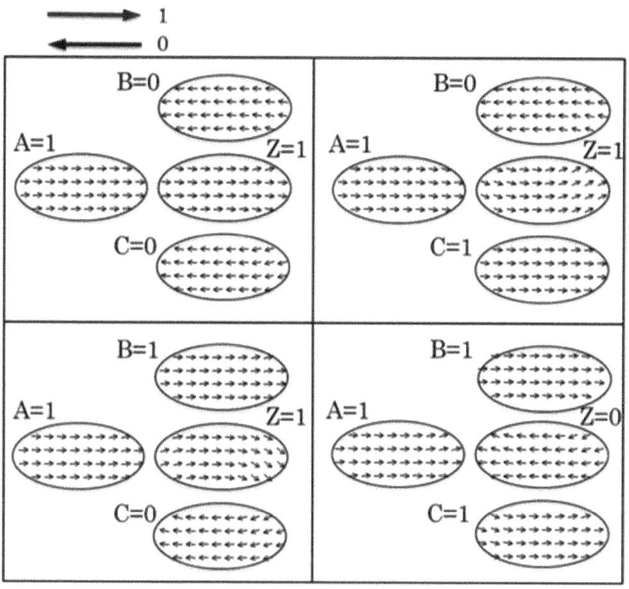

Fig. 20.12 Simulation results for A = 1

Table 20.1 Simulation results

A	B	C	Z	
0	0	0	1	N
0	0	1	0	O
0	1	0	0	R
0	1	1	0	
1	0	0	1	N
1	0	1	1	A
1	1	0	1	N
1	1	1	0	D

is 10 nm. The small arrows indicate the magnetization directions of local areas. The directions of the small arrows are almost parallel in each cell. Figure 20.12 shows the results of the micromagnetics simulation for input A = 1. The directions of the small arrows are almost parallel in each cell as shown in Fig. 11.12.

Table 20.1 shows the results indicated in Figs. 20.11 and 20.12. As shown in the table, the magnetic logic device shows the NOR operation when the input A is “0”. On the other hand, the magnetic logic device shows the NAND operation when the input A is “1”.

Figure 20.13 shows the experimental results of the observation using a magnetic force microscope (MFM). The results perfectly correspond to those of the simulation results indicated in Table 20.1. So that these results indicate the magnetic logic devices will be realized in near future.

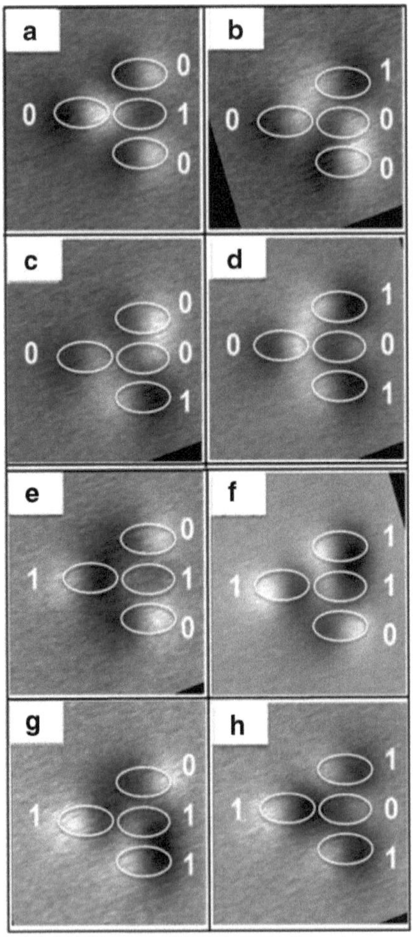

Fig. 20.13 Results of the logic operation confirmed by MFM. (**a**–**d**) NOR operations, (**e**–**h**) NAND operations [16] (©2011, The Japan Society of Applied Physics)

20.4 Summary

Using the magnetic storage systems (hard disk drives), the magnetic memories and the magnetic logic devices, the magnetic computers will be realized. The magnetic computers are thought to be very strong systems for the electromagnetic field, high-energy particles and radiation. Therefore, the magnetic computers should be the most reliable system in outer space and near nuclear reactors.

References

1. Tsang C, Fontana RE, Lin T, Heim DE, Speriosu VS, Gurney BA, Williams ML (1994) IEEE Trans Magn 30:3801–3806
2. Heim DE, Fontana RE, Tsang C, Speriosu VS, Gurney BA, Williams ML (1994) IEEE Trans Magn 30:316–321

3. Rippard WH, Pufall MR, Kaka S, Russek SE, Silva TJ (2004) Phys Rev Lett 92:27201
4. Tulapurkar AA, Suzuki Y, Fukushima A, Kubota H, Maehara H, Tsunekawa K, Djayaprawira DD, Watanabe N, Yuasa S (2005) Nature 438:339–342
5. Yuda M, Kuroda K, Nakano J (1987) Jpn J Appl Phys 26:L166–L168
6. Moriwaki K, Masuda N, Aritome H, Namba S (1980) Jpn J Appl Phys 19:491–494
7. Spencer EG, Schmidt PH, Fischer RF (1970) Appl Phys Lett 17:328–332
8. Ranmuthu KTM, Ranmuthu IW, Pohm AV, Comstock CS, Hassoun M (1992) IEEE Traans Magn 28:2359–2361
9. Tehrani S, Slaughter JM, Chen E, Durlam M, Shi J, DeHerrera M (1999) IEEE Trans Magn 35:2814–2819
10. Fukamichi K, Umetsu RY, Sakuma A, Mitsumata C (2006) Magnetic and electrical properties of practical antiferromagnetic Mn alloys. In: Buschow KHJ (ed) Handbook of magnetic materials, vol 16. Elsevier, Amsterdam (Chapter 4)
11. Nakatani R, Yoshida T, Endo Y, Kawamura Y, Yamamoto M, Takenaga T, Aya S, Kuroiwa T, Beysen S, Kobayashi H (2004) J Appl Phys 95:6714–6716
12. Nakatani R, Yamamoto M (2003) Jpn J Appl Phys 42:100–101
13. Nakatani R, Yoshida T, Endo Y, Kawamura Y, Yamamoto M, Takenaga T, Aya S, Kuroiwa T, Beysen S, Kobayashi H (2005) J Magn Magn Mater 286:31–36
14. Sasaki I, Nakatani R, Yoshida T, Otaki K, Endo Y, Kawamura Y, Yamamoto M, Takenaga T, Aya S, Kuroiwa T, Beysen S, Kobayashi H (2006) Mater Sci Forum 512:171–176
15. Sasaki I, Nakatani R, Endo Y, Kawamura Y, Yamamoto M, Takenaga T, Aya S, Kuroiwa T, Beysen S, Kobayashi H (2006) J Appl Phys 99:08G303
16. Nomura H, Nakatani R (2011) Appl Phys Express 4:013004
17. Haque SA, Yamamoto M, Nakatani R, Endo Y (2004) J Magn Magn Mater 282:380–384
18. Cowburn RP, Welland ME (2000) Science 287:1466–1468
19. Nakatani R, Nomura H, Endo Y (2009) J Phys Conf Ser 165:012030

Chapter 21
Advanced Materials Design of Rare-Earth-Doped Semiconductors by Organometallic Vapor Phase Epitaxy

Yasufumi Fujiwara, Yoshikazu Terai, and Atsushi Nishikawa

Abstract Much attention has been paid to rare-earth (RE)-doped semiconductors as a promising new class of materials that can emit light from the RE 4*f*-shell by electrical injection. We have grown Er,O-codoped GaAs and Eu-doped GaN by atomically controlled organometallic vapor phase epitaxy (OMVPE), and demonstrated light-emitting diodes (LEDs) with the materials, operating at room temperature under current injection. The LEDs exhibit a characteristic emission due to the intra-4*f* shell transitions of trivalent RE ions that are effectively excited by the energy transfer from the hosts.

Keywords Rare-earth-doped semiconductor • Er,O-codoped GaAs • Eu-doped GaN • Organometallic vapor phase epitaxy • Intra-4*f* shell transition • Ultrafast energy transfer • Excitation cross section • External quantum efficiency • Light-emitting diode

21.1 Introduction

A set of 17 chemical elements in the periodic table, particularly the 15 lanthanides plus Sc and Y, are called the rare-earth (RE) elements. The RE elements are frequently used in various fields. For example, Eu-doped Y_2O_3 is a well-known red phosphor for a fluorescence tube. On the other hand, $Nd_2Fe_{14}B$ is known as a strong magnet for an electric vehicle. In these applications, however, either the luminescent or magnetic property of the RE elements has been independently used. Furthermore, research on RE-doped materials has been based on experience

Y. Fujiwara (✉) • Y. Terai • A. Nishikawa
Division of Materials and Manufacturing Science, Graduate School of Engineering, 2-1 Yamadaoka, Suita, Osaka 565-0871, Japan
e-mail: fujiwara@mat.eng.osaka-u.ac.jp

T. Kakeshita (ed.), *Progress in Advanced Structural and Functional Materials Design*, DOI 10.1007/978-4-431-54064-9_21, © Springer Japan 2013

obtained through trial and error, not on material design by the precise control of RE doping and the understanding of the energy transfer mechanism.

RE-doped semiconductors are a new class of materials with various promising potentials (for example [1]). RE ions doped in semiconductors exhibit a characteristic emission due to the intra-4*f* shell transitions of RE ions. The intra-4*f* shell transitions give rise to sharp emission lines whose wavelengths are largely independent of both the host material and temperature. This stability occurs because the filled outer 5*s* and 5*p* electron shells screen transitions within the inner 4*f* electron shell from the interaction with the host. We have intensively investigated RE-doped III–V semiconductors grown by atomically controlled organometallic vapor phase epitaxy (OMVPE) and fabricated new types of light-emitting diodes (LEDs) with the materials. In this chapter, the OMVPE growth and LED application of Er,O-codoped GaAs (GaAs:Er,O) and Eu-doped GaN (GaN:Eu) are reviewed.

21.2 Er,O-Codoped GaAs

Particular attention has been paid to Er-doped III–V semiconductors because the intra-4*f* shell transitions from the first excited state ($^4I_{13/2}$) to the ground state ($^4I_{15/2}$) of Er^{3+} ions result in sharp luminescence lines near 1.5 μm. They have a large impact on optical communication systems operating near 1.5 μm, which is in the range of minimum transmission loss in silica-based fibers.

We have intensively investigated Er-doped III–V semiconductors grown by OMVPE [2]. In Er-doped InP, it has been found that there is a threshold growth temperature between 550 and 580°C for Er incorporation to InP. The majority of Er atoms substitute the In sublattice in the lower-temperature-grown InP, exhibiting a high luminescence efficiency [3]. The threshold growth temperature depends on the host material. In Er-doped GaP, the temperature is higher, and the majority of Er atoms are incorporated into Ga sites in the GaP lattice even in samples grown at 650°C and 700°C [4].

Oxygen has been recognized to influence strongly Er-related luminescence in semiconductors. Er ions doped in Czochralski-grown (CZ) Si containing O atoms of 10^{18} cm^{-3} exhibit a luminescence intensity of more than 100 times higher than that of Er ions doped in float-zone (FZ) Si with higher purity [5]. In Er-doped GaAs, the introduction of O_2 into the OMVPE growth ambient produces a sharp, simple PL spectrum of Er^{3+} [6]. The PL spectrum is dominated by eight emission lines under host-excited conditions at a low temperature. The Er center has been identified as an Er atom located at the Ga sublattice with two adjacent O atoms (hereafter referred to as Er–2O) [7].

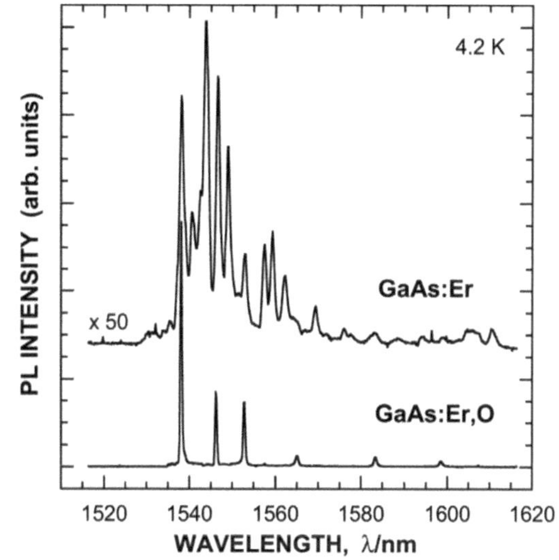

Fig. 21.1 Comparison of Er-related PL spectra of Er-doped and Er,O-codoped GaAs. In Er,O-codoped GaAs, the PL spectrum is dominated by strong emission lines from an Er–2O center

21.2.1 OMVPE Growth of Er,O-Codoped GaAs

A low-pressure growth system having a specially designed reactor with a vertical 4-barrel structure was utilized in this work. The advantages of this growth system were described previously [8]. The reactor pressure was kept at 76 Torr. The samples were grown on (0 0 1)-just semi-insulating GaAs or (0 0 1) Si-doped GaAs substrates, misoriented 2° off to the ⟨1 1 0⟩ direction. Triethylgallium (TEGa) and tertiarybutylarsine (TBAs) were used as source materials for GaAs growth. Er was doped with tris(isopropylcyclopentadienyl)erbium (Er(*i*-PrCp)$_3$). The Er source was maintained at a constant temperature of 90°C under 76 Torr and introduced into the reactor by H_2 flow through a source cylinder. $^{18}O_2$ of 38.4 ppm in Ar gas was used as an O_2 source. The O_2 content in the growth ambient was set at 0.2 ppm. H_2S and diethylzinc (DEZn) were also used as p- and n-type doping sources, respectively.

21.2.2 Photoluminescence of Er,O-Codoped GaAs

Figure 21.1 shows the Er-related photoluminescence (PL) spectrum of GaAs:Er,O, which is compared with that of Er-doped GaAs. An Ar^+ laser operating at 515 nm was used as an excitation source. In Er-doped GaAs, there are many emission lines, reflecting the coexistence of various unknown Er centers. In GaAs:Er,O, the Er-related PL spectrum reveals strong emission lines from an Er–2O center as reported previously [9].

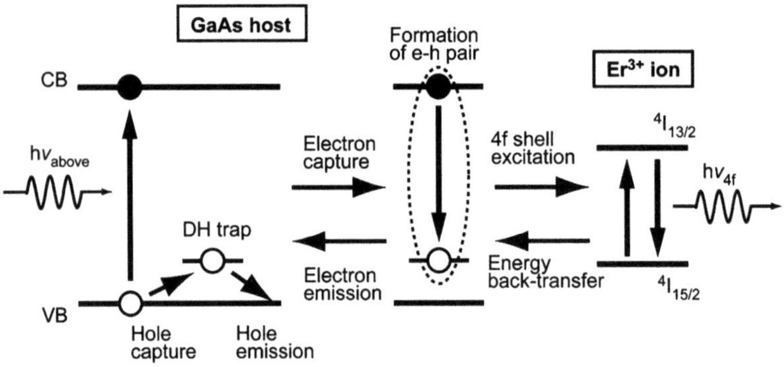

Fig. 21.2 Schematic drawing of excitation mechanism of Er ions in GaAs. The energy transfer between photogenerated free carriers and the Er 4*f*-shell plays an important role in the excitation of the 4*f* shell

The excitation mechanism of Er^{3+} ions in GaAs is schematically shown in Fig. 21.2. It is well known that a RE atom doped in semiconductors produces a bound state similar to an isoelectronic trap in the bandgap [10]. It is assumed in the figure that an Er-related luminescence center forms a donor-like hole trap in the bandgap of GaAs, because the energy level of the trap due to Er doped in GaAs is not clear at present. The energy transfer mechanism under above-bandgap excitation is as follows: optical excitation generates a free electron and a free hole. The trap captures a hole to become positively charged. The charged trap attracts an electron by Coulombic interaction and creates an electron–hole pair, or an exciton at a low temperature. The electron–hole pair recombines and part of the recombination energy is transferred to the Er 4*f*-shell, resulting in a 4*f*-shell excitation. The excited Er 4*f*-shell relaxes by emitting a photon, creating the Er intra-4*f* shell luminescence.

21.2.3 1.5 μm LED with Er,O-Codoped GaAs

We fabricated a GaInP/GaAs:Er,O/GaInP double-heterostructure (DH) LED [11]. Figure 21.3 shows a schematic drawing of the cross-sectional structure of the GaInP/GaAs:Er,O/GaInP DH LED. The growth sequence was as follows: it was initiated by the growth of a 100-nm-thick, n-GaAs (2×10^{18} cm^{-3}) buffer layer at 610°C. Then, the substrate temperature was decreased to 540°C, which was followed by the successive growth of a 900-nm-thick n-GaInP (8×10^{17} cm^{-3}) cladding layer and a 300-, 600- or 1,200-nm-thick GaAs:Er,O active layer. 50-nm-thick undoped GaAs layers were grown on top and at the bottom of the active layer. A p-GaInP (1×10^{18} cm^{-3}) cladding layer was also 900 nm thick and a 1,800-nm-thick p-GaAs (2×10^{19} cm^{-3}) contact layer was grown on top of the p-type cladding layer.

Figure 21.4 shows the room-temperature Er-related electroluminescence (EL) spectrum of the DH LED under forward bias. The EL spectrum exhibits only the

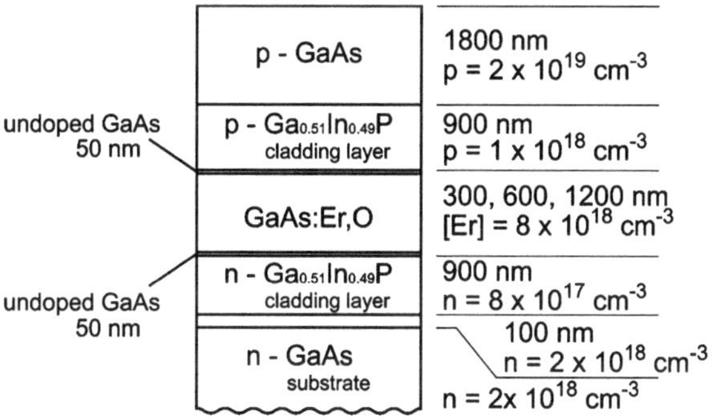

Fig. 21.3 Schematic drawing of cross-sectional structure of GaInP/GaAs:Er,O/GaInP DH LED. 50-nm-thick undoped GaAs layers were grown on *top* and at the *bottom* of the GaAs:Er,O active layer

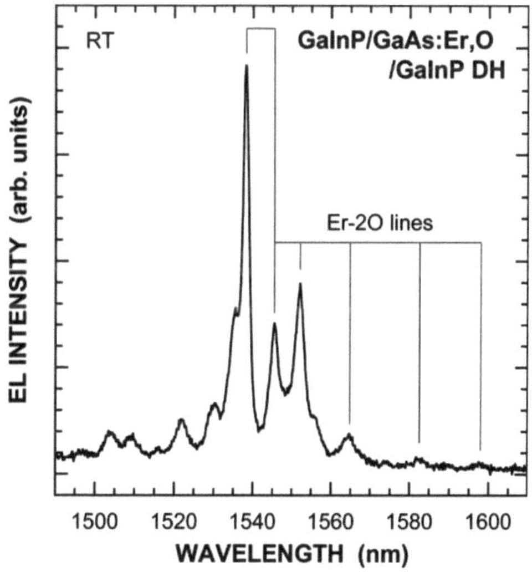

Fig. 21.4 Room-temperature EL spectrum of DH LED under forward bias. The spectrum is dominated by emission lines due to the Er–2O center

emission lines originating from the Er–2O center. Moreover, GaAs band-edge emission was not observed under the measurement conditions. These results indicate that the injected carriers contribute effectively to the excitation of the Er^{3+} ions rather than to the band-edge emission. This observation is due to the ultrafast energy transfer from the GaAs host to the Er ions, which is confirmed directly by pump and probe reflection measurements on photoexcited carriers in GaAs:Er,O [12, 13] and indirectly by the behavior of the Er–2O intensity under the GaAs band-edge lasing in a laser diode (LD) with an GaAs:Er,O active layer [14].

We also investigated the dependence of EL properties on injection current density [15]. At low current densities, EL intensity increased linearly with current

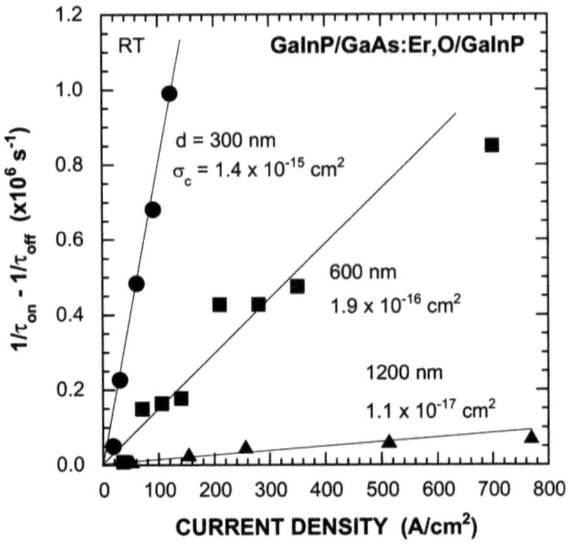

Fig. 21.5 Dependence of $1/\tau_{on}-1/\tau_{off}$ on current density as a function of GaAs:Er,O active layer thickness in DH LEDs. The Er excitation cross section σ_c decreases with increasing active layer thickness

density. At current densities higher than 10 A/cm^2, on the other hand, the intensity tended to saturate because of the long excited-state lifetime of Er^{3+}. The saturation of the intensity implies that the concentration of optically active Er centers is a limiting parameter for EL intensity under forward bias. The saturated EL intensity depended on the thickness of the GaAs:Er,O active layer. The saturated EL intensity of a DH LED with an active layer thickness of 1,200 nm was approximately 20 times higher than that of the 300-nm-thick LED and approximately 50 times higher than that of a homostructure GaAs:Er,O LED [16].

The excitation cross section of Er obtained by current injection was estimated in the DH LEDs [17]. For this estimation, the following equation is used [16]:

$$\frac{1}{\tau_{on}} = \sigma_c \frac{J}{q} + \frac{1}{\tau_{off}} \qquad (21.1)$$

where σ_c is the excitation cross section. τ_{on} is the rising time of Er-related intensity obtained after switching on the pulse current with the density J, and τ_{off} the falling time after switching off in time-resolved measurements.

Figure 21.5 shows the dependence of $1/\tau_{on}-1/\tau_{off}$ on current density as a function of GaAs:Er,O active layer thickness in the DH LEDs. The excitation cross section of the 300-nm-thick DH LED is 1.4×10^{-15} cm^2, which is well comparable to that of the homostructure LED [$(1\text{–}2) \times 10^{-15}$ cm^2] [16] and is five orders in magnitude larger than the optical excitation cross section of a conventional Er-doped fiber amplifier (10^{-20} to 10^{-21} cm^2) [18]. However, it decreases with increasing active layer thickness. This observation also originates from the reduced diffusion lengths of the injected carriers due to ultrafast carrier trapping by Er-related traps.

21.3 Eu-Doped GaN

RE-doped GaN has been identified as a promising candidate for the realization of white LEDs, displays, and lasers. Eu^{3+} ions have been widely used as red-emitting phosphors for cathode ray-tube and plasma display panels. In these applications, the ions are doped into an insulator and red emission is obtained mainly by optical excitation. GaN is an attractive host material for Eu doping because its wide bandgap allows visible wavelength emission from Eu ions and reduces the thermal quenching effect for the emission intensity. We have grown GaN:Eu by OMVPE and observed successfully bright red emission due to the intra-4*f* shell transitions of Eu^{3+} ions from a LED with GaN:Eu as an active layer [19]. However, the output power of 1.3 μW at a dc current of 20 mA was insufficient for practical use (~mW). An improved output power is strongly desired.

21.3.1 OMVPE Growth of Eu-Doped GaN

GaN:Eu was grown on a 2-in. sapphire substrate by OMVPE. Trimethylgallium (TMGa) and ammonia (NH_3) were used as starting sources. Eu was doped using tris (dipivaroylmethanate)europium ($Eu(DPM)_3$). The Eu source and transfer lines were maintained at 135°C and 145°C, respectively, to prevent Eu source condensation during transportation.

The growth sequence of a sample for PL measurements was initiated by the low-temperature growth of a 30-nm-thick GaN buffer layer on a sapphire (0 0 0 1) substrate, which was followed by the successive growth of a 2–3-μm-thick undoped GaN layer, a 400-nm-thick GaN:Eu layer and a 10-nm-thick GaN capping layer.

21.3.2 Photoluminescence of Eu-Doped GaN

In PL measurements with a He–Cd laser as an excitation source, bright red emission was observed over the 2-in. substrate at room temperature. Figure 21.6 shows the room-temperature PL spectrum of the GaN:Eu layer [19]. The emission peaks observed at 543, 600, 621, 633, and 663 nm are associated with the intra-4*f* shell transitions of $^5D_1$–$^7F_1$, $^5D_0$–$^7F_1$, $^5D_0$–$^7F_2$, $^5D_1$–$^7F_4$, and $^5D_0$–$^7F_3$, respectively, in Eu^{3+} ions. It should be noted that neither GaN band-edge emission (which was typically observed at 361 nm for undoped GaN) nor defect-related blue/yellow band luminescence was observed in this wavelength range. The fact that a negligible GaN-related luminescence was observed indicates that the excitation energy of the GaN host material was also effectively transferred to the Eu^{3+} ions for the Eu-related luminescence. The Eu intensity depended strongly on growth conditions [20–22]. Figure 21.7 shows the PL spectra of the samples grown at 10 and 100 kPa [21]. The growth temperature was 1,050°C. The dominant luminescence peak at

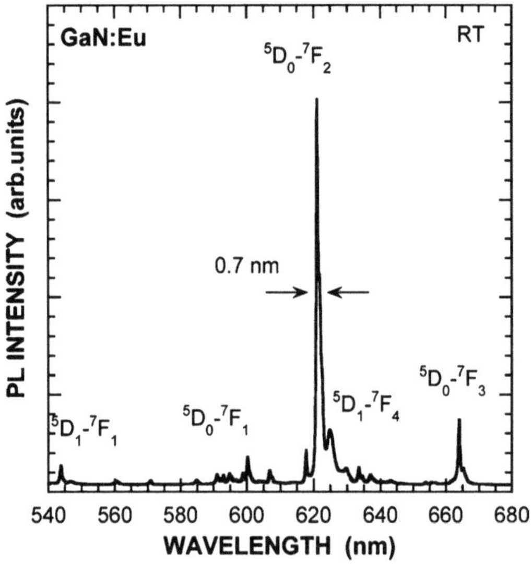

Fig. 21.6 Room-temperature PL spectrum of GaN:Eu layer. Emission peaks are associated with the intra-4*f* shell transitions in Eu^{3+} ions

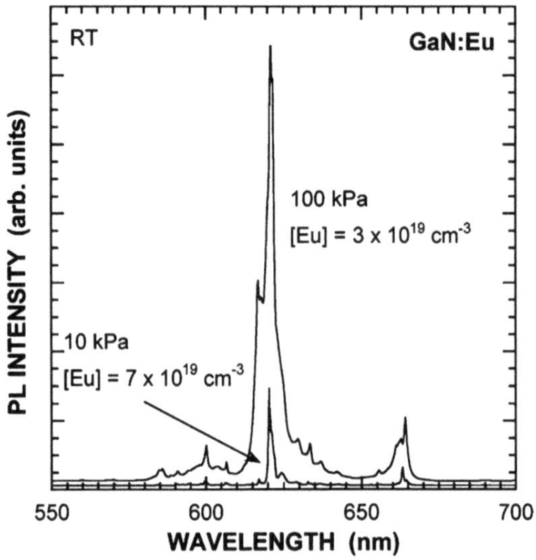

Fig. 21.7 Reactor pressure dependence of PL spectra in GaN:Eu. The dominant peak intensity of the 100 kPa sample is about four times higher than that of the 10 kPa sample

621 nm in each spectrum is assigned to the transition from the $^5D_0$ state to the $^7F_2$ state in the Eu^{3+} ion. The dominant peak intensity of the 100 kPa sample is about four times higher than that of the 10 kPa sample. Moreover, the luminescence peak becomes broader such that the integrated PL intensity is about ten times higher. SIMS measurements revealed that the Eu concentration of the 100 kPa sample is 3×10^{19} cm^{-3}, which is lower than that of the 10 kPa sample (7×10^{19} cm^{-3}). Thus, the luminescence peak intensity does not only depend on the Eu concentration of the GaN:Eu layer.

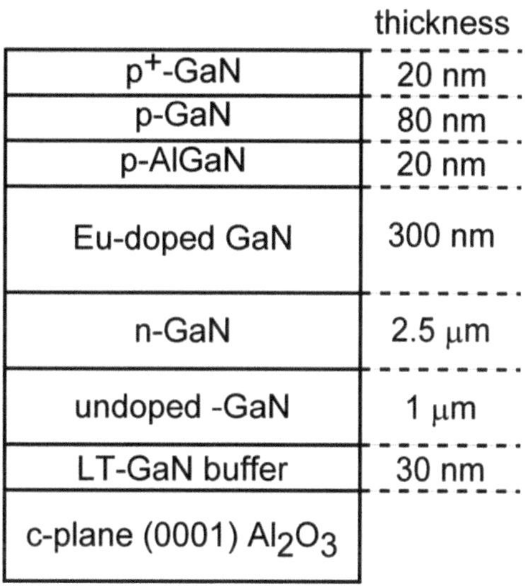

Fig. 21.8 Schematic drawing of GaN:Eu LED structure. The structure is similar to the conventional blue/green LEDs except for the active layer

21.3.3 Red LED with Eu-Doped GaN

We fabricated a red LED with GaN:Eu [19, 21]. The LED structure consisted of a 20-nm-thick Mg-doped GaN contact layer, an 80-nm-thick Mg-doped GaN layer with a Mg doping concentration of 7×10^{19} cm^{-3}, a 20-nm-thick Mg-doped $Al_{0.1}Ga_{0.9}N$ electron-blocking layer, a 300-nm-thick GaN:Eu layer and a 2.5-μ m-thick n-type Si-doped GaN layer with a Si-doping concentration of 4×10^{18} cm^{-3}, which is schematically shown in Fig. 21.8. The reactor pressure was maintained at 10 and 100 kPa when the GaN:Eu layer was grown.

Figure 21.9 shows the room-temperature EL spectrum of a GaN:Eu LED with a forward bias of about 5 V [21]. The main emission line with a half-width of less than 1 nm is observed at 621 nm, which can be assigned to the $^5D_0$–$^7F_2$ transition of Eu^{3+} ions. Notably, no band-edge and defect luminescence was observed under the bias condition, indicating that the Eu luminescence is caused by the ultrafast energy transfer from the GaN host to the Eu^{3+} ions.

The atmospheric-pressure growth of GaN:Eu drastically increased the Eu intensity, which is due to the increased number of optically active Eu centers and efficient energy transfer by the reduced non-radiative processes in the GaN host. In the LED doped with Eu at atmospheric pressure, the output power integrated over the $^5D_0$–$^7F_2$ transition region (around 621 nm) was 17 μW at a dc current of 20 mA; the corresponding external quantum efficiency, which is the ratio of the extracted photons to the injected electrons, was 4.0×10^{-2} % [21].

We have also investigated the EL properties of the LEDs with different active layer thicknesses [23]. With increasing active layer thickness, the light output power increased monotonically. The maximum light output power of 50 μW was obtained in the LED with a 900 nm active layer thickness with an injected current of

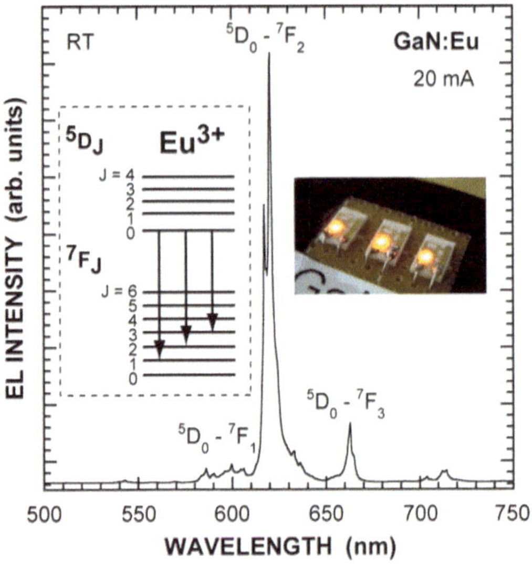

Fig. 21.9 EL spectrum of GaN:Eu LED. The LED shows *red* emission whose wavelength is independent of environmental temperature

20 mA, which is the highest value ever reported. The corresponding external quantum efficiency was 0.13 %, which is comparable to that of a commercially available N-doped GaP green LED.

21.4 Summary

The current status of OMVPE-grown GaAs:Er,O and GaN:Eu was reviewed. In GaAs:Er,O, the codoping of oxygen with Er selectively produced the Er–2O center, resulting in the drastic increase in the Er^{3+} luminescence intensity. A LED with GaAs:Er,O exhibited Er–2O luminescence at around 1.54 μm under current injection at room temperature. The injected current dependence of the EL property revealed Er ions with an extremely large excitation cross section. In GaN:Eu, on the other hand, bright red emission due to the Eu^{3+} ions was successfully observed at room temperature under optical pumping. The LED with GaN:Eu as an active layer also exhibited red emission under current injection. This result suggests a novel method of realizng GaN-based red LEDs, which are an alternative to conventional toxic As-containing AlGaInP/GaAs red LEDs, and to realize a monolithic device composed of red, green and blue GaN-based LEDs for full-color display or lighting technology.

Acknowledgements This work was supported, in part, by a Grant-in-Aid for Creative Scientific Research No. 19GS1209 from the Japan Society for the Promotion of Science, and by the Global Centre of Excellence Program "Advanced Structural and Functional Materials Design" from the Ministry of Education, Culture, Sports, Science and Technology, Japan.

References

1. Dierolf V, Fujiwara Y, Hommerich U, Ruterana P, Zavada JM (eds) (2009) Materials Research Society symposium proceedings, rare-earth doping of advanced materials for photonic applications, vol 1111. Materials Research Society, Pennsylvania
2. Fujiwara Y, Ofuchi H, Tabuchi M, Takeda Y (2000) In: Manasreh MO (ed) InP and related compounds—materials, applications and devices, optoelectronic properties of semiconductors and superlattices, vol 9. Gordon and Breach Science, Amsterdam, p 251
3. Fujiwara Y, Matsubara N, Tsuchiya J, Ito T, Takeda Y (1997) Effects of growth temperature on Er-related photoluminescence in Er-doped InP and GaAs grown by organometallic vapor phase epitaxy with tertiarybutylphosphine and tertiarybutylarsine. Jpn J Appl Phys 36:2587
4. Fujiwara Y, Curtis AP, Stillman GE, Matsubara N, Takeda Y (1998) Low-temperature photoluminescence study on Er-doped GaP grown by organometallic vapor phase epitaxy. J Appl Phys 83:4902
5. Favennec PN, L'Haridon H, Moutonnet D, Salve M, Gauneau M (1990) Optical activation of Er^{3+} implanted in silicon by oxygen impurities. Jpn J Appl Phys 29:L524
6. Takahei K, Taguchi A (1993) Selective formation of an efficient Er-0 luminescence center in GaAs by metalorganic chemical vapor deposition under an atmosphere containing oxygen. J Appl Phys 74:1979
7. Takahei K, Taguchi A, Horikoshi Y, Nakata J (1994) Atomic configuration of the Er-O luminescence center in Er-doped GaAs with oxygen codoping. J Appl Phys 76:4332
8. Fujiwara Y, Nonogaki Y, Oga R, Koizumi A, Takeda Y (2003) Reactor structure dependence of interface abruptness in GaInAs/InP and GaInP/GaAs grown by organometallic vapor phase epitaxy. Appl Surf Sci 216:564
9. Fujiwara Y, Kawamoto T, Koide T, Takeda Y (1999) Luminescence properties of Er, O-codoped III-V semiconductors by organometallic vapor phase epitaxy. Physica B 273–274:770
10. Taguchi A, Takahei K, Horikoshi Y (1994) Multiphonon-assisted energy transfer between Yb 4f shell and InP host. J Appl Phys 76:7288
11. Koizumi A, Fujiwara Y, Inoue K, Urakami A, Yoshikane T, Takeda Y (2003) Room-temperature 1.54 μm light emission from Er, O-codoped GaAs/GaInP LEDs grown by low-pressure organometallic vapor phase epitaxy. Jpn J Appl Phys 42:2223
12. Fujiwara Y, Takemoto S, Nakamura K, Shimada K, Suzuki M, Hidaka K, Terai Y, Tonouchi M (2007) Ultrafast carrier-trapping in Er-doped and Er, O-codoped GaAs revealed by pump and probe technique. Physica B 401–402:234
13. Shimada K, Terai Y, Takemoto S, Hidaka K, Fujiwara Y, Suzuki M, Tonouchi M (2008) Terahertz radiation from Er, O-codoped GaAs surface grown by organometallic vapor phase epitaxy. Appl Phys Lett 92:111115
14. Terai Y, Hidaka K, Fujii K, Takemoto S, Tonouchi M, Fujiwara Y (2008) Ultrafast carrier-capturing in GaInP/Er, O-codoped GaAs/GaInP laser diodes grown by organometallic vapor phase epitaxy. Appl Phys Lett 93:231117
15. Fujiwara Y, Koizumi A, Urakami A, Yoshikane T, Inoue K, Takeda Y (2003) Room-temperature 1.5 μm electroluminescence from GaInP/Er, O-codoped GaAs/GaInP double heterostructure injection-type light emitting diodes grown by organometallic vapor phase epitaxy. Mater Sci Eng B 105:57
16. Koizumi A, Fujiwara Y, Urakami A, Inoue K, Yoshikane T, Takeda Y (2003) Room-temperature electroluminescence properties of Er, O-codoped GaAs injection-type light emitting diodes grown by organometallic vapor phase epitaxy. Appl Phys Lett 83:4521
17. Koizumi A, Fujiwara Y, Urakami A, Inoue K, Yoshikane T, Takeda Y (2003) Effects of active layer thickness on Er excitation cross section in GaInP/GaAs:Er, O/GaInP DH structure light-emitting diodes. Physica B 340–342:309
18. Priolo F, Franzo G, Coffa S, Carnera A (1998) Excitation and nonradiative deexcitation processes of Er^{3+} in crystalline Si. Phys Rev B 57:4443

19. Nishikawa A, Kawasaki T, Furukawa N, Terai Y, Fujiwara Y (2009) Room-temperature red emission from p-type/europium-doped/n-type gallium nitride light-emitting diodes under current injection. Appl Phys Exp 2:071004
20. Kawasaki T, Furukawa N, Nishikawa A, Terai Y, Fujiwara Y (2010) Effect of growth temperature on Eu-doped GaN layers grown by organometallic vapor phase epitaxy. Phys Status Solidi C 7:2040
21. Nishikawa A, Furukawa N, Kawasaki T, Terai Y, Fujiwara Y (2010) Improved luminescence properties of Eu-doped GaN light-emitting diodes grown by atmospheric-pressure organometallic vapor phase epitaxy. Appl Phys Lett 97:051113
22. Furukawa N, Nishikawa A, Kawasaki T, Terai Y, Fujiwara Y (2011) Atmospheric pressure growth of Eu-doped GaN by organometallic vapor phase epitaxy. Phys Status Solidi A 208:445
23. Nishikawa A, Furukawa N, Lee D, Kawabata K, Matsuno T, Harada R, Terai Y, Fujiwara Y (2012) Electroluminescence properties of Eu-doped GaN-based light-emitting diodes grown by organometallic vapor phase epitaxy. In: Dierolf V, Fujiwara Y, Gregorkiewicz T, Jadwisienczak W (eds) Materials Research Society symposium proceedings, rare-earth doping of advanced materials for photonic applications, vol 1342. Cambridge University Press, New York, pp. 9–13

Chapter 22
Advanced Analysis of Defect Formations and Phase Transformations in Nanoparticles by In Situ Transmission Electron Microscopy

Hidehiro Yasuda

Abstract Researches on specific structural properties in nanoparticles are introduced as examples of advanced analyses by a combination of in situ transmission electron microscopy (TEM) observation and nanoprocessing utilizing an electron beam. The structural properties which are different from those in the corresponding bulk materials appear in nanoparticles, which are a small many-body system, since the free energy can greatly change by solute concentrations or atomic arrangements. The chemical free energy by the interaction between the different atoms plays an important role in the structural properties of alloy or compound nanoparticles, and their artificial control will make it possible to form specific structures. As an example, the electronic-excitation-induced defect formations and phase transformations in nanoparticles are reviewed based on the results obtained by in situ TEM.

Keywords Electronic excitation • In situ transmission electron microscopy • Lattice defect • Nanoparticle • Phase transformation

22.1 In Situ Transmission Electron Microscopy for Space- and Time-Resolved Analysis

In materials research, observation techniques of atomic arrangements are required for appropriate nanostructural characterizations of materials. Transmission Electron Microscopy (TEM) is one of the effective techniques for advanced analysis in materials. We can observe images in real space and the corresponding electron diffraction patterns from a selective nanometer-scale area in a millimeter-scale

H. Yasuda (✉)
Research Center for Ultra-High Voltage Electron Microscopy, Osaka University, 7-1 Mihogaoka, Ibaraki, Osaka 567-0047, Japan
e-mail: yasuda@uhvem.osaka-u.ac.jp

T. Kakeshita (ed.), *Progress in Advanced Structural and Functional Materials Design*, DOI 10.1007/978-4-431-54064-9_22,

observation region. Additionally, analyses of chemical compositions and electronic structures can be carried out under a high spatial resolution condition, such as analytical electron microscopy. Such an observation technique in the wide spatial range from all over an area to a local one is essential to estimate macroscopic properties based on the nanostructure of materials. On the other hand, dynamics of atoms in materials is also one of the important factors in advanced analysis. In situ observation by TEM is extremely effective in characterizations of defect formation, phase transformation, reaction, and so on.

From different points of view, materials may transform distinctively by energies given from an electron beam to the atomic or electronic states in materials. Recently, nanoprocessing by electron beam irradiation for nanomaterial formations has attracted a great deal of attention, and is expected for next frontier in nanomaterial science.

In this chapter, researches on specific structural properties in nanoparticles will be introduced as examples of advanced analyses by a combination of in situ TEM observation and nanoprocessing utilizing an electron beam.

22.2 In Situ Observations of Specific Structural Properties in Nanoparticles

Nanoparticles in the size range of from a few to several nanometers often exhibit structures and properties which are significantly different from those of the corresponding bulk materials, and are of interest in both materials science and applications [1, 2]. TEM is an attractive technique to characterize nanomaterials. The research topics obtained from in situ TEM observations which are useful for nanoparticles researches, will be reviewed below.

In nanoparticles, which are small many-body systems, the free energy in the systems can be changed greatly by solute concentrations or atomic arrangements [3–8]. The chemical free energy by the interaction between the different atoms plays an important role in the structural properties of multicomponent nanoparticles, and their artificial control will make it possible to form specific structures [9–11]. The electronic-excitation-induced structural and morphological changes in GaSb nanoparticles are herein reviewed based on the results obtained by in situ TEM.

22.2.1 Phase Transformations Induced by Electronic Excitation in GaSb Nanoparticles

Structural stability in materials under electronic excitation is different from that at the ground state. It is expected that electronic excitation affecting the structural

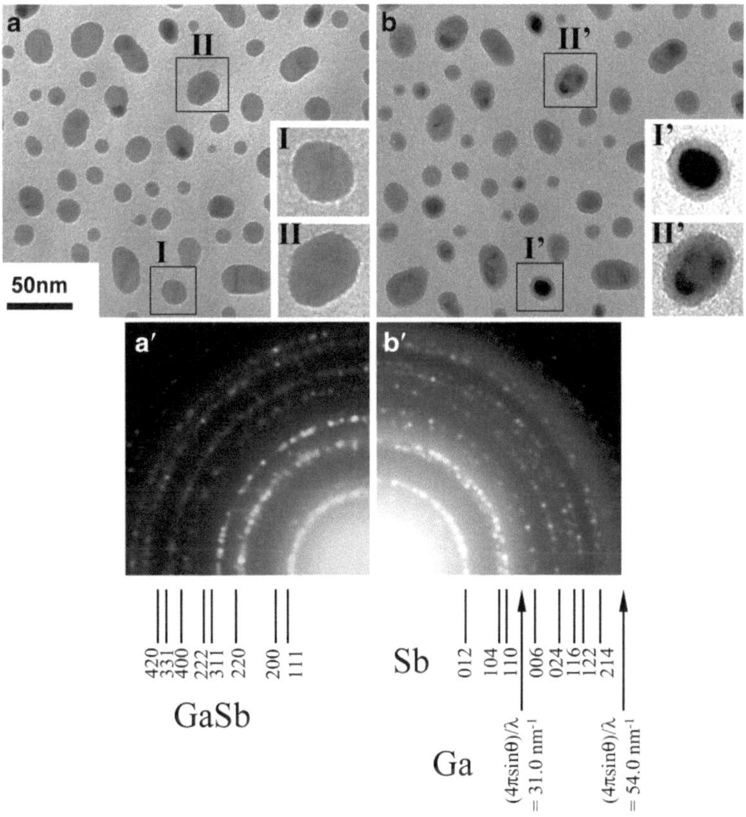

Fig. 22.1 A typical example of the structural changes in GaSb nanoparticles at 423 K by 75 keV electron excitation. (**a** and **a**′) A BFI and the corresponding SAED before excitation. (**b** and **b**′) The same area after excitation for 240 s and the corresponding SAED

stability will be enhanced in nanoparticles which have a high surface to volume ratio and high atomic mobility. Recently, it was found that when GaSb nanoparticles are excited by electrons, phase transformations take place.

Electronic excitation experiments and observations were carried out using a double-source evaporator installed in the specimen chamber of a transmission electron microscope. The microscopes used were operating at accelerating voltages of 75 and 25 kV. The values of electron flux used for excitations were in the range of from approximately 1.0×10^{20} to 1.5×10^{21} m^{-2} s^{-1}.

A typical example of structural changes associated with 75 keV electron excitation in GaSb nanoparticles kept at 423 K is shown in Fig. 22.1. Figure 22.1a, a′ shows a BFI of approximately 20 nm-sized particles before excitation and the corresponding selected-area electron diffraction (SAED) pattern, respectively. The insets in the BFIs show framed enlargements of parts. As shown in Fig. 22.1a′, Debye–Scherrer rings can be consistently indexed as those of GaSb which has the

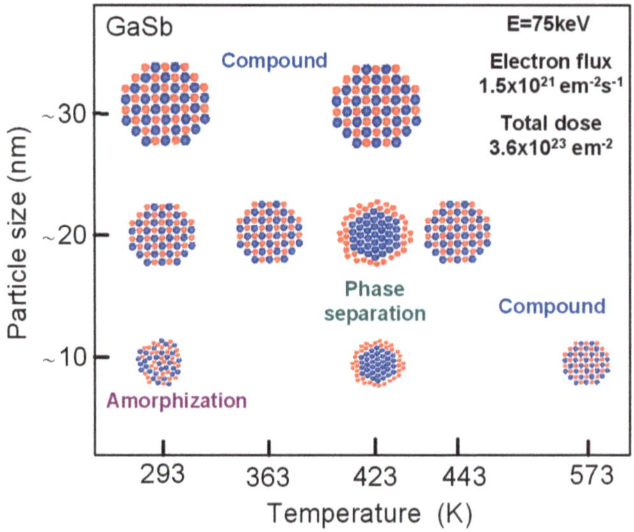

Fig. 22.2 Summary of the results on phase transformations induced by electronic excitation as functions of specimen temperature and the particle size. Total electron dose is fixed at 3.6×10^{23} e m^{-2}

zincblende structure. The same area after excitation for 240 s is shown in Fig. 22.1b. In the interior of the nanoparticles after excitation there appears a nanostructure consisting of a core with dark contrast and a shell with bright contrast. An SAED taken from the excited region is shown in Fig. 22.1b′. In the SAED, Debye–Scherrer rings are recognized, superimposed on halo rings. The Debye–Scherrer rings can be indexed consistently as those of crystalline antimony, which has the hexagonal structure. The values of the scattering vector ($K = (4\pi \sin\theta)/\lambda$) of the halo rings are approximately 31.0 and 54.0 nm^{-1}, which correspond to those from liquid gallium. It was confirmed by dark-field microscopy that nanoparticles after excitation have a two-phase structure consisting of a crystalline antimony core and a liquid gallium shell. From the experiment, it is evident that when 75 keV electron excitation is carried out on approximately 20 nm-sized particles kept at 423 K, a phase separation in the GaSb compound is induced to form a two-phase structure consisting of a crystalline antimony core and a liquid gallium shell [12, 13].

22.2.2 Nonlinear Responses of Phase Transformations

The results on the phase transformations induced by electronic excitation are summarized as functions of particle size and temperature in Fig. 22.2. Total electron dose was fixed at 3.6×10^{23} e m^{-2}. From the results, it is evident that the phase transformations are suppressed with increasing particle size and/or

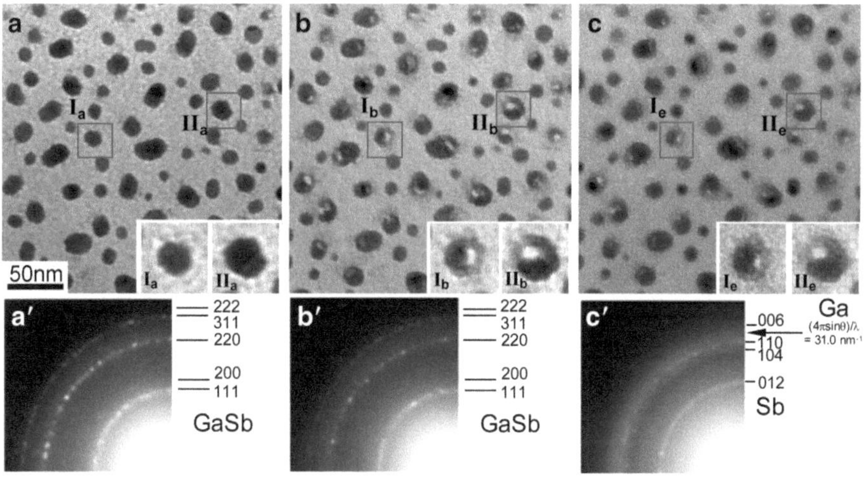

Fig. 22.3 An example of the structural changes in GaSb nanoparticles kept at 430 K by 25 keV electron excitation. (**a** and **a**′) before excitation, (**b** and **b**′) after 60 s, (**c** and **c**′) after 480 s

temperature. The other points noted here are that, in approximately 20 nm-sized particles, the phase transformation is again suppressed with decreasing temperature, but, in approximately 10 nm-sized particles, the phase transformation behavior varies from phase separation to amorphization with decreasing temperature. Such nonlinear responses of phase transformations, that is, competitive formations of four kinds of phases such as crystalline antimony, liquid gallium, amorphous and compound phase with decreasing particle size and/or temperature were observed by the 75 keV electron excitation. It is suggested that such nonlinear responses of the phase transformations may arise from synergistic effects of bond instability by electronic excitation, lifetime of the excited states, enhanced atomic mobility causing the lattice softening characteristic in nanoparticles or thermal equilibrium and kinetics in the reactions [14].

22.2.3 *Formation of Nanoporous Structures in GaSb Nanoparticles*

Excitation-energy-dependent behaviors are important to understand the detailed mechanisms of phase transformations because the excitation energy is closely related to the excitation cross-section of the constituent atoms. We can carry out atomic species-selective excitation by lower energy excitations.

An example of the structural changes in GaSb nanoparticles by 25 keV electron excitation is shown in Fig. 22.3. Figure 22.3a, a′ shows the BFI of nanoparticles with a mean diameter of approximately 20 nm before excitation and the corresponding SAED, respectively. As shown in Fig. 22.3a′, Debye–Scherrer

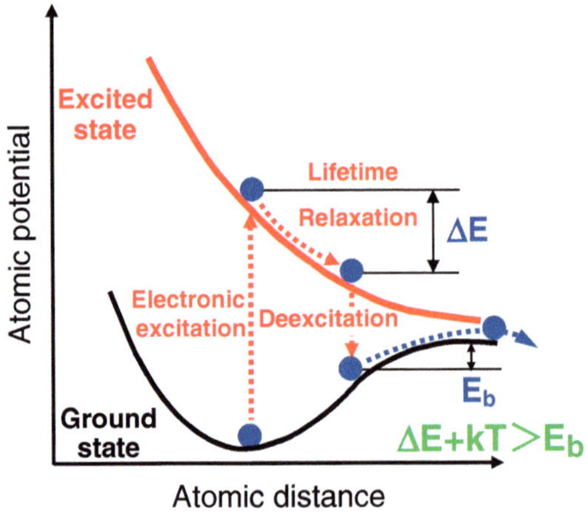

Fig. 22.4 A model of electronic-excitation-induced atom displacements illustrated schematically by atomic potential-distance diagram

rings can be consistently indexed as those of GaSb, which has the zincblende structure. The same area after excitation for 60 s is shown in Fig. 22.3b. In the interior of the particles after the excitation, there appear voids with bright contrast. As seen from a comparison of the magnified images I_a and II_a in (a) with I_b and II_b in (b), the diameter of nanoparticles after the excitation increased by up to 15% compared with those of before excitation. In the SAED taken after the excitation, as shown in Fig. 22.3b′, Debye–Scherrer rings of the zincblende structure are recognized again, but the lattice constant increased by up to 1.8% compared with that of before excitation. The same area after excitation for 480 s is shown in Fig. 22.3c. The voids in the individual particles change in the shape and size, as seen from a comparison of the magnified images I_b and II_b in (b) with I_c and II_c in (c). In the SAED taken after the excitation, as shown in Fig. 22.3c′, Debye–Scherrer rings are recognized, superimposed on a weak halo ring. The Debye–Scherrer rings can be indexed consistently as those of crystalline antimony, which has the hexagonal structure. The value of the scattering vector ($K = (4\pi\sin\theta)/\lambda$) for the halo ring is approximately 31.0 nm^{-1}, which corresponds to the first halo of liquid gallium. This result indicates that a two-phase mixture consisting of a crystalline antimony core and a liquid gallium shell was formed in nanoparticles again. From these results, it is evident that when GaSb particles kept at 430 K are excited by 25 keV electrons, a two-phase separation takes place via void formation [15].

22.2.4 Defect Formations by Electronic-Excitation-Induced Atom Displacements and the Nano-size Effects

A model of atom displacement induced by electronic excitation is shown in Fig. 22.4. From the schematic illustration of the atomic potential-distance diagram, when an atom at the ground state is promoted to the excited state, the instable atom at the excited states displaces to relax for a short lifetime and deexcitation takes place by the athermal process. After the deexcitation, if the summation of relaxation energy accumulated during the excitation and thermal energy is larger than the activation energy for diffusion, the atom displaces to the neighbor site by the athermal and thermal process.

Such atomic displacements are enhanced by nano-size effects. One of the reasons is due to the high atomic mobility caused by the low activation energy in nano systems. It was confirmed that the shallow interatomic potentials by the lattice softening in nanoparticles reduce the activation energy for atomic diffusion [16]. The other is a large relaxation energy caused by the long life time at the excited states. In nanoparticles, electronic excitation effects become remarkably efficient. The exited states which have short lifetimes of the order of 10^{-15} s decay by the scattering of electrons in the solid. The valence densities of states in nanoparticles become lower than those in the corresponding bulk material, because of the discreteness of the valence and conduction band due to the Kubo effect [2]. The low electron densities make the lifetime of the excited states formed in nanoparticles longer in comparison with that in the bulk material. The long lifetime of the excited states increases the energy gain during the relaxation and the resultant atom displacements are enhanced. The increase of the energy gain by the long excitation lifetime and the low activation energy for the diffusion will make it easy to displace the excited atoms in nanoparticles.

22.2.5 Excited States Related to Atom Displacements

The excitation by incident electrons with energies from 25 to 75 keV strongly interacts with the core electrons of the atoms in GaSb nanoparticles. The binding energies of 1*s* core electrons of gallium and antimony atoms are 10.4 and 30.5 eV, respectively. On the other hand, the electron binding energies in the L, M, N and O shell are relatively low in the range from 1.1 to 4.7 keV.

Under 25 keV excitation, the excitation cross-section of the gallium 1*s* electrons which satisfy the resonant excitation condition is largest in all the elementary excitations, because the primary excitation energy by the incident electrons of 25 keV ranges roughly double the binding energy of Ga 1*s*, 10.4 eV. However, the antimony atoms cannot be excited because the binding energy of Sb 1*s* is lower than the excitation energy. After the excitation, nearly half of the competitive relaxation processes (i.e., Auger emission and X-ray fluorescence) to the primary Ga 1*s* excitation is the Auger transition in which the transition probability is 0.47 [17]. Consequently, the final two-hole states in the gallium valence band are formed by the predominant primary K-shell Auger transitions. The bonding states under the presence of the two-hole in the valence band of gallium atoms become anti-bonding. A gallium atom, which has a minimum energy at the electronic ground state, is excited to a high energy state due to the increase in the adiabatic inter-atomic potential under the anti-bonding states [18]. The excited gallium atom is

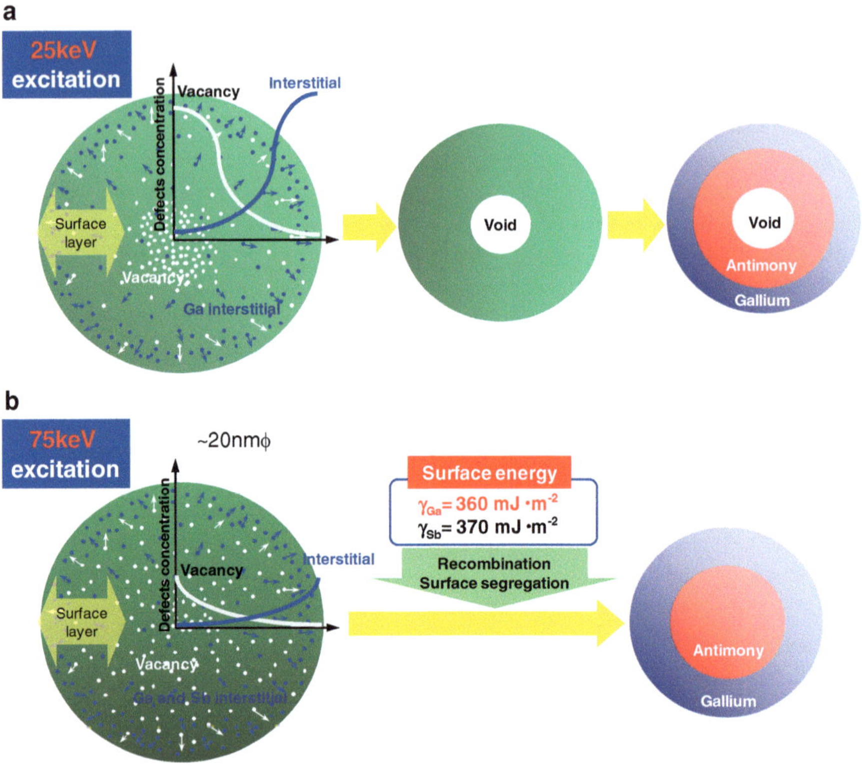

Fig. 22.5 Schematic illustrations of defect migrations and defect concentrations as a function of distance from the center of a nanoparticle and the behaviors of structural changes by electron excitations. (**a**) 25 keV excitation, (**b**) 75 keV excitation

displaced by the model shown in Fig. 22.4. The displaced gallium atom can form a vacancy and gallium interstitial in the crystal. On the other hand, under the 75 keV excitation, both of the displaced gallium and antimony atoms can form vacancies and, gallium and antimony interstitials by the same process. These point defects will recombine or form anti-site defects.

22.2.6 Mechanisms of Electronic-Excitation-Induced Structural Changes

A mechanism of the void formation and phase separation in GaSb nanoparticles will be discussed bellow. Figure 22.5 shows schematic illustrations of defect migrations and defect concentrations as a function of the distance from the center of a nanoparticle and the structural changes by 25 and 75 keV electron excitations.

Under the 25 keV electron excitation, as shown in Fig. 22.5a, when vacancies and gallium interstitials become mobile and apart from annihilation by recombination, they contribute to the growth of defect clusters. The interstitials and their clusters have a strong compressive strain field and the compressive strain field interacts more strongly with a tensile strain field of the surface layer of the nanoparticle than a strain field of an individual defect or its clusters. The surface layer of the nanoparticle will act as a preferential sink for interstitials and their clusters over the whole of the nanoparticles. The result of this greater capture cross-section of the surface layer for interstitials and their clusters is to create a situation where the vacancies are the dominant species in the nanoparticle. On the other hand, the capture cross-section of the surface layer for vacancies and their clusters is smaller than that for interstitials and their clusters. The vacancies and their clusters interact weakly with those of the surface layer. In nanoparticles, only the vacancies in the surface layer which is finite in thickness can disappear toward the top of the surface. Consequently, the vacancy concentration in the nanoparticle core is higher than that in the surface layer, but interstitial concentration increases toward the surface. Under the condition of vacancy supersaturation in the nanoparticle core, the vacancy clusters will grow to form a void, and the subsequent surface segregation of interstitial clusters will lead to the separation to the two-phase structure.

Under the 75 keV electron excitation, as shown in Fig. 22.5b, when vacancies and both of gallium and antimony interstitials become mobile, the probability of recombinations becomes larger. Then, the vacancy clustering will be suppressed. The surface energy of gallium is lower than that of antimony in the solid state. Consequently, surface segregation of gallium driven by surface energy induces the formation of two-phase nanoparticles consisting of a crystalline antimony core and a liquid gallium shell without void formation.

22.3 Summary

Electronic-excitation-induced defect formations and phase transformations in GaSb nanoparticles were by in situ TEM in order to see the structural stabilities under excited states in nanometer-sized systems. When GaSb nanoparticles were excited by electrons, the compound transformed into a two-phase consisting of an antimony core and a gallium shell or an amorphous phase, or remained the original compound phase, depending on particle size and/or temperature. It is suggested that such nonlinear responses of the phase transformations may arise from synergistic effects of bond instability, long excitation lifetime, enhanced diffusivity, or thermal equilibrium in reactions.

We hope that nanomaterials science and processing by electron irradiation or excitation effects will evolve utilizing effective TEM techniques in the future.

References

1. Andres RP et al (1989) J Mater Res 4:704
2. Halperin WP (1986) Rev Mod Phys 58:533
3. Yasuda H, Mori H (1992) Phys Rev Lett 69:3747
4. Yasuda H, Mori H, Komatsu M, Takeda K (1992) App Phys Lett 61:2173
5. Yasuda H, Mori H (1994) Z Phys D 31:131
6. Yasuda H, Furuya K (2000) Eur Phys J D 10:279
7. Yasuda H, Mori H (1997) Z Phys D 40:144
8. Yasuda H, Mori H (1997) Z Phys D 40:140
9. Yasuda H, Mitsuishi K, Mori H (2001) Phys Rev B 64:094101
10. Lee JG, Mori H, Yasuda H (2002) Phys Rev B 65:1321061
11. Lee JG, Mori H, Yasuda H (2002) Phys Rev B 66:0121051
12. Yasuda H, Mori H, Lee JG (2004) Phys Rev B 70:214105
13. Yasuda H, Tanaka A, Usui H, Mori H, Lee JG (2006) Eur Phys J D 37:231
14. Yasuda H, Mori H, Lee JG (2004) Phys Rev Lett 92:135501
15. Yasuda H, Tanaka A, Matsumoto K, Nitta N, Mori H (2008) Phys Rev Lett 100:105506
16. Harada J, Ohshima K (1981) Surf Sci 106:51
17. Bambynek W et al (1972) Rev Mod Phys 44:716
18. Sumi H (1991) Surf Sci 248:382

Index

A
Ablation, 43–46, 48
Absorbed energy, 64
A_{C1} point, 63
Ac susceptibility, 246
Activation energy, 279
Advanced analyse, 274
Advancing side, 61
Agglomeration, 101
Al–Cu alloy, 65
Alpha-Cr_2O_3, 222
Amorphization, 141–144, 151, 277
Amorphous, 137–151
Anisotropic, 156, 157, 161, 164
Anti-bonding states, 279
Antiferromagnetism, 221, 238, 251
Antiphase boundary, 183
Anti-site defects, 280
Apatite, 155–157, 160, 162
Arc plasma, 30–39, 41
Arc welding process, 27–41
Arrott-plot, 240
Athermal process, 279
Atom displacement, 278
Atomic diffusion, 279
Atomic mobility, 277
Atomic potential, 278
Atomic species-selective excitation, 277
Attenuation length, 72, 73, 79, 80
Auger emission, 279
Auger transitions, 279

B
Binding energy, 70, 79, 279
Biological apatite (BAp), 155–157, 159–166
Biomaterial, 164–166
Blocking temperature, 218
BMD. *See* Bone mineral density (BMD)
B_2O_3, 122
Bonding states, 279
Bond instability, 277
Bone, 155–166
Bone mineral density (BMD), 155, 162, 163
Bone quality, 155, 156, 159, 163
Bone quantity, 155
Bravais lattice, 157
Brillouin zone, 199
Bulk materials, 274, 279

C
Calvarial, 160–162
Canted-antiferromagnetism, 239
Carbon, 43, 47, 48, 50
Characterizations, 273
Chemical free energy, 274
Chemical shift, 79
Clausius–Clapeyron equation, 170
Coarsening, 98
Cobalt oxide, 238
Collagen (Col), 156, 157, 165, 166
Compound, 277
Conduction band, 279
Continuous casting techniques, 20–22, 26
Convection, 38, 39
Corrosion, 69–72, 74
Crystal grain, 86
Crystallization, 144–148, 150, 151
Cu-Kα, 160, 259
Curie temperature, 175, 238

T. Kakeshita (ed.), *Progress in Advanced Structural and Functional Materials Design*,
DOI 10.1007/978-4-431-54064-9,

D
Dark field microscopy, 276
Debye–Scherrer rings, 275
Deexcitation, 279
Defect, 137–141, 144, 151
  clusters, 281
  formation, 274
Degree of orientation, 160
Dendrite, 98
Dendritic growth, 94
Diamond, 47–50
Diamond structure, 199, 201–210
Dilatancy, 101
Dipole interaction, 219
Disagglomeration, 101
Dislocations, 183
Disorder-order transformation, 114
Double-heterostructure (DH), 265
Driving force, 171
Dynamic recrystallization, 61
Dynamics of atoms, 274

E
Easy axis, 178
Eco-friendly, 119–126
Electrical conductivity, 31–33, 41
Electroluminescence (EL), 265
Electromagnetic force, 31, 38
4*f* Electron, 262
Electron backscattered pattern-orientation imaging microscopy (EBSP-OIM), 86
Electron beam irradiation, 274
Electronic excitation, 274
Electron spectroscopy for chemical analysis (ESCA), 72
Electrostatic coupling, 228–230
Energy transfer mechanism, 264
Epitaxial growth, 218
Equilibrium temperature, 170
Er, 262–266, 270
Er-doped GaP, 262
Er-doped InP, 262
Er–2O, 262
Er,O-Codoped GaAs, 262–263
Eu, 261, 262, 267–270
Eu-Doped GaN, 267
Exchange anisotropy, 221–222
Exchange bias, 221
Exchange bias field, 251
Exchange coupling, 251
Excitation cross section, 266, 277
Excited states, 277
Exergy, 121, 122
External quantum eficiency, 270

F
Faraday's law, 227
Fatigue, 83
Femtosecond laser, 43–55
Fe–Rh system, 175
Ferrimagnetism, 238
Ferromagnet, 221
Ferromagnetic shape memory alloy, 178
Ferromagnetism, 238
Field-cooled magnetization, 218
Finite element method, 84
First order transformation, 170
Flexible devices, 226, 234, 235
Fluid flow, 38, 41
Fluorapatite, 157
Forced volume magnetostriction, 171
Forging, 6
Formability, 9
Forming, 4
Frank van Merwe growth, 215
Free energy, 274
Free volume, 138, 151
Friction stir powder processing (FSPP), 65
Friction Stir Welding (FSW), 59, 64

G
GaAs, 262–266, 270
GaN, 262, 267–271
Gene-defected, 156, 163
Glass, 119–126
Groove geometry, 28
Ground state, 278

H
Halo ring, 278
Hard disk drive, 220
Heat affected zone (HAZ), 61
Heat input, 29, 32, 36–39, 41
Hexagonal, 156, 157, 160
High carbon steel, 62
High-Entropy (HE) material, 139
High nickel alloy, 70
High pressure, 43, 47, 50–55
High-voltage electron microscopy (HVEM), 138, 141, 148

H_2O, 120–125
Hydrogen, 16, 17, 19–24, 26
Hydrothermal, 120–126

I
ICP. *See* Inductively coupled plasma (ICP)
IEDF. *See* Ion energy distribution function (IEDF)
Implants, 156, 164, 166
Inductively coupled plasma (ICP), 227–231, 234, 235
Inelastic mean free path (IMFP), 79
Inorganic organichybridmaterials, 226
In situ observation, 93
In situ transmission electron microscopy (TEM), 274, 281
Interatomic potentials, 279
Interface, 219
Interface magnetic anisotropy, 221
Intermetallic compound, 141–145, 148–150, 183
Interparticle interactions, 219
Interstitials, 138, 151, 280
Intra-4*f* shell transitions, 262
Invar alloys, 172
Ion bombardment, 226, 232–235
Ion energy distribution, 227, 232, 234, 235
Ion energy distribution function (IEDF), 230–232, 234
Iron, 43, 47, 50–55
Irradiation, 137–151

K
Kinetic energy, 72, 78, 79
Kinetics, 277
Kubo effect, 279

L
Laser diode (LD), 265
Latent heat, 177
Lattice, 156, 157
Lattice softening, 277
Layer-by-layer growth, 215
Lifetime, 277
Lift-off method, 250, 253
Light-emitting diodes (LEDs), 262
Lighting technology, 271
Lightweight materials, 3
Lithography, 249–258
Localized mode, 206–210
Low-damage plasma, 225–235
Low-inductance antenna (LIA), 227, 229–231, 234, 235

M
Macrophage colony-stimulatingfactor (M-CSF), 163
Magnesium, 6
Magnetic anisotropy energy, 108
Magnetic computers, 258
Magnetic field, 169
Magnetic layer, 251
Magnetic logic devices, 255–258
Magnetic memories, 251–255, 258
Magnetic moment, 238, 251
Magnetic random access memory (MRAM), 220, 251, 253
Magnetization curve, 115
Magnetocrystalline anisotropy, 109, 114, 178
Magneto-crystalline anisotropy, 220
Magneto crystalline anisotropy energy, 241
Magneto-electric effect, 222
Magneto-optic Kerr effect, 222
Magnetostatic interaction, 255
Martensitic transformation, 172, 182
Maxwell's equation, 199
Mechanical function, 155–157
Membranous ossification, 160, 163
Metallic foams, 9
Metallic glasses, 138, 144–148
Microbeam X-ray, 155–166
Microbeam XRD, 157
Micromagnetics simulation, 255
Microstructure, 4, 107
Mineral, 155
Mineral apposition rate (MAR), 163
Mo, 61
Modeling, 163
Molecular beam epitaxy, 215
Multiscale, 156
Multi-scale analysis, 86

N
Nano-indentation, 156
Nanoparticles, 274–281
Nanoprocessing, 274
Nano-size effects, 279
Nanostructure, 213–215, 223, 274
N-doped GaP, 270

Neutron diffraction, 242
Ni_2MnGa, 178
Nitrogen, 19, 20
Nonlinear responses, 277
Nucleation, 115
Numerical model, 28–33

O
Op/op mouse, 163
Optimum band gap, 203, 206
Ordered domain structure, 184
Organometallic vapor phase, 262
Organometallic vapor phase epitaxy (OMVPE), 262
Osteoclasts, 163, 164
Osteocyte (OCYs), 163–165
Osteopetrotic (op/op) mouse, 163
Osteoporosis, 163
Output power, 267

P
Paramagnetic, 177
Passive film, 69–72, 74–79
Passivity, 79, 80
Penetration shape, 28, 29, 38
Peritectic reaction, 94, 98
Permalloy, 255
Perovskite, 238
Perpendicular exchange bias, 221
Perpendicular magnetic anisotropy, 220–221
Phase contrast, 97
Phase separation, 276
Phase transformation, 274
Phenyl group, 231, 233, 234
Photoionization cross section, 72, 78, 80
Photoluminescence (PL), 263
Photonic band gap, 196, 197, 201, 208, 210
Photonic band iagram, 201
Photonic crystals, 195–210
π-conjugated, 231
π-π^* shake-up satellite, 233, 234
Plane wave expansion method, 199
Plasma processes, 225–235
Point defects, 280
Pores, 15–26
Porosity, 17–21, 23–26
Porous, 120, 122, 126
Porous materials, 3
Porous metals, 15–26
Principal stress, 160, 164
Probe, 60
Pseudoelasticity, 182
Pure iron, 173

Q
Quantitative analysis, 72–80

R
Rare-earth (RE)-doped semiconductors, 262
Rare-earth (RE) elements, 261
Reaction, 274
Recombination, 281
Recycling, 119–126
Red LED, 270
Reflection high-energy electron diffraction, 215
Regenerated, 156, 162, 163, 166
Regeneration, 162
Relaxation energy, 279
Remodeling, 163
Residual stress, 83–90
Retreating side, 61
Rolling, 4

S
Scattering vector, 278
Secondary arm, 98
Semisolids, 94
Servo presses, 11
Shape memory alloys, 182
Shape memory effect, 182
Shock, 43, 46–55
Shoulder, 60
Si, 262
Simulation software, 28, 29, 41
Slag, 119–121, 126
Small many-body systems, 274
Soft-material, 226, 227, 231–235
Solid, 60
Solidification, 15–18, 20, 22–26, 93
Solute, 274
Spin electronic, 250–251
Spin glass, 245
Spin-orbit interaction, 220
Spontaneous magnetization, 178, 238
Stainless steel, 70–71, 74, 75, 78, 79
Steel, 61–64
Stereolithography, 195–210
Stir zone (SZ), 61

Stranski-Krastanov growth, 215
Stray fields, 253
Stress corrosion cracking (SCC), 83
Structuralization, 83
Structural stability, 274
Sulfur content, 38–41
Supercooling, 171
Superheating, 171
Superparamagnetism, 216
Supersaturation, 281
Surface, 219
  energy, 281
  layer, 281
  segregation, 281
  tension, 38, 39
Synchrotron, 93
Synergistic effects, 277

T
Temperature, 28–36, 38–41
Terahertz wave, 197–199
Tetragonal distortion, 110
Thermal elastic plastic analysis, 84
Thermal equilibrium, 277
Thermal process, 279
Thermomechanically affected zone (TMAZ), 61
Thixotropic, 101
III–V semiconductors, 262
TIG arc, 32–39, 41
Tool, 60
Tool steel, 64
Tooth, 160
Transformation, 62
Transmission electron microscope (TEM), 183
Tungsten carbide, 64
Turnover, 163
Twinning plane, 112
Twinning shear, 112
Two-hole states, 279

U
Ultrahigh vacuum, 214
Ultrathin film, 213–223

V
Vacancy, 138, 151, 280
Valence, 279
Variants, 108
Virtual work principle, 84
Voids, 278
Volmer-Weber growth, 215

W
Waste, 119, 120, 122, 125
Weiss mean field theory, 173
Welded structures, 89
Welding, 83
Weld pool, 29, 33, 38–41

X
XPS. *See* X-rayphoto electron spectroscopy (XPS)
X-ray, 158–160, 166
  fluorescence, 279
  imaging, 93
X-ray photo electron spectroscopy (XPS), 69–80, 231–235

Y
Young's modulus, 163–165

Z
Zero-field-cooled magnetization, 218
Zincblende structure, 277

MIX
Papier aus verantwortungsvollen Quellen
Paper from responsible sources
FSC® C105338

If you have any concerns about our products,
you can contact us on
ProductSafety@springernature.com

In case Publisher is established outside the EU,
the EU authorized representative is:
Springer Nature Customer Service Center GmbH
Europaplatz 3, 69115 Heidelberg, Germany

Printed by Libri Plureos GmbH
in Hamburg, Germany